Comparative Effectiveness Review
Number 118

Treatment Strategies for Patients With Peripheral Artery Disease

Prepared for:
Agency for Healthcare Research and Quality
U.S. Department of Health and Human Services
540 Gaither Road
Rockville, MD 20850
www.ahrq.gov

Contract No. 290-2007-10066-I

Prepared by:
Duke Evidence-based Practice Center
Durham, NC

Investigators:
W. Schuyler Jones, M.D.
Kristine M. Schmit, M.D., M.P.H.
Sreekanth Vemulapalli, M.D.
Sumeet Subherwal, M.D., M.B.A.
Manesh R. Patel, M.D.
Victor Hasselblad, Ph.D.
Brooke L. Heidenfelder, Ph.D.
Megan M. Chobot, M.S.L.S.
Rachael Posey, M.S.L.S.
Liz Wing, M.A.
Gillian D. Sanders, Ph.D.
Rowena J. Dolor, M.D., M.H.S.

AHRQ Publication No. 13-EHC090-EF
May 2013

This report is based on research conducted by the Duke Evidence-based Practice Center (EPC) under contract to the Agency for Healthcare Research and Quality (AHRQ), Rockville, MD (Contract No. 290-2007-10066-I). The findings and conclusions in this document are those of the authors, who are responsible for its contents; the findings and conclusions do not necessarily represent the views of AHRQ. Therefore, no statement in this report should be construed as an official position of AHRQ or of the U.S. Department of Health and Human Services.

The information in this report is intended to help health care decisionmakers—patients and clinicians, health system leaders, and policymakers, among others—make well-informed decisions and thereby improve the quality of health care services. This report is not intended to be a substitute for the application of clinical judgment. Anyone who makes decisions concerning the provision of clinical care should consider this report in the same way as any medical reference and in conjunction with all other pertinent information, i.e., in the context of available resources and circumstances presented by individual patients.

This report may be used, in whole or in part, as the basis for development of clinical practice guidelines and other quality enhancement tools, or as a basis for reimbursement and coverage policies. AHRQ or U.S. Department of Health and Human Services endorsement of such derivative products may not be stated or implied.

This document is in the public domain and may be used and reprinted without permission except those copyrighted materials that are clearly noted in the document. Further reproduction of those copyrighted materials is prohibited without the specific permission of copyright holders.

Persons using assistive technology may not be able to fully access information in this report. For assistance contact EffectiveHealthCare@ahrq.hhs.gov.

> None of the investigators have any affiliations or financial involvement that conflicts with the material presented in this report.

Suggested citation: Jones WS, Schmit KM, Vemulapalli S, Subherwal S, Patel MR, Hasselblad V, Heidenfelder BL, Chobot MM, Posey R, Wing L, Sanders GD, Dolor RJ. Treatment Strategies for Patients With Peripheral Artery Disease. Comparative Effectiveness Review No. 118. (Prepared by the Duke Evidence-based Practice Center under Contract No. 290-2007-10066-I.) AHRQ Publication No. 13-EHC090-EF. Rockville, MD: Agency for Healthcare Research and Quality; May 2013. www.effectivehealthcare.ahrq.gov/reports/final.cfm.

Preface

The Agency for Healthcare Research and Quality (AHRQ), through its Evidence-based Practice Centers (EPCs), sponsors the development of systematic reviews to assist public- and private-sector organizations in their efforts to improve the quality of health care in the United States. These reviews provide comprehensive, science-based information on common, costly medical conditions, and new health care technologies and strategies.

Systematic reviews are the building blocks underlying evidence-based practice; they focus attention on the strength and limits of evidence from research studies about the effectiveness and safety of a clinical intervention. In the context of developing recommendations for practice, systematic reviews can help clarify whether assertions about the value of the intervention are based on strong evidence from clinical studies. For more information about AHRQ EPC systematic reviews, see www.effectivehealthcare.ahrq.gov/reference/purpose.cfm

AHRQ expects that these systematic reviews will be helpful to health plans, providers, purchasers, government programs, and the health care system as a whole. Transparency and stakeholder input are essential to the Effective Health Care Program. Please visit the Web site (www.effectivehealthcare.ahrq.gov) to see draft research questions and reports or to join an email list to learn about new program products and opportunities for input.

We welcome comments on this systematic review. They may be sent by mail to the Task Order Officer named below at: Agency for Healthcare Research and Quality, 540 Gaither Road, Rockville, MD 20850, or by email to epc@ahrq.hhs.gov.

Carolyn M. Clancy, M.D.
Director
Agency for Healthcare Research and Quality

Jean Slutsky, P.A., M.S.P.H.
Director, Center for Outcomes and Evidence
Agency for Healthcare Research and Quality

Stephanie Chang, M.D., M.P.H.
Director
Evidence-based Practice Program
Center for Outcomes and Evidence
Agency for Healthcare Research and Quality

Elisabeth U. Kato, M.R.P.
Task Order Officer
Center for Outcomes and Evidence
Agency for Healthcare Research and Quality

Acknowledgments

The authors thank Megan von Isenburg, M.S.L.S., for help with the literature search and retrieval.

Key Informants

In designing the study questions, the EPC consulted several Key Informants who represent the end-users of research. The EPC sought the Key Informant input on the priority areas for research and synthesis. Key Informants are not involved in the analysis of the evidence or the writing of the report. Therefore, in the end, study questions, design, methodological approaches, and/or conclusions do not necessarily represent the views of individual Key Informants.

Key Informants must disclose any financial conflicts of interest greater than $10,000 and any other relevant business or professional conflicts of interest. Because of their role as end-users, individuals with potential conflicts may be retained. The TOO and the EPC work to balance, manage, or mitigate any conflicts of interest.

The list of Key Informants who participated in developing this report follows:

Peter Alagona, M.D.
Penn State Hershey Heart and Vascular Institute
Hershey, PA

Mike S. Conte, M.D.
Codirector, Heart and Vascular Center
University of California San Francisco Medical Center
San Francisco, CA

Mark Creager, M.D.
Director, Vascular Center
Brigham and Women's Hospital, Cardiovascular Division
Boston, MA

Mary McDermott, M.D.
Professor of Medicine and Preventive Medicine
Northwestern University Feinberg School of Medicine
Chicago, IL

Sanjay Misra, M.D.
Associate Professor of Radiology
Mayo Clinic
Rochester, MN

Erin O'Connell Peiffer
Spokesperson
WomenHeart
Baltimore, MD

Jeffrey Olin, M.D.
Professor of Medicine, Cardiology
Mount Sinai School of Medicine
New York, NY

Diane Reid, M.D.
Division of Heart and Vascular Diseases
National Heart, Lung, and Blood Institute
Bethesda, MD

Diane Treat-Jacobsen, Ph.D., R.N.
Associate Professor and Chair, Adult & Gerontological Health Cooperative
University of Minnesota School of Nursing
Minneapolis, MN

Christopher White, M.D.
Director, John Ochsner Heart & Vascular Institute
Ochsner Medical Center
New Orleans, LA

Technical Expert Panel

In designing the study questions and methodology at the outset of this report, the EPC consulted several technical and content experts. Broad expertise and perspectives were sought. Divergent and conflicted opinions are common and perceived as healthy scientific discourse that results in a thoughtful, relevant systematic review. Therefore, in the end, study questions, design, methodologic approaches, and/or conclusions do not necessarily represent the views of individual technical and content experts.

Technical Experts must disclose any financial conflicts of interest greater than $10,000 and any other relevant business or professional conflicts of interest. Because of their unique clinical or content expertise, individuals with potential conflicts may be retained. The TOO and the EPC work to balance, manage, or mitigate any potential conflicts of interest identified.

The list of Technical Experts who participated in developing this report follows:

Mike S. Conte, M.D.
Codirector, Heart and Vascular Center
University of California San Francisco
Medical Center
San Francisco, CA

Mark Creager, M.D.
Director, Vascular Center
Brigham and Women's Hospital,
Cardiovascular Division
Boston, MA

Mary McDermott, M.D.
Professor of Medicine and Preventive
Medicine
Northwestern University Feinberg School of
Medicine
Chicago, IL

David Moher
Senior Scientist, Clinical Epidemiology
Ottawa Hospital Research Institute
Ottawa, Ontario, Canada

Sanjay Misra, M.D.
Associate Professor of Radiology
Mayo Clinic
Rochester, MN

Jeffrey Olin, M.D.
Professor of Medicine, Cardiology
Mount Sinai School of Medicine
New York, NY

Diane Reid, M.D.
Division of Heart and Vascular Diseases
National Heart, Lung, and Blood Institute
Bethesda, MD

Diane Treat-Jacobsen, Ph.D., R.N.
Associate Professor and Chair, Adult &
Gerontological Health Cooperative
University of Minnesota School of Nursing
Minneapolis, MN

David Vanness, Ph.D.
Associate Professor of Population Health
Sciences
Affiliate, Center for Demography and
Ecology
University of Wisconsin School of Medicine
and Public Health
Madison, WI

Christopher White, M.D.
Director, John Ochsner Heart & Vascular
Institute
Ochsner Medical Center
New Orleans, LA

Peer Reviewers

Prior to publication of the final evidence report, EPCs sought input from independent Peer Reviewers without financial conflicts of interest. However, the conclusions and synthesis of the scientific literature presented in this report does not necessarily represent the views of individual reviewers.

Peer Reviewers must disclose any financial conflicts of interest greater than $10,000 and any other relevant business or professional conflicts of interest. Because of their unique clinical or content expertise, individuals with potential non-financial conflicts may be retained. The TOO and the EPC work to balance, manage, or mitigate any potential non-financial conflicts of interest identified.

The list of Peer Reviewers follows:

John White, M.D.
Advocate Lutheran General Hospital
Niles, IL

Thomas Tsai, M.D.
Director, Interventional Cardiology
Denver VA Medical Center
Denver, CO

Deepak L. Bhatt, M.D., M.P.H.
Senior Physician
Brigham and Women's Hospital
Boston, MA

Ken Cavanaugh, Ph.D.
Supervisory Biomedical Engineer
U.S. Food and Drug Administration
Silver Spring, MD

Treatment Strategies for Patients With Peripheral Artery Disease

Structured Abstract

Objectives. For patients with peripheral artery disease (PAD), the optimal treatment for cardiovascular protection, symptom relief, preservation of walking and functional status, and prevention of amputation is not known. This review assessed the comparative effectiveness of antiplatelet therapy, medical therapy, exercise, and endovascular and surgical revascularization in PAD patients with intermittent claudication (IC) or critical limb ischemia (CLI).

Data sources. We searched PubMed®, Embase®, and the Cochrane Database of Systematic Reviews for relevant English-language studies published since January 1995.

Review methods. Two investigators screened each abstract and full-text article for inclusion, abstracted the data, and performed quality ratings and evidence grading. Random-effects models were used to compute summary estimates of effects. A meta-analysis of direct comparisons was supplemented by a mixed-treatment analysis to incorporate data from placebo comparisons, head-to-head comparisons, and multiple treatment arms.

Results. A total of 83 studies contributed evidence. Eleven studies—10 randomized controlled trials (RCTs), 1 observational study—evaluated the comparative effectiveness of antiplatelet agents. In asymptomatic PAD patients, there was no difference between aspirin and placebo for all-cause mortality, cardiovascular mortality, myocardial infarction (MI), or stroke. In patients with IC, one RCT suggests that aspirin may reduce MI and composite vascular events compared with placebo but was inconclusive for other outcomes of interest. Another RCT involving IC patients suggests that clopidogrel is more effective than aspirin for reducing cardiovascular mortality, nonfatal MI, and composite vascular events. Clopidogrel and aspirin appear to be equivalent for prevention of nonfatal stroke, but the confidence interval was wide, making this conclusion less certain. In symptomatic (92% IC) and asymptomatic (8%) PAD patients, dual antiplatelet therapy (DAPT)—clopidogrel plus aspirin—had no impact on composite or individual outcomes. Similarly, in IC or CLI patients after unilateral bypass graft, one RCT showed no difference between DAPT and aspirin alone on nonfatal stroke and composite vascular events and was inconclusive for other outcomes. In patients with IC or CLI after an endovascular procedure, one RCT showed no difference between DAPT and aspirin alone in cardiovascular events or mortality at 6 months but was underpowered for those outcomes. Four additional studies assessed other antiplatelet comparisons but were too small to make any meaningful conclusions about effectiveness. Seven RCTs reported different types of bleeding events, and the use of antiplatelet agents was associated with higher rates of minor and moderate bleeding compared with placebo.

Thirty-five studies (27 RCTs, 8 observational) evaluated the comparative effectiveness of cilostazol, pentoxifylline, exercise therapy, endovascular revascularization, or surgical revascularization in IC patients, with the majority of the studies comparing one intervention with either placebo or one other intervention. In order to place all treatments in a common framework for comparison, we created a network meta-analysis. Although the data were still too sparse to definitively conclude which treatment is most effective, we were able to depict relative effect sizes and identify which treatments are clearly superior to placebo for which outcomes. No specific treatment had a statistically significant effect on all-cause mortality (12 RCTs). Exercise training improved maximal walking distance (16 RCTs), and exercise training and endovascular intervention improved initial claudication distance (12 RCTs) compared with usual care. Quality-of-life scores (10 RCTs) showed a significant improvement from cilostazol, exercise training, endovascular intervention, and surgical intervention compared with usual care. Seventeen RCTs reported safety concerns. Cilostazol was associated with higher rates of headache, dizziness, and diarrhea, while endovascular interventions were associated with more transfusions, arterial dissections/perforations, and hematomas compared with the usual care groups.

Twenty-three studies (1 RCT, 22 observational) in CLI patients and 12 studies (2 RCTs, 10 observational) in IC or CLI patients evaluated the comparative effectiveness of endovascular or surgical treatments. Long-term amputation-free survival and all-cause mortality were not different between the two treatments in the CLI population. Primary patency varied, but secondary patency rates appeared to favor endovascular interventions in the CLI population. In four observational studies comparing endovascular interventions with usual care, there was insufficient evidence on the comparative effect for all clinical outcomes. In observational studies of the IC-CLI population, there were fewer periprocedural complications from endovascular interventions, while RCTs showed lower rates in the surgical intervention arm.

Conclusions. From a limited number of studies, it appears that aspirin has no benefit over placebo in the asymptomatic PAD patient; clopidogrel monotherapy is more beneficial than aspirin in the IC patient; and DAPT is not significantly better than aspirin at reducing cardiovascular events in patients with IC or CLI. For IC patients, exercise therapy, cilostazol, and endovascular intervention all had an effect on improving functional status and quality of life; the impact of these therapies on cardiovascular events and mortality is uncertain. The comparisons of endovascular and surgical revascularization in CLI are primarily from observational studies, and the heterogeneity of the results makes conclusions for all clinical outcomes less certain. Several advances in care in both medical therapy and invasive therapy have not been rigorously tested and thus provide an impetus for further research.

Contents

Executive Summary ES-1
Introduction 1
  Background 1
    Epidemiology of Peripheral Artery Disease (PAD) 1
    Diagnostic Tests 2
    Classification Schemes 2
    Outcome Measures for PAD 3
      Cardiovascular Events 3
      Functional Capacity 3
      Quality of Life 3
      Limb Outcomes 3
    Therapies for PAD 4
      Reducing Cardiovascular Morbidity and Mortality in All Patients With PAD 4
      Improving Functional Status in Patients With IC 4
      Improving Functional Status and Reducing Leg Amputation in Patients With CLI ... 6
  Scope and Key Questions (KQs) 7
    Scope of the Review 7
    KQs 7
      Analytic Framework 8
Methods 10
  Topic Refinement and Review Protocol 10
  Literature Search Strategy 11
    Sources Searched 11
    Inclusion and Exclusion Criteria 11
    Study Selection 13
    Data Extraction 14
  Quality Assessment of Individual Studies 14
  Data Synthesis 15
  Strength of the Body of Evidence 18
  Applicability 19
  Peer Review and Public Commentary 19
Results 20
  Results of Literature Searches 20
  KQ 1. Comparative Effectiveness and Safety of Antiplatelet Therapy in Adults With PAD ... 21
    Key Points 22
      Effectiveness of Interventions 22
      Modifiers of Effectiveness 22
      Safety Concerns 23
    Description of Included Studies 23
    Detailed Synthesis 23
      Effectiveness of Interventions 23
      Modifiers of Effectiveness 33
      Safety Concerns 34
    SOE Ratings for KQ 1 36

KQ 2. Comparative Effectiveness and Safety of Exercise, Medications, and Endovascular and Surgical Revascularization for IC 41
   Key Points 41
      Effectiveness of Interventions 41
      Modifiers of Effectiveness 42
      Safety Concerns 43
   Description of Included Studies 43
   Detailed Synthesis 44
      Description of Comparisons 44
      Effectiveness of Interventions 46
      Modifiers of Effectiveness 73
      Safety Concerns 75
   SOE Ratings for KQ 2 80
KQ 3. Comparative Effectiveness and Safety of Usual Care and Endovascular and Surgical Revascularization for CLI 87
   Key Points 87
      Effectiveness of Interventions 87
      Modifiers of Effectiveness 87
      Safety Concerns 88
   Description of Included Studies 88
   Detailed Synthesis 89
      Effectiveness of Interventions 89
      Modifiers of Effectiveness 114
      Safety Concerns 124
   SOE Ratings for KQ 3 127

Discussion 135
   Key Findings and SOE 135
      KQ 1. Comparative Effectiveness and Safety of Antiplatelet Therapy in Adults With PAD 135
      KQ 2. Comparative Effectiveness and Safety of Exercise, Medications, and Endovascular and Surgical Revascularization for IC 140
      KQ 3. Comparative Effectiveness and Safety of Usual Care and Endovascular and Surgical Revascularization for CLI 147
   Findings in Relation to What Is Already Known 152
   Challenges in Evaluating the Existing Literature in PAD Patients 154
   Applicability 155
   Implications for Clinical and Policy Decisionmaking 155
   Limitations of the Review Process 156
   Limitations of the Evidence Base 156
   Research Gaps 157
      KQ 1 Research Gaps 157
      KQ 2 Research Gaps 157
      KQ 3 Research Gaps 158
      Underreporting of Subgroup Results Across All KQs 158
   Conclusions 159
References 161

Abbreviations 171

Tables
Table A. Summary SOE for KQ 1: Comparative effectiveness and safety of antiplatelet therapy for adults with PAD ES-10
Table B. Summary SOE for KQ 2: Comparative effectiveness and safety of treatments for IC ES-18
Table C. Summary SOE for KQ 3: Comparative effectiveness and safety of treatments for CLI ES-24
Table D. Research Gaps ES-31
Table 1. Fontaine classification 2
Table 2. Rutherford classification..2
Table 3. Inclusion and exclusion criteria 12
Table 4. Definitions of overall quality ratings 15
Table 5. Example effect size calculation 17
Table 6. SOE in required domains...18
Table 7. Calculated hazard ratios for aspirin versus placebo or no antiplatelet 24
Table 8. Calculated hazard ratio for clopidogrel with or without aspirin versus placebo with aspirin...28
Table 9. Results of other antiplatelet comparisons 33
Table 10. Studies reporting subgroup results of antiplatelet therapy (modifiers of effectiveness)...34
Table 11. Studies reporting harms of antiplatelet therapy 35
Table 12. Detailed SOE for aspirin versus placebo in adults with asymptomatic or symptomatic PAD at 2 or more years...36
Table 13. Detailed SOE for clopidogrel versus aspirin in adults with intermittent claudication at 2 years (CAPRIE) 38
Table 14. Detailed SOE for clopidogrel + aspirin versus aspirin monotherapy in adults with PAD at 2 years 39
Table 15. Mortality analysis for all treatment comparisons 47
Table 16. Calculated effect size: maximal walking measures 51
Table 17. Calculated effect size: claudication onset measures 59
Table 18. Calculated effect size: quality-of-life measures...64
Table 19. Studies reporting subgroup results (modifiers of effectiveness) in the IC population 74
Table 20. Studies reporting harms of therapies in the IC population 76
Table 21. Detailed strength of evidence for IC therapies by comparator 81
Table 22. Endovascular intervention versus usual care 90
Table 23. Endovascular versus surgical revascularization: all-cause mortality 92
Table 24. Endovascular versus surgical revascularization: lower-extremity amputation..............98
Table 25. Endovascular versus surgical revascularization: amputation-free survival.................103
Table 26. Endovascular versus surgical revascularization: vessel patency 107
Table 27. Endovascular versus surgical revascularization: hospital length of stay 112
Table 28. Modifiers of effectiveness for KQ 3 115
Table 29. Safety concerns in the IC-CLI population 125
Table 30. Detailed SOE for endovascular intervention versus usual care in CLI and IC-CLI populations 127

Table 31. Detailed SOE for endovascular versus surgical revascularization in CLI
and IC-CLI populations 129
Table 32. Summary SOE for KQ 1: Comparative effectiveness and safety of antiplatelet therapy
for adults with PAD 136
Table 33. Summary SOE for KQ 2: Comparative effectiveness and safety of treatments
for IC 142
Table 34. Summary SOE for KQ 3: Comparative effectiveness and safety of treatments
for CLI 148
Table 35. Research gaps 159

Figures
Figure A. Analytic framework ES-4
Figure B. Literature flow diagram ES-8
Figure C. Network meta-analysis of treatment effects versus usual care and each other
on mortality in IC patients ES-14
Figure D. Network meta-analysis of treatment effects versus usual care on walking distance
in IC patients ES-14
Figure E. Network sensitivity meta-analysis of treatment effects versus usual care
on walking distance in IC patients ES-15
Figure F. Network meta-analysis of treatment effects versus each other on walking distance
in IC patients ES-15
Figure G. Network sensitivity meta-analysis of treatment effects versus each other
on walking distance in IC patients ES-15
Figure H. Network meta-analysis of treatment effects versus usual care and each other
on claudication distance in IC patients ES-16
Figure I. Network meta-analysis of treatment effects versus usual care on quality of life
in IC patients ES-16
Figure J. Network meta-analysis of treatment effects versus each other on quality of life
in IC patients ES-17
Figure 1. Analytic framework 9
Figure 2. Steps of a systematic review 10
Figure 3. Literature flow diagram 21
Figure 4. Forest plot for RCTs of aspirin versus placebo: nonfatal MI at 2 or more years ...25
Figure 5. Forest plot for RCTs of aspirin versus placebo: nonfatal stroke at 2 or more years 26
Figure 6. Forest plot for RCTs of aspirin versus placebo: cardiovascular mortality at 2 or more
years 27
Figure 7. Forest plot for RCTs of aspirin versus placebo: composite vascular events at 2 or more
years 27
Figure 8. Clopidogrel versus aspirin for all outcomes in PAD subgroup of CAPRIE RCT 30
Figure 9. Dual antiplatelet versus aspirin outcomes in CHARISMA and CASPAR RCTs 32
Figure 10. Dual antiplatelet versus aspirin outcomes in MIRROR RCT 32
Figure 11. Network meta-analysis of treatment effects versus usual care and each other on
mortality in IC patients 49
Figure 12. Network meta-analysis of treatment effects versus usual care on walking distance in
IC patients 55
Figure 13. Network sensitivity meta-analysis of treatment effects versus usual care on walking
distance in IC patients 56

Figure 14. Network meta-analysis of treatment effects versus each other on walking distance in IC patients 57
Figure 15. Network sensitivity meta-analysis of treatment effects versus each other on walking distance in IC patients 57
Figure 16. Network meta-analysis of treatment effects versus usual care and each other on claudication distance in IC patients 63
Figure 17. Network meta-analysis of treatment effects versus usual care on quality of life in IC patients 72
Figure 18. Network meta-analysis of treatment effects versus each other on quality of life in IC patients 72
Figure 19. Forest plot for meta-analysis of cilostazol versus placebo on headache complications in the IC population 78
Figure 20. Forest plot for meta-analysis of cilostazol versus placebo on diarrhea complications in the IC population 79
Figure 21. Forest plot for meta-analysis of cilostazol versus placebo on palpitation complications in the IC population 79
Figure 22. Forest plot for meta-analysis of mortality at 6 or more months in the CLI and IC-CLI populations 96
Figure 23. Forest plot for meta-analysis of mortality at 1 to 2 years in the CLI and IC-CLI populations 97
Figure 24. Forest plot for meta-analysis of mortality at 3 or more years in the CLI and IC-CLI populations 97
Figure 25. Forest plot for meta-analysis of amputation at less than 2 years in the CLI and IC-CLI populations 101
Figure 26. Forest plot for meta-analysis of amputation at 2 to 3 years in the CLI and IC-CLI populations 102
Figure 27. Forest plot for meta-analysis of amputation after 5 years in the CLI population.......102
Figure 28. Forest plot for meta-analysis of amputation-free survival at 1 year in the CLI population 104
Figure 29. Forest plot for meta-analysis of amputation-free survival at 2 to 3 years in the CLI population 105
Figure 30. Forest plot for meta-analysis of amputation-free survival after 5 years in the CLI population 106
Figure 31. Forest plot for meta-analysis of primary patency at 1 year in the CLI and IC-CLI populations 110
Figure 32. Forest plot for meta-analysis of primary patency at 2 to 3 years in the CLI and IC-CLI populations 111
Figure 33. Forest plot for meta-analysis of secondary patency at 1 year in the CLI and IC-CLI populations 111
Figure 34. Forest plot for meta-analysis of secondary patency at 2 to 3 years in the CLI population 112
Figure 35. Forest plot for meta-analysis of surgical versus endovascular revascularization on periprocedural complications by 30 days in the IC-CLI population..126
Figure 36. Forest plot for meta-analysis of surgical versus endovascular revascularization on infections by 30 days in the IC-CLI population..127

Appendixes
Appendix A. Exact Search Strings
Appendix B. Data Abstraction Elements
Appendix C. Study Characteristics Tables
Appendix D. Included Studies
Appendix E. Excluded Studies

Executive Summary

Background

Peripheral artery disease (PAD) refers to chronic narrowing or atherosclerosis of the lower extremities[1] and represents a spectrum of disease severity from asymptomatic disease to intermittent claudication (IC), to critical limb ischemia (CLI). PAD has a similar atherosclerotic process to coronary artery disease and shares similar risk factors: male gender, age, diabetes, smoking, hypertension, high cholesterol, and renal insufficiency.[2] PAD is known to be associated with a reduction in functional capacity and quality of life as well as an increased risk for myocardial infarction (MI), stroke, and death; it is also a major cause of limb amputation.[3-7] Therefore, the general goals of treatment for PAD are cardiovascular protection, relief of symptoms, preservation of walking and functional status, and prevention of amputation. The optimal treatment for PAD—with specific emphasis on the comparative effectiveness of treatment options—is not known.[8]

The backbone of treatment for PAD is smoking cessation, risk factor modification, dietary modification, and increased physical activity. There are three main treatment options for improving functional status and other clinical outcomes in patients with PAD: (1) medical therapy, (2) exercise training, and (3) revascularization. The treatment options offered to PAD patients depend on whether the patient is asymptomatic or symptomatic (with either IC or CLI).

Medical Therapy

The goal of medical therapy in patients with PAD is to reduce the risk of future cardiovascular morbidity and mortality in patients with high ischemic risk, and/or to improve walking distance and functional status in patients with IC. Secondary prevention includes the use of antiplatelet agents and angiotensin-converting enzyme (ACE) inhibitors and the management of other risk factors such as tobacco use, diabetes, LDL levels, and hypertension. With respect to antiplatelet therapy, there is clinical uncertainty. It is not clear which antiplatelet strategy—aspirin versus clopidogrel, monotherapy versus dual antiplatelet therapy (DAPT)—is of most benefit. Further, the role of these agents in patients with asymptomatic PAD also is unclear.

Selected medical therapies have been shown to improve walking distance in patients with PAD, compared with placebo. Cilostazol and pentoxifylline both work by increasing blood flow to the limb, preventing blood clots, and widening the blood vessels. Common side effects of cilostazol include headache and diarrhea, and its use is contraindicated in patients with congestive heart failure; however, pentoxifylline has fewer side effects of nausea and diarrhea.[9]

Exercise Training

Over the past 30 years, research efforts within PAD have focused on the potential benefits of noninvasive therapy, such as exercise, for patients with IC. Most studies investigate differences between supervised exercise training and standard home exercise training. More recently, supervised exercise training has also been compared with endovascular revascularization.

Revascularization

Historically, patients with IC have been treated conservatively for their leg symptoms with medical therapy, lifestyle modification, and exercise programs.[10] When IC patients continue to have symptoms despite conservative, noninvasive treatment, then revascularization becomes a treatment option. For patients with CLI, revascularization is often attempted to restore blood flow, improve wound healing, and prevent amputation. Decisions about whether to revascularize and how to revascularize patients with PAD depend on a number of factors, including patient-specific characteristics, anatomic characteristics, severity of symptoms, need for possible repeat revascularization in the future, and patient and physician preferences. Clinical guidelines remain vague regarding the absolute indications for and the appropriate use of revascularization strategies in patients with PAD.[11] Ultimately, clinicians must weigh risks and benefits in determining which patients have the greatest chance for success with revascularization. Multiple strategies for revascularization include surgery, angioplasty (cryoplasty, drug-coated, cutting, and standard angioplasty balloons are available for use in peripheral arteries), stenting (self-expanding and balloon-expandable stents are available, but drug-eluting stents are not currently approved for treating peripheral arteries in the United States), and atherectomy (laser, directional, orbital, and rotational atherectomy devices are approved for use in the United States). With improvements in endovascular techniques and equipment, the use of balloon angioplasty, stenting, and atherectomy has led to the application of endovascular revascularization to a wider range of patients over the past decade, both among those with more severe symptoms and those with less severe symptoms.[12] Very few large clinical trials have been performed in patients with IC or CLI that aim to determine the best revascularization strategy; however, many questions remain, as newer endovascular therapies are applied to a broader population of patients.

Scope and Key Questions (KQs)

This comparative effectiveness review was funded by the Agency for Healthcare Research and Quality (AHRQ). The review was designed to evaluate the effectiveness of available strategies—exercise, medications, revascularization—used to treat patients with PAD. With input from our Technical Expert Panel (TEP), we constructed KQs using the general approach of specifying the population of interest, interventions, comparators, outcomes, timing of outcomes, and settings (PICOTS). The KQs considered in this comparative effectiveness review were:

- **KQ 1.** In adults with PAD, including asymptomatic patients and symptomatic patients with atypical leg symptoms, IC, or CLI:
    a. What is the comparative effectiveness of aspirin and other antiplatelet agents in reducing the risk of adverse cardiovascular events (e.g., all-cause mortality, myocardial infarction, stroke, cardiovascular death), functional capacity, and quality of life?
    b. Does the effectiveness of treatments vary according to the patient's PAD classification or by subgroup (age, sex, race, risk factors, or comorbidities)?
    c. What are the significant safety concerns associated with each treatment strategy (e.g., adverse drug reactions, bleeding)? Do the safety concerns vary by subgroup (age, sex, race, risk factors, comorbidities, or PAD classification)?
- **KQ 2.** In adults with symptomatic PAD (atypical leg symptoms or IC):
    a. What is the comparative effectiveness of exercise training, medications (cilostazol, pentoxifylline), endovascular intervention (percutaneous transluminal angioplasty,

atherectomy, or stents), and/or surgical revascularization (endarterectomy, bypass surgery) on outcomes including cardiovascular events (e.g., all-cause mortality, myocardial infarction, stroke, cardiovascular death), amputation, quality of life, wound healing, analog pain scale score, functional capacity, repeat revascularization, and vessel patency?
  b. Does the effectiveness of treatments vary by use of exercise and medical therapy prior to invasive management or by subgroup (age, sex, race, risk factors, comorbidities, or anatomic location of disease)?
  c. What are the significant safety concerns associated with each treatment strategy (e.g., adverse drug reactions, bleeding, contrast nephropathy, radiation exposure, infection, exercise-related harms, and periprocedural complications causing acute limb ischemia)? Do the safety concerns vary by subgroup (age, sex, race, risk factors, comorbidities, anatomic location of disease)?
- **KQ 3.** In adults with CLI due to PAD:
  a. What is the comparative effectiveness of endovascular intervention (percutaneous transluminal angioplasty, atherectomy, or stents) and surgical revascularization (endarterectomy, bypass surgery) for outcomes including cardiovascular events (e.g., all-cause mortality, myocardial infarction, stroke, cardiovascular death), amputation, quality of life, wound healing, analog pain scale score, functional capacity, repeat revascularization, and vessel patency?
  b. Does the effectiveness of treatments vary by subgroup (age, sex, race, risk factors, comorbidities, or anatomic location of disease)?
  c. What are the significant safety concerns associated with each treatment strategy (e.g., adverse drug reactions, bleeding, contrast nephropathy, radiation exposure, infection, and periprocedural complications causing acute limb ischemia)? Do the safety concerns vary by subgroup (age, sex, race, risk factors, comorbidities, or anatomic location of disease)?

Figure A shows the analytic framework for this comparative effectiveness review.

Figure A. Analytic framework

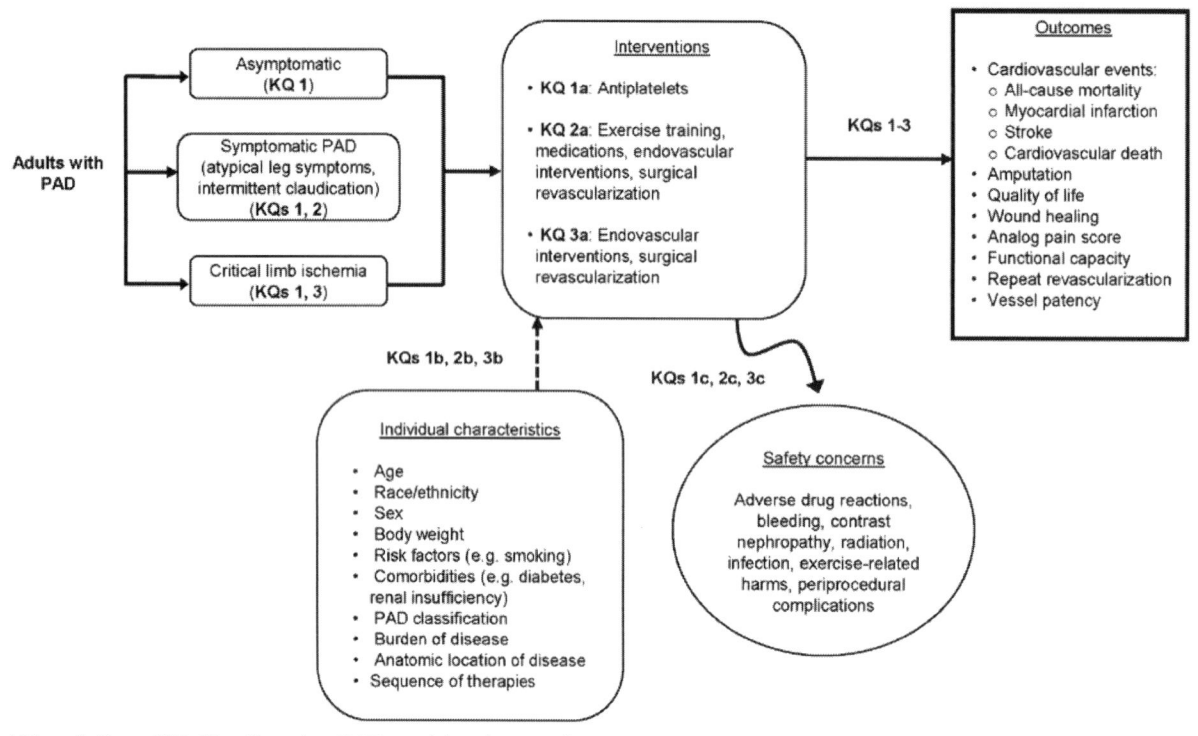

Abbreviations: KQ=Key Question; PAD=peripheral artery disease.

Methods

The methods for this comparative effectiveness review follow those suggested in the AHRQ "Methods Guide for Effectiveness and Comparative Effectiveness Reviews" (www.effectivehealthcare.ahrq.gov/methodsguide.cfm; hereafter referred to as the Methods Guide).[13] During the topic refinement stage, we solicited input from Key Informants (KIs) representing clinicians (cardiology, radiology, vascular surgery, general medicine, and nursing), patients, scientific experts, and Federal agencies to help define the KQs. The KQs were then posted for public comment for 30 days, and the comments received were considered in the development of the research protocol. We next convened a TEP comprising clinical, content, and methodological experts to provide input in defining populations, interventions, comparisons, or outcomes as well as in identifying particular studies or databases to search.

The KIs and members of the TEP were required to disclose any financial conflicts of interest greater than $10,000 and any other relevant business or professional conflicts of interest. Any potential conflicts of interest were balanced or mitigated. Of the 10 TEP members, four held positions on scientific advisory boards representing 14 entities, of which 2 members overlapped on 2 entities; thus there was not majority interest in any particular company or institute. Neither KIs nor members of the TEP did analysis of any kind and did not contribute to the writing of the report. Members of the TEP were invited to provide feedback on an initial draft of the review protocol, which was then refined based on their input, reviewed by AHRQ, and posted for public access at the AHRQ Effective Health Care Program Web site.[14]

Literature Search Strategy

To identify the relevant published literature, we searched PubMed®, Embase®, and the Cochrane Database of Systematic Reviews. An experienced search librarian guided all searches. Exact search strings and dates are included in the Appendix of the full report. We date-limited our search to articles published since 1995, corresponding with the time period when contemporary studies on antiplatelet therapy, exercise training, endovascular interventions, and surgical revascularization were published. We supplemented the electronic searches with a manual search of references from a key set of primary and systematic review articles. All citations were imported into an electronic database (EndNote® X4; Thomson Reuters: Philadelphia, PA).

We searched the grey literature of study registries and conference abstracts for relevant articles from completed studies, including ClinicalTrials.gov; metaRegister of Controlled Trials; WHO International Clinical Trials Registry Platform Search Portal; and ProQuest COS Conference Papers Index. Scientific information packets were requested from the manufacturers of medications and devices and reviewed for relevant articles.

Inclusion and Exclusion Criteria

Criteria used to screen articles for inclusion/exclusion at both the title-and-abstract and full-text screening stages are detailed in the full report. English-language randomized controlled trials (RCTs) or observational studies with relevant treatment comparisons and outcomes were included. For KQ 1, this consisted of studies of all PAD populations comparing antiplatelet medications (aspirin or clopidogrel). For KQ 2, this consisted of studies of PAD patients with IC comparing exercise therapy, medications (cilostazol, pentoxifylline), endovascular intervention (percutaneous transluminal angioplasty, atherectomy, or stents), and/or surgical revascularization (endarterectomy, bypass surgery). For KQ 3, this consisted of studies of PAD patients with CLI or the combination of patients with IC or CLI comparing endovascular interventions, surgical revascularization, and/or usual care. The following outcomes were considered: cardiovascular events, (e.g., all-cause mortality, MI, stroke, cardiovascular death), amputation, quality of life, wound healing, functional capacity, repeat revascularization, vessel patency, and adverse effects of therapy.

Study Selection

Using the prespecified inclusion and exclusion criteria, titles and abstracts were examined independently by two reviewers for potential relevance to the KQs. Articles included by any reviewer underwent full-text screening. At the full-text screening stage, two independent reviewers read each article to determine if it met eligibility criteria. At the full-text review stage, paired researchers independently reviewed the articles and indicated a decision to include or exclude the article for data abstraction. When the paired reviewers arrived at different decisions about whether to include or exclude an article, we reconciled the difference through a third-party arbitrator. Relevant review articles, meta-analyses, and methods articles were flagged for hand-searching and cross-referencing against the library of citations identified through electronic database searching. All screening decisions were made and tracked in a DistillerSR database (Evidence Partners, Inc.: Manotick, Ontario, Canada).

Data Extraction

The investigative team created data abstraction forms and evidence table templates for the KQs. The design and piloting of the data abstraction forms is described in detail in the full report. Based on clinical and methodological expertise, two investigators were assigned to the research questions to abstract data from the eligible articles. One investigator abstracted the data, and the second reviewed the completed abstraction form alongside the original article to check for accuracy and completeness. Disagreements were resolved by consensus or by obtaining a third reviewer's opinion if consensus could not be reached.

Quality Assessment of Individual Studies

We evaluated the quality of individual studies by using the approach described in the Methods Guide.[13] To assess quality, we used the strategy to (1) classify the study design, (2) apply predefined criteria for quality and critical appraisal, and (3) arrive at a summary judgment of the study's quality. For RCTs, criteria included adequacy of randomization and allocation concealment; the comparability of groups at baseline; blinding; the completeness of followup and differential loss to followup; whether incomplete data were addressed appropriately; the validity of outcome measures; and conflict of interest. For observational studies, additional elements such as methods for selection of participants, measurement of interventions, addressing any design-specific issues, and controlling for confounding were considered. We used the summary ratings of good, fair, or poor based on the study's adherence to well-accepted standard methodologies and adequate reporting.[13]

Data Synthesis

We began our data synthesis by summarizing key features of the included studies for each KQ. We then determined the feasibility of completing a quantitative synthesis (i.e., meta-analysis). Feasibility depended on the volume of relevant literature, conceptual homogeneity of the studies, and completeness of the reporting of results. We considered meta-analysis for comparisons where at least three studies reported the same outcome at similar followup intervals.

Meta-analyses were based on the nature of the outcome variable, but random-effects models were used for all outcomes because of the heterogeneity of the studies. Continuous outcome measures comparing two treatments that used a similar scale were combined without transformation using a random-effects model as implemented in Comprehensive Meta-Analysis Version 2 (Biostat: Englewood, New Jersey). Continuous outcome measures comparing two treatments made on different scales (such as quality-of-life measures) were combined using a random-effects model on the effect sizes as implemented in Comprehensive Meta-Analysis. Dichotomous outcome measures comparing two treatments were combined and odds ratios were computed using a random-effects model as implemented in Comprehensive Meta-Analysis.

For KQ 2, there were a limited number of studies available for each treatment comparison, and some studies had multiple treatment arms; therefore, direct comparative analysis could not be performed. Instead, we employed the methods of indirect comparative meta-analysis. RCTs reporting continuous outcome measures on different scales (such as functional capacity and quality-of-life measures) were combined using a random-effects meta-regression model on the effect sizes as implemented in the SAS procedure NLMIXED (SAS Institute: Cary, North Carolina). Effect size interpretation is based on Cohen's d, whereby zero equates to no effect, 0.2 equates to a small effect, 0.5 equates to a medium effect, 0.8 equates to a large effect, and effects larger than 1.0 equate to very large effects.[15] The p-value is an indication of the significance of the effect, which is also reflected by the confidence interval around the summary estimate. Factors influencing the significance of the effect (or p-value) include the number of studies contributing to the estimate, the standard error of each individual study, and the heterogeneity of the individual study results.

Studies reporting dichotomous outcome measures were combined using a random-effects, multiple logistic model as implemented in EGRET (Cytel Software Corporation: Cambridge, Massachusetts). We tested for statistical heterogeneity between studies (Q and I^2 statistics) while recognizing that the power to detect such heterogeneity may be limited. Potential clinical heterogeneity between studies was reflected through the confidence intervals of the summary statistics obtained from a random-effects approach. We present summary estimates, standard errors, and confidence intervals in our data synthesis.

Strength of the Body of Evidence

We rated the strength of evidence (SOE) for each KQ and outcome using the approach described in the Methods Guide.[16,17] In brief, this approach requires assessment of four domains: risk of bias, consistency, directness, and precision. Additionally, when appropriate, the observational studies were evaluated for the presence of confounders that would diminish an observed effect, the strength of association (magnitude of effect), and publication bias. These domains were considered qualitatively, and a summary rating of high, moderate, or low SOE was assigned after discussion by two reviewers. In some cases, high, moderate, or low ratings were impossible or imprudent to make; for example, when no evidence was available or when evidence on the outcome was too weak, sparse, or inconsistent to permit any conclusion to be drawn. In these situations, a grade of insufficient was assigned.

Applicability

We assessed applicability across our KQs using the method described in the Methods Guide.[13,18] In brief, this method uses the PICOTS format as a way to organize information relevant to applicability. We used these data to evaluate the applicability to clinical practice, paying special attention to study eligibility criteria; demographic features of the enrolled population (such as age, ethnicity, and sex) in comparison with the target population; version or characteristics of the intervention used in comparison with therapies currently in use (such as specific components of treatments considered to be "optimal medical therapy," plus advances over time in endovascular and surgical revascularization techniques); and clinical relevance and timing of the outcome measures. We summarized issues of applicability qualitatively.

Results

Figure B depicts the flow of articles through the literature search and screening process for the review. Searches of PubMed®, Embase®, and the Cochrane Database of Systematic Reviews from January 1995 to August 2012 yielded 5,908 citations, 1,082 of which were duplicates. Manual searching and contacts to drug manufacturers identified 47 additional citations, for a total of 4,873. After applying inclusion/exclusion criteria at the title-and-abstract level, 626 full-text articles were retrieved and screened. Of these, 521 were excluded at the full-text screening stage, leaving 105 articles (representing 83 unique studies) for data abstraction.

Figure B. Literature flow diagram

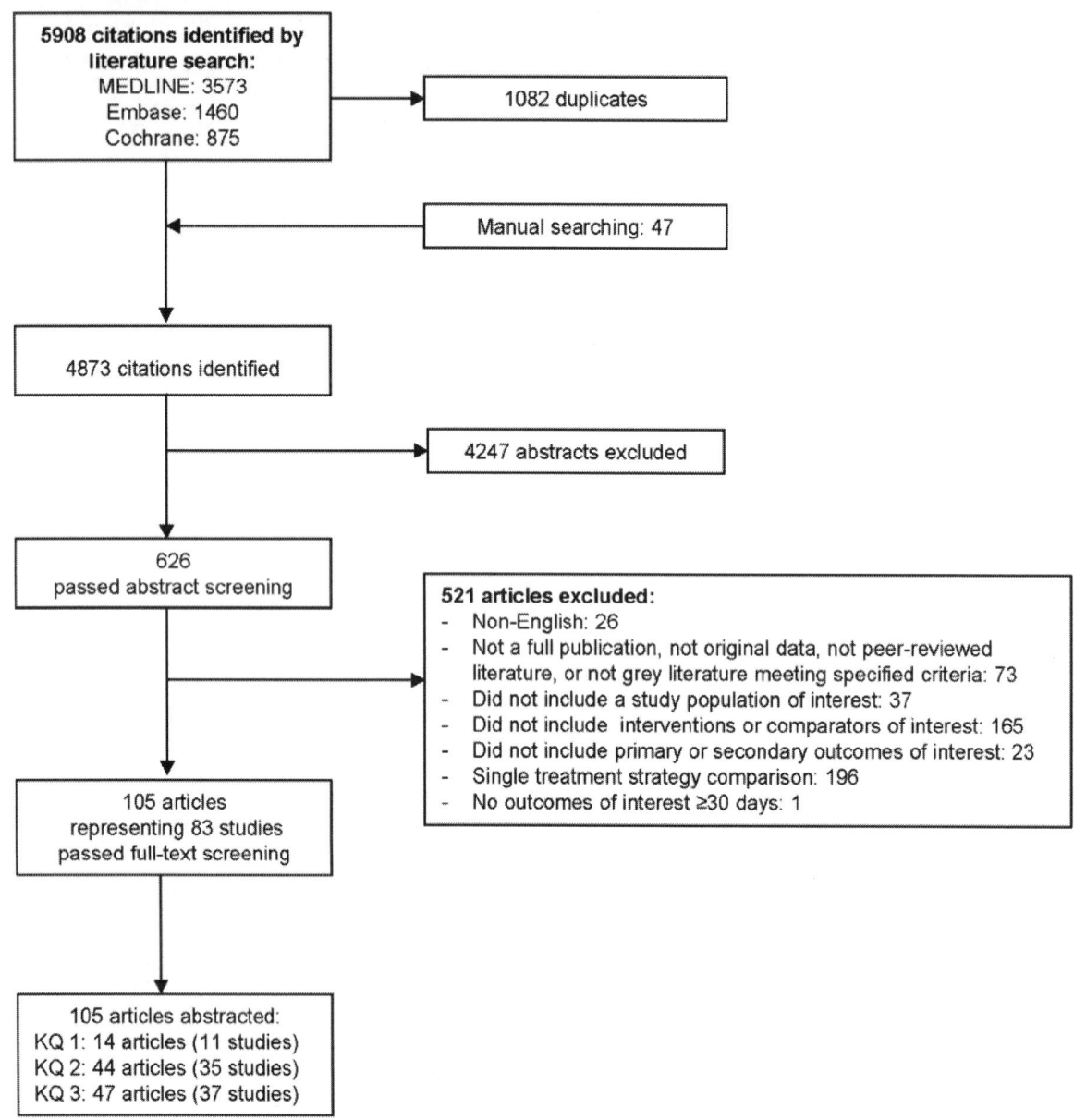

```
┌─────────────────────────────┐
│ 5908 citations identified by│
│    literature search:       │──────▶ 1082 duplicates
│    MEDLINE: 3573            │
│    Embase: 1460             │
│    Cochrane: 875            │
└─────────────────────────────┘
               │
               │         ◀──────── Manual searching: 47
               ▼
┌─────────────────────────────┐
│  4873 citations identified  │
└─────────────────────────────┘
               │
               │────────▶ 4247 abstracts excluded
               ▼
┌─────────────────────────────┐
│           626               │
│  passed abstract screening  │
└─────────────────────────────┘
               │
               │────────▶ 521 articles excluded:
               │           - Non-English: 26
               │           - Not a full publication, not original data, not peer-reviewed
               │             literature, or not grey literature meeting specified criteria: 73
               │           - Did not include a study population of interest: 37
               │           - Did not include interventions or comparators of interest: 165
               │           - Did not include primary or secondary outcomes of interest: 23
               │           - Single treatment strategy comparison: 196
               ▼           - No outcomes of interest ≥30 days: 1
┌─────────────────────────────┐
│       105 articles          │
│   representing 83 studies   │
│  passed full-text screening │
└─────────────────────────────┘
               │
               ▼
┌─────────────────────────────┐
│    105 articles abstracted: │
│  KQ 1: 14 articles (11 studies) │
│  KQ 2: 44 articles (35 studies) │
│  KQ 3: 47 articles (37 studies) │
└─────────────────────────────┘
```

Abbreviations: KQ=Key Question; RCT=randomized controlled trial.

KQ 1. Comparative Effectiveness and Safety of Antiplatelet Therapy for Adults With PAD

We identified 11 unique studies (10 RCTs, 1 observational) that evaluated the comparative effectiveness of aspirin and antiplatelet agents in 15,150 patients with PAD. (Please refer to the full report for references to included studies.)

The key points are:

- For asymptomatic PAD patients, there appears to be no benefit of aspirin over placebo for all-cause mortality, cardiovascular mortality, MI, or stroke (high SOE for all outcomes except cardiovascular mortality, which was rated moderate based on two good-quality RCTs).

- For IC patients, one small, fair-quality RCT suggests with low SOE that aspirin compared with placebo may reduce MI (fatal and nonfatal) and composite vascular events (MI/stroke/pulmonary embolus), but there was insufficient SOE for all other outcomes due to study quality and imprecision.
- For IC patients, the PAD subgroup analysis of the CAPRIE RCT suggests that clopidogrel is more effective than aspirin for reducing cardiovascular mortality, nonfatal MI, and composite vascular events (moderate SOE for all outcomes). Clopidogrel and aspirin appear to be equivalent for prevention of nonfatal stroke, but the confidence interval was wide, making this conclusion less certain (low SOE).
- In patients with symptomatic or asymptomatic PAD, the PAD subgroup analysis of the CHARISMA RCT showed no difference between aspirin and dual therapy (clopidogrel plus aspirin) for outcomes of all-cause mortality (moderate SOE), nonfatal stroke (low SOE), cardiovascular mortality (low SOE), or composite vascular events (moderate SOE). There was a statistically significant benefit favoring dual therapy compared with aspirin for reducing nonfatal MI (low SOE).
- In patients with IC or CLI after unilateral bypass, the CASPAR RCT showed that DAPT resulted in no difference in nonfatal stroke and composite vascular events (low SOE), but there was insufficient SOE for other outcomes.
- In patients with IC or CLI after endovascular procedure, the MIRROR RCT showed no difference between dual therapy and aspirin in cardiovascular events or mortality at 6 months but was insufficiently powered for those outcomes (insufficient SOE).

Four RCTs reported subgroup analyses of demographic or clinical factors that modify the effect of antiplatelet agents in PAD and involved 5,053 patients. Two of these RCTs included asymptomatic or high-risk patients and two included patients with either IC or CLI. Subgroups analyzed included diabetes (one RCT), age (one RCT), sex (two RCTs), and PAD characteristics (two studies assessing ABI or type of bypass graft). The small number of and variation in subgroup analyses precluded the calculation of any overall estimate.

One RCT of patients with IC or CLI showed a benefit of clopidogrel plus aspirin for reducing composite vascular events in patients with a prosthetic bypass graft compared with those with a venous bypass graft. Clinical outcomes were similar in men and women treated with antiplatelet agents. Given the heterogeneity of the subgroups, interventions, and clinical outcomes, the SOE for modifiers of effectiveness was insufficient.

Seven RCTs reported safety concerns from antiplatelet treatment in the PAD population and involved 8297 patients. All seven RCTs reported bleeding as a harm. In general, use of antiplatelet agents was associated with higher rates of minor and moderate bleeding compared with placebo, ranging from 2 to 4 percent with aspirin, 2 percent with dual antiplatelet (no procedure), and 2.5 to 16.7 percent with dual antiplatelet (after percutaneous transluminal angioplasty or bypass grafting). Some RCTs reported adverse events such as rash and wound leak. The SOE of evidence for safety concerns is insufficient.

Table A shows summary SOE ratings for KQ 1. The full report contains detailed SOE tables with ratings for risk of bias, consistency, directness, and precision for each outcome and comparison.

Table A. Summary SOE for KQ 1: Comparative effectiveness and safety of antiplatelet therapy for adults with PAD[a]

Comparison	Population	Outcome SOE	Results or Effect Estimate (95% Confidence Interval)
Aspirin vs. placebo in adults with asymptomatic or symptomatic PAD at 2+ years	*Asymptomatic population*	All-cause mortality **SOE=High**	2 RCTs, 3,986 patients HR 0.93 (0.71 to 1.24) HR 0.95 (0.77 to 1.16) No difference
		Nonfatal MI **SOE=High**	2 RCTs, 3,986 patients HR 0.98 (0.68 to 1.42) HR 0.91 (0.65 to 1.29) No difference
		Nonfatal stroke **SOE=High**	2 RCTs, 3,986 patients HR 0.71 (0.44 to 1.14) HR 0.97 (0.62 to 1.53) No difference
		Cardiovascular mortality **SOE=Moderate**	2 RCTs, 3,986 patients HR 1.23 (0.79 to 1.92) HR 0.95 (0.77 to 1.17) No difference
		Composite vascular events **SOE=High**	2 RCTs, 3,986 patients HR 0.98 (0.76 to 1.26) HR 1.00 (0.85 to 1.17) No difference
		Functional outcomes Quality of life Safety concerns (subgroups) **SOE=Insufficient**	0 studies
		Modifiers of effectiveness (subgroups) **SOE=Insufficient**	2 RCTs, 3,986 patients Inconclusive evidence due to imprecision, with 1 study reporting similar rates of cardiovascular outcomes by age, sex, or baseline ABI and 1 study reporting similar rates of cardiovascular mortality and stroke by diabetic status.
		Safety concerns **SOE=Insufficient**	2 RCTs, 3,986 patients Inconclusive evidence due to heterogeneous results between aspirin and placebo in regard to major hemorrhage and GI bleeding rates.
	IC population	Nonfatal MI **SOE=Low**	1 RCT, 181 patients HR 0.18 (0.04 to 0.82) Favors aspirin.
		Nonfatal stroke **SOE=Insufficient**	1 RCT, 181 patients HR 0.54 (0.16 to 1.84) Inconclusive evidence due to imprecision.
		Cardiovascular mortality **SOE=Insufficient**	1 RCT, 181 patients HR 1.21 (0.32 to 4.55) Inconclusive evidence due to imprecision.
		Composite vascular events **SOE=Low**	1 RCT, 181 patients HR 0.35 (0.15 to 0.82) Favors aspirin.
		Functional outcomes Quality of life Safety concerns (subgroups **SOE=Insufficient**	0 studies

Table A. Summary SOE for KQ 1: Comparative effectiveness and safety of antiplatelet therapy for adults with PAD[a] (continued)

Comparison	Population	Outcome SOE	Results or Effect Estimate (95% Confidence Interval)
Aspirin vs. placebo in adults with asymptomatic or symptomatic PAD at 2+ years (continued)		Modifiers of effectiveness (subgroups) SOE=Insufficient	1 RCT, 216 patients Inconclusive evidence due to imprecision, with 1 study reporting similar rates in vessel patency by sex.
		Safety concerns SOE=Insufficient	1 RCT, 181 patients Inconclusive evidence due to imprecision, with 1 study reporting a bleeding rate of 3% in aspirin group and 0% in placebo group.
	CLI population	Nonfatal MI SOE=Insufficient	1 observational study, 113 patients Inconclusive evidence due to imprecision, with 1 study reporting MI rate of 1.2% in aspirin group and 5.9% in no-aspirin group.
		Nonfatal stroke SOE=Insufficient	1 observational study, 113 patients Inconclusive evidence due to imprecision, with 1 study reporting stroke rate of 2.5% in aspirin group and 8.8% in no-aspirin group.
		Cardiovascular mortality SOE=Insufficient	1 observational study, 113 patients Inconclusive evidence due to imprecision, with 1 study reporting cardiovascular mortality rate of 33% in aspirin group and 26% in no-aspirin group..
		Functional outcomes Quality of life Modifiers of effectiveness (subgroups) Safety concerns Safety concerns (subgroups) SOE=Insufficient	0 studies
Clopidogrel vs. aspirin in adults with IC at 2 years (CAPRIE)		Nonfatal MI SOE=Moderate	1 RCT, 6,452 patients HR 0.62 (0.43 to 0.88) Favors clopidogrel.
		Nonfatal stroke SOE=Low	1 RCT, 6,452 patients HR 0.95 (0.68 to 1.31) No difference.
		Cardiovascular mortality SOE=Moderate	1 RCT, 6,452 patients HR 0.76 (0.64 to 0.91) Favors clopidogrel.
		Composite cardiovascular events SOE=Moderate	1 RCT, 6,452 patients HR 0.78 (0.65 to 0.93) Favors clopidogrel.
		All-cause mortality Functional outcomes Quality of life Modifiers of effectiveness (subgroups) Safety concerns Safety concerns (subgroups) SOE=Insufficient	0 studies

Table A. Summary SOE for KQ 1: Comparative effectiveness and safety of antiplatelet therapy for adults with PAD[a] (continued)

Comparison	Population	Outcome SOE	Results or Effect Estimate (95% Confidence Interval)
Clopidogrel vs. aspirin in adults with IC at 2 years (CAPRIE) (continued)	Symptomatic–asymptomatic population (CHARISMA)	All-cause mortality SOE=Moderate	1 RCT, 3,096 patients HR 0.89 (0.68 to 1.16) No difference.
		Nonfatal MI SOE=Low	1 RCT, 3,096 patients HR 0.63 (0.42 to 0.95) Favors dual antiplatelet.
		Nonfatal stroke SOE=Low	1 RCT, 3,096 patients HR 0.79 (0.51 to 1.22) No difference.
		Cardiovascular mortality SOE=Low	1 RCT, 3,096 patients HR 0.92 (0.66 to 1.29) No difference.
		Composite cardiovascular events SOE=Moderate	1 RCT, 3,096 patients HR 0.85 (0.66 to 1.09) No difference.
		Functional outcomes Quality of life Safety concerns (subgroups) Modifiers of effectiveness (subgroups) SOE=Insufficient	0 studies
		Safety concerns SOE=Insufficient	1 RCT, 3,096 patients Inconclusive evidence due to low rates of severe and moderate bleeding, although minor bleeding was significantly higher with DAPT (34.4%) vs. ASA (20.8%).
	IC–CLI population (CASPAR, MIRROR, Cassar)	All-cause mortality SOE=Insufficient	2 RCTs, 931 patients CASPAR, HR 1.44 (0.77 to 2.69) MIRROR, OR 0.33 (0.01 to 8.22) Inconclusive evidence due to imprecision.
		Nonfatal MI SOE=Insufficient	1 RCT, 851 patients CASPAR, HR 0.81 (0.32 to 2.06) Inconclusive evidence due to imprecision.
		Nonfatal stroke SOE=Low	1 RCT, 851 patients CASPAR, HR 1.02 (0.41 to 2.55) No difference.
		Cardiovascular mortality SOE=Insufficient	1 RCT, 851 patients CASPAR, HR 1.44 (0.77 to 2.69) Inconclusive evidence due to imprecision.
		Composite cardiovascular events SOE=Low (CASPAR) SOE=Insufficient (MIRROR)	2 RCTs, 931 patients CASPAR, HR 1.09 (0.65 to 1.82), No difference MIRROR, OR 0.71 (0.28 to 1.81), Inconclusive evidence due to imprecision.
		Functional outcomes Quality of life Safety concerns (subgroups) SOE=Insufficient	0 studies

Table A. Summary SOE for KQ 1: Comparative effectiveness and safety of antiplatelet therapy for adults with PAD[a] (continued)

Comparison	Population	Outcome SOE	Results or Effect Estimate (95% Confidence Interval)
Clopidogrel vs. aspirin in adults with IC at 2 years (CAPRIE) (continued)		Modifiers of effectiveness (subgroups) SOE=Insufficient	1 RCT, 851 patients Inconclusive evidence due to imprecision, with 1 study reporting that patients with prosthetic graft had lower cardiovascular events on DAPT.
		Safety concerns SOE=Insufficient	3 RCTs, 1,034 patients Inconclusive evidence due to inconsistent results from individual studies: CASPAR study showed statistically significant higher rates of moderate and minor bleeding with DAPT; Cassar study showed more bruising with DAPT but no significant difference in gastrointestinal bleeding or hematoma; MIRROR study showed no significant difference in bleeding.

[a]Grey background indicates insufficient SOE.
Abbreviations: ABI=ankle-brachial index; CLI=critical limb ischemia; DAPT=dual antiplatelet therapy; HR=hazard ratio; IC=intermittent claudication; OR=odds ratio; RCT=randomized controlled trial; SOE=strength of evidence.

KQ 2. Comparative Effectiveness and Safety of Exercise, Medications, and Endovascular and Surgical Revascularization for IC

We identified 35 unique studies (27 RCTs, 8 observational) that evaluated the comparative effectiveness of exercise training, medications, endovascular intervention, and/or surgical revascularization in 7475 patients who have PAD with IC. (Please refer to the full report for references to included studies.)

The following comparisons were assessed in the included studies: (1) medical therapy (cilostazol) versus placebo (10 RCTs; 4,103 total patients); (2) exercise training versus usual care (10 RCTs, two observational; 754 total patients); (3) endovascular intervention versus usual care (five RCTs, four observational; 1,593 total patients); (4) surgical revascularization versus usual care (1 observational; 427 total patients); (5) endovascular intervention versus exercise training (Nine RCTs; 1,005 total patients); (6) surgical revascularization versus exercise plus medical therapy (1 observational; 127 total patients); and (7) endovascular versus surgical revascularization (three observational studies; 836 total patients).

A majority of the endovascular procedures consisted of percutaneous transluminal angioplasty with or without stent placement; and the type of stent was not specified. Differences in treatment comparisons, measures, and followup time points reduced the number of studies that could be pooled for analysis of direct comparisons. When this occurred, we constructed an effect size for each relevant arm of each study. We used a random-effects model that was a generalization of the standard random-effects model used in the meta-analysis of effect sizes.

The Key Points are:
- In a random-effects network meta-analysis of 12 RCTs that assessed the effect of 6 comparisons on all-cause mortality, no specific treatment was found to have a statistically significant effect (low SOE for all comparisons) (See Figure C).

Figure C. Network meta-analysis of treatment effects versus usual care and each other on mortality in IC patients

Treatment comparison	Odds ratio	Lower limit	Upper limit	p-Value
Cilostazol vs. Control	0.91	0.62	1.35	0.65
Exercise vs. Control	0.84	0.34	2.07	0.70
Exercise vs. Cilostazol	0.65	0.27	1.55	0.33
Endovascular vs. Control	0.91	0.34	2.45	0.86
Endovascular vs. Cilostazol	0.71	0.27	1.84	0.48
Endovascular vs. Exercise	0.77	0.39	1.54	0.47

Favors first treatment — Favors second treatment

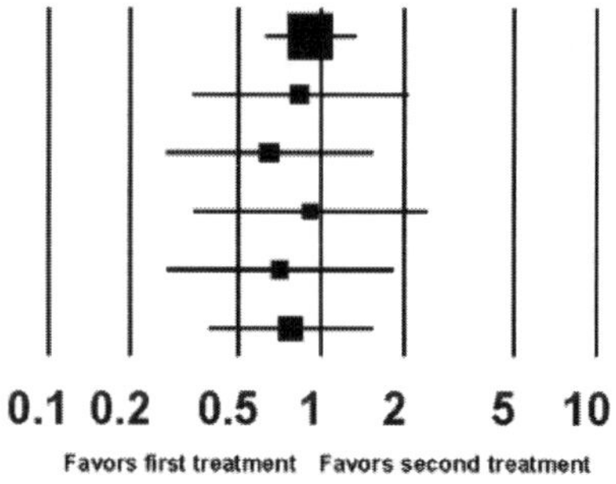

Abbreviation: CI=confidence interval.

- A random-effects meta-analysis of 16 RCTs compared the effect of multiple treatments on maximal walking distance (MWD) or absolute claudication distance (ACD). Exercise training, pentoxifylline, and the combination of endovascular treatment with exercise were associated with large effects, while cilostazol and endovascular intervention were associated with moderate effects when compared with usual care (Figure D). A sensitivity analysis that removed the pentoxifylline studies (due to inconsistent and imprecise results) is shown in Figure E, with effect size estimates that are slightly increased for the remaining treatment modalities. None of the other treatments were found to have a statistically significant effect when compared against each other (Figures F and G). We observed similar results in studies that were excluded due to measurement of peak walking time rather than distance. SOE was rated *moderate* for exercise; *low* for cilostazol, endovascular treatment, and the combination of endovascular treatment with exercise; and *insufficient* for pentoxifylline.

Figure D. Network meta-analysis of treatment effects versus usual care on walking distance in IC patients

Treatment	Std diff in means	Lower limit	Upper limit	p-Value
Exercise training	0.89	0.06	1.71	0.04
Cilostazol	0.62	-0.21	1.45	0.14
Pentoxifylline	1.70	0.36	3.04	0.01
Endovascular intervention	0.41	-0.54	1.36	0.40
Endovascular intervention & exercise	1.08	-0.37	2.53	0.14

Favors Usual Care — Favors Treatment

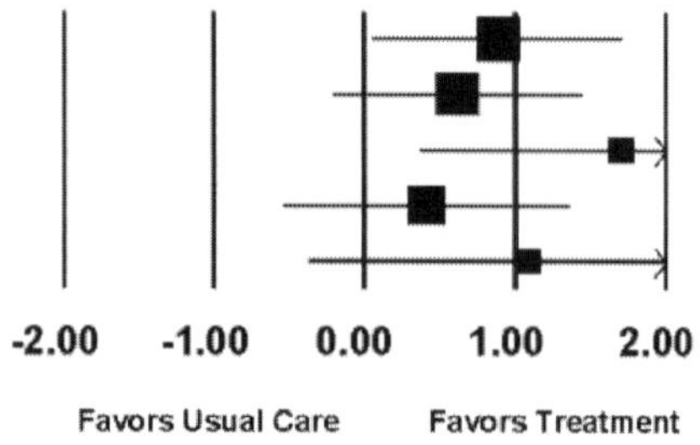

Abbreviation: CI=confidence interval.

Figure E. Network sensitivity meta-analysis of treatment effects versus usual care on walking distance in IC patients

Treatment	Std diff in means	Lower limit	Upper limit	p-Value
Exercise training	0.98	0.23	1.74	0.01
Cilostazol	0.61	-0.20	1.42	0.14
Endovascular intervention	0.51	-0.35	1.37	0.25
Endovascular intervention & exercise	1.20	-0.11	2.50	0.07

Abbreviation: CI=confidence interval.

Figure F. Network meta-analysis of treatment effects versus each other on walking distance in IC patients

Treatment comparison	Std diff in means	Lower limit	Upper limit	p-Value
Cilostazol vs Pentoxifylline	1.08	-0.35	2.52	0.14
Cilostazol vs Endovascular	-0.21	-1.33	0.92	0.72
Cilostazol vs Endovascular & exercise	0.46	-1.10	2.03	0.56
Pentoxifylline vs Endovascular	-1.29	-2.84	0.26	0.10
Pentoxifylline vs Endovascular & exercise	-0.62	-2.51	1.27	0.52
Exercise vs Cilostazol	-0.27	-1.29	0.76	0.61
Exercise vs Pentoxifylline	0.82	-0.67	2.30	0.28
Exercise vs Endovascular	-0.47	-1.40	0.46	0.32
Exercise vs Endovascular & exercise	0.20	-1.23	1.63	0.79
Endovascular vs Endovascular & exercise	0.67	-0.71	2.05	0.34

Abbreviation: CI=confidence interval.

Figure G. Network sensitivity meta-analysis of treatment effects versus each other on walking distance in IC patients

Treatment comparison	Std diff in means	Lower limit	Upper limit	p-Value
Cilostazol vs Endovascular	-0.10	-1.16	0.96	0.85
Cilostazol vs Endovascular & exercise	0.58	-0.84	2.01	0.42
Exercise vs Cilostazol	-0.37	-1.34	0.60	0.45
Exercise vs Endovascular	-0.47	-1.31	0.36	0.27
Exercise vs Endovascular & exercise	0.22	-1.05	1.50	0.73
Endovascular vs Endovascular & exercise	0.68	-0.55	1.91	0.28

Abbreviation: CI=confidence interval.

- In a random-effects meta-analysis of 12 RCTs that compared the effect of multiple treatments on initial claudication distance or pain-free walking distance, cilostazol was associated with a statistically nonsignificant improvement when compared with usual care; however, exercise training and endovascular revascularization were associated with moderate to large effects and a statistically significant improvement when compared with usual care (Figure H). When directly compared in head-to-head studies, there was no difference between the three treatments. Similar results were observed in studies excluded due to measurement of claudication onset time rather than distance. SOE was rated low across all comparisons.

Figure H. Network meta-analysis of treatment effects versus usual care and each other on claudication distance in IC patients

Treatment comparison	Std diff in means	Lower limit	Upper limit	p-Value
Usual Care vs Cilostazol	0.631	-0.024	1.286	0.059
Usual Care vs Exercise training	0.691	0.230	1.152	0.003
Usual Care vs Endovascular intervention	0.789	0.292	1.286	0.002
Cilostazol vs Exercise training	0.059	-0.668	0.786	0.874
Cilostazol vs Endovascular intervention	0.158	-0.593	0.909	0.680
Exercise vs Endovascular intervention	0.098	-0.376	0.572	0.685

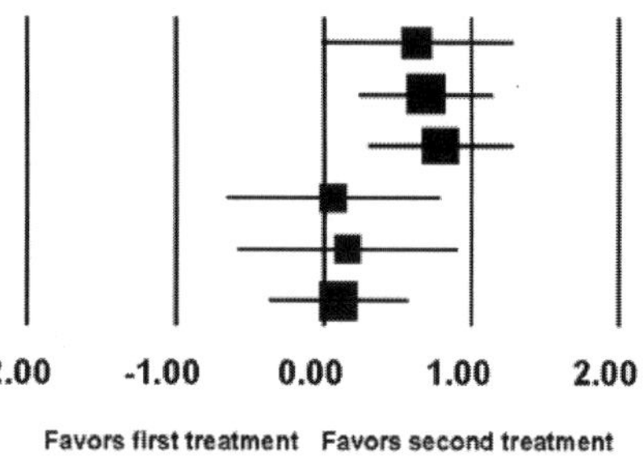

Favors first treatment   Favors second treatment

Abbreviation: CI=confidence interval.

- A random-effects meta-analysis of 10 studies examining the difference in the SF-36 measure of physical functioning assessed between 3 months and 6 months showed a significant improvement in quality of life from cilostazol, exercise training, endovascular intervention, and surgical intervention—ranging from moderate to large effects compared with usual care (Figure I). However, the comparisons of all active treatments with each other showed that none of the treatments are significantly different from each other (Figure J). SOE was rated low for all comparisons.

Figure I. Network meta-analysis of treatment effects versus usual care on quality of life in IC patients

Treatment comparison	Std diff in means	Lower limit	Upper limit	p-Value
Cilostazol	0.4400	0.0479	0.8321	0.0278
Exercise	0.5630	0.2559	0.8701	0.0003
Endovascular	0.6120	0.2989	0.9251	0.0001
Surgical	0.8230	0.2560	1.3900	0.0044

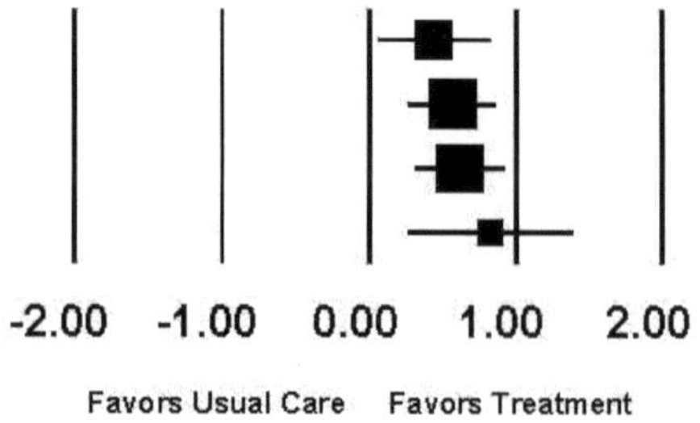

Favors Usual Care   Favors Treatment

Abbreviation: CI=confidence interval.

Figure J. Network meta-analysis of treatment effects versus each other on quality of life in IC patients

Treatment comparison	Std diff in means	Lower limit	Upper limit
Cilostazol vs exercise training	0.12	-0.32	0.56
Cilostazol vs endovascular	0.17	-0.27	0.62
Cilostazol vs surgical	0.38	-0.27	1.03
Exercise training vs endovascular	0.05	-0.24	0.34
Exercise training vs surgical	0.26	-0.31	0.83
Endovascular vs surgical	0.21	-0.34	0.76

Abbreviation: CI=confidence interval.

- Cardiovascular events (e.g., MI, stroke, cardiovascular death), amputation, wound healing, analog pain scale score, repeat revascularization, and vessel patency were infrequently reported. SOE was rated insufficient for all comparisons.
- One observational study of surgical revascularization versus usual care reported mortality and vessel patency results at 5 years. SOE was rated insufficient.

Prior to 1995, many observational studies had been published of surgical revascularization versus usual care, and RCTs of pentoxifylline versus placebo within the IC population. However, to improve the applicability of this report to modern clinical treatment, which includes more aggressive medical therapy with antiplatelet agents and statin medications, these studies published before 1995 were not included in this review.

Six studies (four RCTs, two observational studies) reported variations in the treatment effectiveness by subgroup, including severity of symptoms, functional limitations, anatomic location of disease, and success of revascularization. Despite limited data on which to base definitive conclusions, one observational study reported improvements in quality-of-life measures and ABI in patients with successful endovascular revascularization when compared with patients without successful endovascular revascularization. One other RCT reported a statistically nonsignificant improvement in MWD favoring exercise training over endovascular revascularization in patients with superficial femoral artery stenosis when compared with patients with iliac stenosis. Last, a single observational study reported variability in the patency of surgical revascularization based on anatomic location and graft type.

Seventeen RCTs reported safety concerns. A single RCT of exercise therapy versus usual care did not identify side effects from exercise. RCTs of cilostazol had higher rates of headache, palpitation complications, and diarrhea. RCTs of endovascular interventions reported more transfusions, arterial dissection/perforation, and hematomas compared with the usual care groups, but the complication rates were low (1 to 2 percent). No studies were identified that measured contrast nephropathy, radiation, infection, or exercise-related harms. No studies reported on whether any of the harms vary by subgroup (age, sex, race, risk factors, comorbidities, anatomic location of disease). The SOE for safety concerns by subgroup was insufficient.

Table B shows summary SOE ratings for KQ 2. The full report contains detailed SOE tables with ratings for risk of bias, consistency, directness, and precision for each outcome and comparison.

Table B. Summary SOE for KQ 2: Comparative effectiveness and safety of treatments for IC[a]

Comparison	Outcome SOE	Results or Effect Estimate (95% Confidence Interval)
Medical therapy vs. usual care	All-cause mortality SOE=Low	4 RCTs, 2732 patients OR 0.91 (0.62 to 1.35) No difference.
	Nonfatal MI SOE=Insufficient	2 RCTs, 497 patients Inconclusive evidence due to low event rates in both groups.
	Nonfatal stroke SOE=Insufficient	3 RCTs, 1932 patients Inconclusive evidence due to low event rates in both groups.
	Amputation SOE=Insufficient	2 RCTs, 497 patients Inconclusive evidence due to sparse data, with only 1 patient who underwent amputation in the 2 RCTs.
	Quality of life SOE=Low	2 RCTs, 631 patients ES: 0.44 (0.05 to 0.83) Favors cilostazol.
	MWD or ACD **SOE=Low (cilostazol)** **SOE=Insufficient (pentoxifylline)**	Cilostazol (6 RCTs, 1632 patients) ES: 0.62 (-0.21 to 1.45) full model; 0.61 (-0.20 to 1.42) sensitivity analysis No difference. Pentoxifylline (3 RCTs, 797 patients) ES: 1.70 (0.36 to 3.04) full model Inconclusive evidence due to imprecision.
	Initial claudication distance or pain-free walking distance **SOE=Low (cilostazol)**	5 RCTs, 1255 patients ES: 0.63 (-0.03 to 1.29) No difference.
	Modifiers of effectiveness (subgroups) SOE=Insufficient	2 RCTs, 155 patients Inconclusive evidence due to individual studies reporting different endpoints.
	Safety concerns **SOE=High (headache)** **SOE=Moderate (diarrhea)** **SOE=Moderate (palpitations)**	Higher side effects on cilostazol Headache 10 RCTs, 3485 patients OR 3.00 (2.29 to 3.95) Diarrhea 10 RCTs, 3485 patients OR 2.51 (1.58 to 3.97) Palpitations 10 RCTs, 3485 patients OR 18.11 (5.95 to 55.13)
	Primary patency Secondary patency Composite cardiovascular events Wound healing Analog pain scale Safety concerns (subgroups) **SOE=Insufficient**	0 studies

Table B. Summary SOE for KQ 2: Comparative effectiveness and safety of treatments for IC[a] (continued)

Comparison	Outcome SOE	Results or Effect Estimate (95% Confidence Interval)
Exercise training vs. usual care	All-cause mortality **SOE=Low**	2 RCTs, 238 patients OR 0.84 (0.34 to 2.07) No difference.
	Nonfatal MI **SOE=Insufficient**	1 RCT, 63 patients Inconclusive evidence due to sparse data, with only 1 MI in exercise group.
	Nonfatal stroke **SOE=Insufficient**	1 RCT, 63 patients Inconclusive evidence due to sparse data, with only 1 stroke in each group.
	Amputation **SOE=Insufficient**	1 RCT; 31 patients Inconclusive evidence due to sparse data, with only 1 patient who underwent amputation.
	Quality of life **SOE=Low**	4 RCTs, 1 observational study, 275 patients ES: 0.56 (0.26 to 0.87) Favors exercise.
	MWD or ACD **SOE=Moderate**	9 RCTs, 2 observational studies, 624 patients ES: 0.89 (0.06 to 1.71) full model; 0.98 (0.23 to 1.74) sensitivity analysis Favors exercise.
	Initial claudication distance or pain-free walking distance **SOE=Low**	9 RCTs, 1 observational studies, 396 patients ES: 0.69 (0.22 to 1.15) Favors exercise.
	Safety concerns **SOE=Insufficient**	3 RCTs, 107 patients Inconclusive evidence due to sparse data, with studies reporting no adverse events in exercise or usual care groups.
	Composite cardiovascular events Wound healing Analog pain scale Safety concerns (subgroups) **SOE=Insufficient**	0 studies
Endovascular intervention vs. usual care	All-cause mortality **SOE=Low**	2 RCTs, 3 observational studies, 977 patients OR 0.91 (0.34 to 2.45) No difference.
	Nonfatal MI **SOE=Insufficient**	1 observational study; 479 patients Inconclusive evidence due to imprecision, with 1 study reporting 3.0% in endovascular group and 8.8% in usual care group.
	Nonfatal stroke **SOE=Insufficient**	2 observational studies; 800 patients Inconclusive evidence due to sparse data, with 1 study reporting 4 strokes for total study, and 1 study reporting 1 stroke in endovascular group, 2 strokes in usual care group.
	Amputation **SOE=Insufficient**	1 RCT, 1 observational study, 73 patients Inconclusive evidence due to imprecision, with 1 study reporting similar amputation rates in the endovascular and usual care groups.
	Quality of life **SOE=Low**	2 RCTs, 2 observational studies, 576 patients ES: 0.61 (0.30 to 0.93) Favors endovascular intervention.

Table B. Summary SOE for KQ 2: Comparative effectiveness and safety of treatments for IC[a] (continued)

Comparison	Outcome SOE	Results or Effect Estimate (95% Confidence Interval)
Endovascular intervention vs. usual care (continued)	MWD or ACD SOE=Low	4 RCTs, 285 patients ES: 0.41 (-0.54 to 1.36) full model; 0.51 (-0.35 to 1.37) sensitivity analysis No difference.
	Initial claudication distance or pain-free walking distance SOE=Low	5 RCTs, 281 patients ES: 0.79 (0.29 to 1.29) Favors endovascular intervention.
	Modifiers of effectiveness (subgroups) SOE=Insufficient	1 observational study, 526 patients Inconclusive evidence due to imprecision, with 1 study reporting better quality-of-life scores if ABI improvement was >0.1 after successful revascularization.
	Safety concerns SOE=Insufficient	2 RCTs, 155 patients Inconclusive evidence due to sparse data, with 1 study reporting no events, and 1 study reporting low rates of transfusion, dissection, and perforation in the endovascular group.
	Composite cardiovascular events Wound healing Analog pain scale Safety concerns (subgroups) SOE=Insufficient	0 studies
Surgical revascularization vs. usual care	All-cause mortality SOE=Insufficient	1 observational study, 427 patients Inconclusive evidence due to imprecision, with mortality rates of 10.4% in surgical group and 16.7% in usual care group.
	Quality of life SOE=Low	2 observational studies, 727 patients ES: 0.82 (0.26 to 1.39) Favors surgery.
	Primary patency Secondary patency SOE=Insufficient	1 observational study, 427 patients Inconclusive evidence due to imprecision, with 1 study reporting vessel patency only in patients undergoing revascularization (aortofemoral bypass 95.5%, axillofemoral bypass 83.3%, femorofemoral bypass 95.5%, femoropopliteal bypass [AK] 67.6%, femorofemoral bypass [BK] 45.2%).
	Modifiers of effectiveness (subgroups) SOE=Insufficient	1 observational study, 427 patients Inconclusive evidence due to results from 1 study where patency rates were significantly lower for infrainguinal bypass and synthetic graft vs. suprainguinal and autologous vein graft.
	Nonfatal MI Nonfatal stroke Amputation Composite cardiovascular events Wound healing Analog pain scale Safety concerns (subgroups) SOE=Insufficient	0 studies

Table B. Summary SOE for KQ 2: Comparative effectiveness and safety of treatments for IC[a] (continued)

Comparison	Outcome SOE	Results or Effect Estimate (95% Confidence Interval)
Endovascular intervention vs. exercise training	All-cause mortality **SOE=Low**	5 RCTs, 710 patients OR 0.77 (0.39 to 1.54) No difference.
	Nonfatal MI **SOE=Insufficient**	1 RCT, 106 patients Inconclusive evidence due to sparse data, with no events occurring in either treatment group.
	Nonfatal stroke **SOE=Insufficient**	1 RCT, 106 patients Inconclusive evidence due to sparse data, with only 1 stroke in each group.
	Amputation **SOE=Insufficient**	1 RCT, 149 patients Inconclusive evidence due to sparse data, with 1 amputation in endovascular group and none in exercise group.
	Quality of life **SOE=Low**	4 RCTs, 444 patients ES: 0.05 (-0.24 to 0.34) No difference.
	MWD or ACD **SOE=Moderate**	4 RCTs, 695 patients ES: -0.47 (-1.41 to 0.46) full model; -0.47 (-1.31 to 0.36) sensitivity analysis No difference.
	ICD or PFWD **SOE=Low**	5 RCTs, 448 patients ES: 0.10 (-0.38 to 0.58) No difference.
	Modifiers of effectiveness (subgroups) **SOE=Insufficient**	1 RCT, 56 patients Inconclusive evidence due to indirect results from 1 study reporting a statistically nonsignificant improvement in MWD in patients with SFA disease treated with PTA.
	Safety concerns **SOE=Insufficient**	5 RCTs, 282 patients Inconclusive evidence due to heterogeneity of reporting, with individual studies reporting that endovascular interventions were associated with higher rates of transfusion, dissection/perforation, and hematomas.
	Composite cardiovascular events Wound healing Analog pain scale Safety concerns (subgroups) **SOE=Insufficient**	0 studies
Surgical intervention vs. exercise + medical therapy (pentoxifylline)	MWD or ACD **SOE=Insufficient**	1 observational study, 127 patients Inconclusive evidence due to imprecision, with 1 study reporting that MWT improved to >15 min in surgical group and >11 min in exercise plus medical therapy group.
	Initial claudication distance or pain-free walking distance **SOE=Insufficient**	1 observational study, 127 patients Inconclusive evidence due to imprecision, with 1 study reporting that COT improved to >10 min in surgical group and >7 min in exercise plus medical therapy group.
	Composite cardiovascular events Wound healing Analog pain scale Safety concerns (subgroups) **SOE=Insufficient**	0 studies

Table B. Summary SOE for KQ 2: Comparative effectiveness and safety of treatments for IC[a] (continued)

Comparison	Outcome SOE	Results or Effect Estimate (95% Confidence Interval)
Endovascular intervention vs. surgical revascularization	All-cause mortality SOE=Insufficient	2 observational studies, 305 patients Inconclusive evidence due to inadequate reporting, with neither study reporting results by treatment group; overall mortality rate ranged from 3 to 8%.
	Quality of life SOE=Low	2 observational studies, 242 patients ES: 0.21 (-0.34 to 0.76) No difference.
	MWD or absolute claudication distance SOE=Insufficient	0 studies
	ICD or PFWD SOE=Insufficient	0 studies
	Modifiers of effectiveness (subgroups) SOE=Insufficient	1 RCT, 264 patients Inconclusive evidence due to indirect results from 1 study, with similar patency rates for suprainguinal and infrainguinal reconstruction.
	Nonfatal MI Nonfatal stroke Amputation Primary patency Secondary patency Composite cardiovascular events Wound healing Analog pain scale Safety concerns (subgroups) SOE=Insufficient	0 studies
Endovascular intervention + exercise training vs. usual care	MWD or ACD SOE=Low	2 RCTs, 248 patients ES: 1.08 (-0.37 to 2.53) full model; 1.20 (-0.11 to 2.50) sensitivity analysis Favors endovascular intervention plus exercise training.
	Composite cardiovascular events Wound healing Analog pain scale Safety concerns (subgroups) SOE=Insufficient	0 studies
Exercise training vs. invasive therapy vs. usual care	Primary patency Secondary patency SOE=Insufficient	1 RCT, 225 patients Inconclusive evidence due to biased reporting where vessel patency was only reported in patients undergoing revascularization (endovascular group 59%, surgical group 98%).
	Composite cardiovascular events Wound healing Analog pain scale Safety concerns (subgroups) SOE=Insufficient	0 studies

[a]Grey background indicates insufficient SOE.

Abbreviations: ABI=ankle-brachial index; ACD=absolution claudication distance; COT=claudication onset time; ES=effect size; ICD=initial claudication distance; MI= myocardial infarction; MWD=maximal walking distance; MWT=maximal walking time; OR=odds ratio; PFWD=pain-free walking distance; PTA=percutaneous transluminal angioplasty; RCT=randomized controlled trial; SFA=superficial femoral artery; SOE=strength of evidence.

KQ 3. Comparative Effectiveness and Safety of Usual Care and Endovascular and Surgical Revascularization for CLI

We identified 37 unique studies (3 RCTs, 34 observational) that evaluated the comparative effectiveness of usual care, endovascular intervention, and surgical revascularization in CLI or IC-CLI patients. Of these, four observational studies compared usual care with endovascular intervention. Of the 37 studies, 23 (1 RCT, 22 observational) evaluated the comparative effectiveness of endovascular and surgical revascularization in 12,779 patients with CLI, and 12 (2 RCTs, 10 observational) evaluated the comparative effectiveness of endovascular and surgical revascularization in a *mixed* population of 565,168 PAD patients with either IC or CLI. (Please refer to the full report for references to included studies.)

The Key Points are:
- Four observational studies comparing endovascular interventions with usual care reported on mortality, amputation/limb salvage, amputation-free survival, and hospital length of stay. However, because the results were inconsistent and imprecise, SOE was insufficient.
- All-cause mortality was not different between patients treated with endovascular versus surgical revascularization (low SOE), although endovascular interventions did demonstrate a statistically nonsignificant benefit in all-cause mortality at less than 2 years in the IC-CLI population.
- Amputation-free survival was not different between patients treated with endovascular versus surgical revascularization (low SOE).
- Evidence regarding patency rates varied, but secondary patency rates demonstrated a benefit of endovascular interventions compared with surgical revascularization across followup time points (low SOE).

Variations in treatment effectiveness by subgroup were reported in 14 studies (2 RCTs, 12 observational). Subgroups reported included age (three studies), symptom class (three studies), renal failure (two studies), arterial outflow/runoff (two studies), anatomic factors (two studies), type of vein graft (two studies), diabetes (two studies), and one study each on smoking status, vessel patency, sex, hyperlipidemia, hypertension, coronary artery disease, location of stenosis, and stent graft size. In the single RCT of CLI patients, the use of autologous vein was associated with improved outcomes when compared with prosthetic conduit. Additionally, the performance of subintimal angioplasty was associated with statistically nonsignificant worse outcomes when compared with standard angioplasty. Data derived from the observational studies had a high likelihood of bias but did show that with advanced age, renal failure, and higher Rutherford classification, patients generally fared worse in terms of mortality and amputation.

Only one observational study in the CLI population reported safety concerns. Specifically, this study reported the incidence of thrombosis at 30 days and found that the risk of thrombosis was higher in patients undergoing surgical revascularization than in patients undergoing endovascular revascularization. Six studies (two RCTs, four observational) in the mixed IC-CLI population reported harms of bleeding, infection, renal dysfunction, or periprocedural complications causing acute limb ischemia. There were conflicting results in the summary estimates for periprocedural complications in the IC-CLI population, with the observational studies showing lower rates in patients who received an endovascular intervention and RCTs showing lower rates in the surgical population. However, the wide confidence intervals make the differences nonsignificant. Infection was more common in the surgical intervention arm based on three studies.

We found few studies that assessed functional outcomes, quality of life, or cardiovascular outcomes (cardiovascular mortality, nonfatal stroke, nonfatal MI, or composite events); therefore, the evidence base is insufficient to draw any conclusions on these outcomes. Like the other KQs, few studies reported modifiers of effectiveness or safety outcomes.

Table C shows summary SOE ratings for KQ 3. The full report contains detailed SOE tables with ratings for risk of bias, consistency, directness, and precision for each outcome and comparison.

Table C. Summary SOE for KQ 3: Comparative effectiveness and safety of treatments for CLI[a]

Comparison	Outcome SOE	Results or Effect Estimate (95% Confidence Interval)
Endovascular intervention vs. usual care in CLI and IC-CLI populations	All-cause mortality **SOE=Insufficient**	CLI-Obs (3 studies, 562 patients) Inconclusive evidence due to imprecision. IC-CLI-Obs (1 study, 107 patients) Inconclusive evidence due to imprecision, with 1 study reporting similar mortality rates.
	Amputation **SOE=Insufficient**	CLI-Obs (3 studies, 562 patients) Inconclusive evidence due to heterogeneity in reporting amputation rates across studies. IC-CLI-Obs (1 study, 107 patients) Inconclusive evidence due to imprecision, with 1 study reporting a nonsignificant difference.
	Amputation-free survival **SOE=Insufficient**	CLI-Obs (1 study, 70 patients) Inconclusive evidence due to imprecision, with 1 study reporting AFS rates (endovascular group 60%, usual care 47%).
	Length of stay **SOE=Insufficient**	CLI-Obs (3 studies, 562 patients) Inconclusive evidence due to inconsistent and imprecise results across studies.
	Nonfatal stroke Nonfatal MI Composite cardiovascular events MWD or absolute claudication distance Initial claudication distance or pain-free walking distance Quality of life Primary patency Secondary patency Wound healing Analog pain scale Modifiers of effectiveness (subgroups) Safety concerns Safety concerns (subgroups) **SOE=Insufficient**	All PAD populations and study design (0 studies)

Table C. Summary SOE for KQ 3: Comparative effectiveness and safety of treatments for CLI[a] (continued)

Comparison	Outcome SOE	Results or Effect Estimate (95% Confidence Interval)
Endovascular vs. surgical revascularization in CLI and IC-CLI populations	All-cause mortality less than or equal to 6 months **SOE=Low**	CLI-Obs (11 studies, 8,249 patients), OR 0.85 (0.57 to 1.27) CLI-RCT (1 study, 452 patients), OR 0.51 (0.20 to 1.35) Favors endovascular. IC-CLI-Obs (2 studies, 823 patients), OR 0.45 (0.18 to 1.09) Favors endovascular.
	All-cause mortality at 1 to 2 years **SOE=Low**	CLI-Obs (12 studies, 7,850 patients), OR 1.01 (0.80 to 1.28) No difference. IC-CLI-Obs (2 studies, 145 patients), OR 0.51 (0.20 to 1.31) IC-CLI-RCT (2 studies, 130 patients), OR 0.81 (0.23 to 2.82) Favors endovascular.
	All-cause mortality at 3 or more years **SOE=Low (CLI)** **SOE=Insufficient (IC-CLI)**	CLI-Obs (7 studies, 7,176 patients), OR 1.05 (0.54 to 2.06) CLI-RCT (1 study, 452 patients), OR 1.07 (0.73 to 1.56) No difference. IC-CLI-RCT (1 study, 58 patients) OR 0.88 (0.28 to 2.73) Inconclusive evidence due to imprecision.
	Nonfatal MI **SOE=Insufficient**	CLI-RCT (1 study, 452 patients) Inconclusive evidence due to imprecision, with 1 study reporting MI rates (endovascular group 3% and surgical group 8%).
	Amputation at <2 years **SOE=Low (CLI)** **SOE=Insufficient (IC-CLI)**	CLI-Obs (11 studies, 4,490 patients), OR 0.73 (0.48 to 1.09) CLI-RCT (1 study, 452 patients), OR 1.23 (0.72 to 2.11) No difference. IC-CLI-Obs (2 studies, 823 patients), OR 1.11 (0.40 to 3.05) IC-CLI-RCT (2 studies, 130 patients), OR 0.22 (0.05 to 1.07) Inconclusive evidence due to imprecision.
	Amputation at 2 to 3 years **SOE=Low (CLI)** **SOE=Insufficient (IC-CLI)**	CLI-Obs (4 studies, 3,187 patients), OR 1.08 (0.62 to 1.89) CLI-RCT (1 study, 452 patients), OR 1.02 (0.64 to 1.63) No difference. IC-CLI-Obs (1 study, 169 patients), OR 1.00 (0.18 to 5.54) IC-CLI-RCT (1 study, 86 patients), OR 0.18 (0.02 to 1.29) Inconclusive evidence due to imprecision.

Table C. Summary SOE for KQ 3: Comparative effectiveness and safety of treatments for CLI[a] (continued)

Comparison	Outcome SOE	Results or Effect Estimate (95% Confidence Interval)
Endovascular vs. surgical revascularization in CLI and IC-CLI populations (continued)	Amputation after 5 years **SOE=Low**	CLI-Obs (7 studies, 3,101 patients), OR 1.06 (0.70 to 1.59) No difference.
	Amputation-free survival at 1 year **SOE=Low**	CLI-Obs (2 studies, 1,881 patients), OR 0.76 (0.48 to 1.21) CLI-RCT (1 study, 452 patients), OR 0.87 (0.58 to 1.30) No difference.
	Amputation-free survival at 2 to 3 years **SOE=Low**	CLI-Obs (3 studies, 1,972 patients), OR 0.75 (0.53 to 1.09) CLI-RCT (1 study, 452 patients), OR 1.22 (0.84 to 1.77) No difference.
	Amputation-free survival after 5 years **SOE=Low**	CLI-Obs (4 studies, 2,190 patients), OR 0.89 (0.59 to 1.34) No difference.
	Wound healing **SOE=Insufficient**	CLI-Obs (1 study, 91 patients) Inconclusive evidence due to imprecision, with 1 study reporting similar rates of wound healing in the surgical revascularization group (83%) and endovascular revascularization group (80%).
	Primary patency at 1 year **SOE=Moderate (CLI)** **SOE=Low (IC-CLI)**	CLI-Obs (5 studies, 890 patients), OR 0.63 (0.46 to 0.86) No difference. IC-CLI-Obs (3 studies, 328 patients), OR 0.71 (0.40 to 1.28) IC-CLI-RCT (2 studies, 130 patients), OR 0.40 (0.08 to 1.93) Favors endovascular intervention.
	Primary patency at 2 to 3 years **SOE=Insufficient**	CLI-Obs (4 studies, 768 patients), OR 0.77 (0.24 to 2.42) Inconclusive evidence due to imprecision. IC-CLI-Obs (2 studies, 231 patients), OR 0.29 (0.15 to 0.55) IC-CLI-RCT (1 study, 86 patients), OR 0.96 (0.42 to 2.16) Inconclusive evidence due to imprecision.
	Secondary patency at 1 year **SOE=Low (CLI)** **SOE=Insufficient (IC-CLI)**	CLI-Obs (4 studies, 759 patients), OR 0.57 to (0.40 to 0.82) Favors endovascular intervention. IC-CLI-RCT (1 study, 44 patients), OR 0.04 (0.00 to 0.73) Inconclusive evidence due to imprecision.
	Secondary patency at 2 to 3 years **SOE=Low**	CLI-Obs (4 studies, 815 patients), OR 0.49 (0.28 to 0.85) Favors endovascular intervention.

Table C. Summary SOE for KQ 3: Comparative effectiveness and safety of treatments for CLI[a] (continued)

Comparison	Outcome SOE	Results or Effect Estimate (95% Confidence Interval)
Endovascular vs. surgical revascularization in CLI and IC-CLI populations (continued)	Length of stay **SOE=Insufficient**	CLI-Obs (8 studies, 1,745 patients) CLI-RCT (1 study, 452 patients) Inconclusive evidence due to inconsistency and imprecision, with individual studies reporting LOS longer in surgical group with large SD in 3 observational studies and no variability reported in 4 observational studies and one RCT. IC-CLI-Obs (3 studies, 563,935 patients) IC-CLI-RCT (2 studies, 130 patients) Inconclusive evidence due to imprecision, with individual studies reporting LOS longer in surgical group with large SD in the observational studies and RCTs.
	Modifiers of effectiveness (subgroups) **SOE=Insufficient**	All PAD populations and study design (14 studies, 572,188 patients) Inconclusive evidence due to heterogeneity in subgroups assessed across individual studies and inability to quantitatively synthesize results. One RCT showed higher survival in autologous vein graft compared with prosthetic graft. An observational study showed worse survival in advanced age, renal failure, and with higher PAD severity.
	Safety concerns: periprocedural complications **SOE=Insufficient**	IC-CLI-Obs (4 studies, 968 patients), OR 1.87 (0.63 to 5.49) IC-CLI-RCT (2 studies, 130 patients), OR 0.57 (0.14 to 2.26) Inconclusive evidence due to inconsistency and imprecision with observational studies favoring endovascular while the RCTs favor surgical revascularization.
	Safety concerns: infection **SOE=Low**	IC-CLI-Obs (2 studies, 823 patients), OR 14.10 (0.43 to 460.70) IC-CLI-RCT (1 study, 44 patients), OR 12.09 (0.61 to 239.54) Favors endovascular intervention.
	Nonfatal stroke Composite cardiovascular events MWD or absolute claudication distance Initial claudication distance or pain-free walking distance Quality of life Analog pain scale Safety concerns (subgroups) **SOE=Insufficient**	All PAD populations and study design (0 studies)

[a] Grey background indicates insufficient SOE.
Abbreviations: CLI=critical limb ischemia; IC=intermittent claudication; Obs=observational; OR=odds ratio; PAD=peripheral artery disease; RCT=randomized controlled trial; SD=standard deviation; SOE=strength of evidence.

Discussion

Key Findings

We identified a total of 83 studies that tested a wide array of pharmacotherapy, exercise training, and endovascular and surgical revascularization in patients with PAD. Our meta-analysis of RCTs comparing the effectiveness of aspirin versus placebo[19-21] shows that aspirin for the primary prevention of vascular events in asymptomatic PAD patients has no clear benefit. For IC patients, one small RCT shows a benefit of aspirin in the reduction of nonfatal MI and combined vascular events.[20] A prior systematic review of aspirin versus placebo in PAD[22] also found a benefit favoring aspirin for these outcomes; however, that review had a mixed population and different background medical therapy. The lack of clinical effectiveness of 100 mg daily of aspirin in addition to better (i.e., aggressive) management of cardiovascular risk factors is of clinical note and consistent with the meta-analysis by Berger et al.[22] when viewed with regard to background therapy.

Our finding that clopidogrel monotherapy is superior or equivalent to aspirin monotherapy in reducing adverse cardiovascular outcomes represents current clinical practice and helps reinforce the current guideline recommendations for patients with PAD. The role of DAPT compared with aspirin monotherapy is less certain. From the subgroup analysis of PAD patients in one large RCT[23] and two smaller RCTs on a postrevascularization population,[24,25] the combination of clopidogrel with aspirin as DAPT did not show a significant benefit in reducing stroke events or cardiovascular mortality in IC or CLI patients. In patients with symptomatic or asymptomatic PAD (92% IC, 8% asymptomatic), the PAD subgroup analysis of the CHARISMA RCT did however show a statistically significant benefit favoring dual therapy (clopidogrel plus aspirin) compared with aspirin for reducing nonfatal MI, but showed no difference between aspirin and dual therapy for other outcomes. Our findings are similar to those of the only other systematic review of antiplatelet agents for IC by the Cochrane group.[26] The main differences between the reviews are: (1) the Cochrane report did not include the results of the CHARISMA, CASPAR, or MIRROR RCTs; and (2) our review did not include other antiplatelet agents such as indobufen, picotamide, ticlopidine, and triflusal, which are not prescribed in the United States. Additionally, several new antiplatelet agents have recently been studied in patients with coronary artery disease, and the effects of these agents in patients with PAD is not known.

For KQ 2, our review found that exercise training improved functional measures for walking distance when indirectly compared with usual care or medical therapy. Endovascular therapy in our review was found to lead to a statistically nonsignificant functional improvement, although these studies again were limited by the multiple comparisons and possibility of bias. Patients treated with a combination of endovascular intervention and exercise training had better outcomes than patients treated with either exercise training or endovascular intervention alone in a study by Frans et al.[27] These findings again highlight the need for more studies when viewed in context of the recent CLEVER RCT of exercise versus endovascular therapy for aortoiliac disease, which found greater functional improvement with exercise and greater quality-of-life improvement with endovascular therapy.[28]

Our findings for KQ 2 are consistent with existing systematic reviews of exercise therapy in patients with IC[29,30] and with the systematic review for the NICE (National Institute for Health and Care Excellence) guidelines[31] of medical therapy, supervised exercise, angioplasty, and surgical bypass for patients with IC. Current practice for patients with symptomatic PAD is to maximize medical and behavioral treatments prior to more invasive endovascular or surgical treatment. To examine the effectiveness of more invasive treatments, this review included any studies that assessed endovascular or surgical treatments versus usual care and that were published since 1995, when more effective medical treatments such as statins, ACE inhibitors, and adequate control of hypertension and diabetes came into use as standard practice. Unfortunately, few surgical studies have been published since 1995. The endovascular studies in this review found mixed results with respect to functional improvement except when combined with exercise training. The few studies since 1995 that compared surgical treatment with usual care provided little information on functional outcomes. The NICE guidelines focused on direct comparisons of specific therapies, and therefore the number of studies identified for each comparison was low and limited the authors' conclusions. In our systematic review, we used an effect size meta-analysis to assess the comparative effectiveness across all treatment strategies—medications, exercise training, endovascular interventions, and surgical revascularization—on the clinical outcomes outlined in KQ 2.

For KQ 3 in the CLI population, the current findings should serve as a call to action for further studies. This review found 1 RCT and 22 observational studies in the CLI population and 2 RCTs and 10 observational studies in a mixed IC-CLI population evaluating endovascular therapy versus surgical revascularization. The RCTs were performed in the balloon angioplasty-only era, and the observational studies suffer from risk of bias based on treatment decisions and patient inclusion. A Cochrane review of bypass surgery for CLI also concluded that there was limited evidence for the effectiveness of bypass surgery compared with angioplasty.[32] The NICE evidence statements for the comparison of angioplasty and bypass surgery are primarily based on the only RCT conducted in the CLI population (i.e., the BASIL study). We understand that the subgroup analysis from the BASIL study found survival benefit of open bypass surgery for patients who survived longer than 2 years, but this subgroup analysis does not provide the level of evidence to make a key point and should instead be considered hypothesis-generating rather than conclusive.[33] Therefore, our findings the current variability and lack of a consistently agreed-upon treatment approach for patients with CLI, as evidenced by the recommendations from current guidelines to perform revascularization based on best clinical judgment.

For assessing same-treatment strategy comparisons, the draft guidelines from NICE in March 2012[31] and a previous AHRQ report on invasive interventions for lower extremity PAD in 2008[17] contain meta-analyses regarding stent versus angioplasty, bare metal stent versus drug-eluting stent, angioplasty with selective stent placement versus angioplasty with primary stent placement, and autologous vein versus prosthetic bypass comparisons. Given these prior results, our review did not assess the comparative effectiveness of same-treatment strategies. Our primary interest was focused on the comparative effectiveness of different treatment strategies.

Limitations

This review and the body of evidence in patients with PAD have many limitations, specifically that (1) there have been no large-scale RCTs comparing the use of antiplatelet agents in PAD patients, unlike other subgroups of patients with atherosclerotic cardiovascular disease (e.g., coronary artery disease); (2) there are few direct comparisons of treatment strategies (medical therapy, exercise training, revascularization) in patients with IC, and no study has evaluated whether exercise training before or after revascularization is superior to either treatment strategy alone; (3) many studies that were identified in this systematic review were same-treatment strategy comparisons that have been studied in prior systematic reviews; (4) there were no studies comparing treatment strategies of medical therapy, exercise training, or revascularization in patients with atypical leg pain; and (5) due to the low number of studies, we were unable to stratify our analyses based on severity of disease, risk, or symptoms; however, most RCTs had a similar entry criteria for PAD and similar baseline ABIs, thus reducing the need to adjust the analysis for covariates. In addition, we were not able to assess the effectiveness of treatment strategies that were delivered if another modality had failed.

Challenges in Evaluating the Existing Literature in PAD Patients

Comparing endovascular with surgical revascularization techniques in published studies presents the following challenges:

1. *Population differences*: Inclusion and exclusion criteria have varied among studies, and stratification based on symptom status and procedural risk is important.
2. *Endpoint differences*: These differences include variable functional endpoints for evaluation of claudication therapies and the surgical literature that defines success by primary and secondary patency, while the endovascular literature measures success by the lack of need for target lesion or target vessel revascularization.
3. *Length of followup*: Studies have been biased toward shorter duration of followup, thus heavily influencing differential ascertainment including the important clinical endpoint of amputation-free survival.
4. *Evolution of revascularization techniques*: Improvements in surgical and endovascular techniques have made direct comparisons between "state-of-the-art" strategies more challenging; we were unable to account for this in our analyses.
5. *Crossover between surgical and endovascular therapies*: Patients often undergo both surgical and endovascular revascularization in studies as well as in clinical practice, either as part of a hybrid approach to revascularization or because of treatment failure.

While these challenges persist, our systematic review is an up-to-date analysis of the current state of literature in PAD. Multiple groups, including the American College of Cardiology, Vascular Surgery working groups, and Peripheral Academic Research Consortium, are currently working on improved definitions of PAD severity, lower extremity anatomy, and clinical outcomes. These efforts should bolster the design of clinical studies and improve the selection of data to be captured and reported.

Applicability

To improve the applicability of the findings to current clinical practice, we used 1995 as the start date for the literature search. The data available for antiplatelet agents in PAD treatment fell into two categories: (1) subgroup analysis of PAD patients in large antiplatelet RCTs and (2) smaller antiplatelet RCTs in patients who recently had an endovascular intervention or bypass surgery. There are no studies that specifically evaluate the role of antiplatelet agents in a population of patients representing the full spectrum of PAD (asymptomatic, IC, and CLI).

In the analysis of treatments for the IC population, there were a number of single-center and multicenter studies conducted outside the United States (primarily in Europe). There were several randomized studies comparing exercise training, medical therapies, and endovascular interventions. Most of the studies comparing endovascular interventions with usual care or surgical revascularization were based on observational studies. Among the studies of treatments for the CLI population, only one RCT of endovascular versus surgical revascularization has been conducted, with the majority of the literature based on observational, single-center studies.

Subsequently, the introduction of stents, drug-eluting stents, and drug-coated balloons has likely changed the definition and results of the endovascular therapy group. Therefore, the available evidence for CLI revascularization is significantly limited with regard to applicability to current practice.

Research Gaps

The current literature search for PAD revealed many single-center, single-modality observational studies that could not be included for this comparative effectiveness review on the basis of our inclusion/exclusion criteria—and, unfortunately, studies that assessed direct comparisons between treatments were limited. Thus there are numerous evidence gaps and areas for potential future research. We used the framework recommended by Robinson[34] to identify gaps in the evidence and classify why these gaps exist (Table D).

Table D. Research gaps

Criteria	Evidence Gap	Reason	Type of Studies To Consider
Patients	Comparative effectiveness of therapies for PAD subpopulations of interest, including subgroups based on age, sex, race, risk factors, comorbidities and PAD classification (all KQs)	Insufficient information	RCTs and potentially patient-level meta-analyses of existing/future RCTs
	Low representation of women and minorities (all KQs)	Insufficient information	RCTs and prospective registries with oversampling of female and minority populations
Interventions/ comparators	Comparative effectiveness of new antiplatelet medications to aspirin or clopidogrel (KQ 1)	Insufficient information	RCTs
	Comparative effectiveness of DAPT to antiplatelet monotherapy (KQ 1)	Imprecise and inconsistent information	RCTs
	Comparative effectiveness of endovascular and surgical revascularization in CLI (KQ 3)	Imprecise and inconsistent information	RCTs
Outcomes	Comparative effectiveness of available therapies on functional capacity, quality of life in IC patients (KQ 2)	Imprecise and inconsistent information	RCTs or prospective cohort studies using standardized measures of patient-centered outcomes
	Comparative effectiveness of available therapies on functional capacity, quality of life in CLI patients (KQ 3)	Insufficient information	RCTs or prospective cohort studies using standardized measures of patient-centered outcomes
	Comparative effectiveness of available therapies on mortality (all-cause or cardiovascular), nonfatal MI, nonfatal stroke, and composite vascular events in the IC and CLI populations (KQ 2 and KQ 3)	Insufficient information	RCTs adequately powered to assess short- and long-term cardiovascular outcomes

Table D. Research gaps (continued)

Criteria	Evidence Gap	Reason	Type of Studies To Consider
Outcomes (continued)	Comparative effectiveness of available therapies in impacting healthcare utilitization (KQ 2 and KQ 3)	Insufficient information	Observational studies
	Comparative safety of available therapies, focusing on harms such as such as bleeding, infection, and adverse drug reactions (KQ 2 and KQ 3, especially the exercise, endovascular, and surgical therapies)	Insufficient information	Reporting from RCTs and observational studies
Settings	Limited settings need larger real world populations represented (all KQs)	Insufficient information	Large, real-world registries

Abbreviations: CLI=critical limb ischemia; IC=intermittent claudication; DAPT=dual antiplatelet therapy; KQ=Key Question; PAD=peripheral artery disease; RCTs=randomized controlled trials.

KQ 1

For KQ 1, the primary limitation of the available evidence is the low number of studies that compare the effectiveness of aspirin, clopidogrel, and new antiplatelet agents. A single RCT has compared clopidogrel with aspirin, and three RCTs have compared clopidogrel plus aspirin to aspirin alone. More RCTs on asymptomatic or symptomatic patients with PAD are needed to allow us to firmly conclude whether antiplatelet monotherapy or DAPT is warranted in this high-risk cardiovascular population. Additionally, newer antiplatelet agents are available that have not been studied in the PAD population. RCTs that focus solely on enrollment of the PAD population are to be encouraged, since much of the existing literature is based on PAD subgroups (often with an inclusion criterion for the main RCT of known coronary artery, cerebrovascular, or PAD), and this makes it harder to apply the findings with confidence specifically to PAD patients. Types of studies to consider include: (a) RCTs and potentially patient-level meta-analyses of existing/future RCTs; (b) RCTs and large, real-world prospective registries with oversampling of female and minority populations, and representative samples of asymptomatic, IC, and CLI PAD populations; and (c) RCTs that compare the safety and effectiveness of novel medical therapies with that of existing treatments.

KQ 2

For KQ 2, the primary limitation of the available evidence is the heterogeneity of the outcome measures used to assess functional capacity in the IC population, such that an effect size analysis had to be performed across the treatment strategies for this report. Some studies failed to report the variability of the mean, median, or percentage change result and so had to be excluded from the random-effects model. Also, the quality-of-life measures varied among five instruments (SF-36, EQ-5D, WIQ, PAQ, and VascuQOL). We focused on the results of the SF-36 physical functioning score since it was most commonly reported. Generic health-related quality-of-life measures, such as the SF-36 physical functioning score, are often thought to be less responsive to change than a disease-specific measure is. From the limited studies we analyzed, it appears that there was a large effect of various therapies on improvement in quality of life. Validation in future research using both general and disease-specific quality-of-life measures is to be encouraged, and treatment studies that compare exercise, medical therapy, and invasive approaches are needed. Types of studies to consider include: (a) RCTs and potentially patient-level meta-analyses of existing/future RCTs; (b) RCTs and large, real-world prospective registries with oversampling of female and minority populations; (c) RCTs or prospective cohort (observational) studies using standardized measures of patient-centered outcomes; (d) RCTs that directly compare available treatment options, and (e) RCTs adequately powered to assess short- and long-term cardiovascular outcomes.

KQ 3

For KQ 3, the primary limitation of the existing evidence is the plethora of observational studies (only one RCT) comparing endovascular with surgical revascularization. A majority of these studies were rated poor quality due to insufficient reporting of study methodology and variability in the reporting of results. Since most of the studies were retrospective studies, there was a lack of assessment of functional capacity or quality-of-life measures. All-cause mortality and amputation (or limb salvage) rates were commonly reported. Newer studies have started to report amputation-free survival, but very few reported other vascular events such as MI, stroke, or minor amputations. The relationship between vessel patency and functional outcomes or quality of life is not well established, so this is viewed more as a surrogate clinical outcome and not a direct clinical outcome. Needed are more RCTs or prospective cohort studies with assessment of functional capacity, quality of life, and additional vascular outcomes. Types of studies to consider include: (a) RCTs and potentially patient-level meta-analyses of existing/future RCTs; (b) RCTs and large, real-world prospective registries with oversampling of female and minority populations; (c) RCTs or prospective cohort (observational) studies using standardized measures of patient-centered outcomes; and (d) RCTs adequately powered to assess short- and long-term cardiovascular outcomes.

All KQs

Across all KQs, underreporting of results for subgroups that may modify the comparative effectiveness was common. Given the limited space in publications, it would be helpful to have online supplementary appendixes that report the outcomes by age, race, sex, PAD classification, and comorbidities. The representation of women and the reporting of race/ethnicity were also low in these studies. Future studies that oversample for women and minority populations are needed to address subpopulation questions.

In addition, the reporting of safety concerns such as bleeding, exercise-related harms, infection, and adverse drug reactions was sparse in these studies. Underreporting may be expected in retrospective observational studies since medical documentation of safety issues is often lacking. However, we would expect that RCTs or prospective cohort studies would make it a priority to measure these harms during the course of the study and to report them in a published manuscript. Harms related to antiplatelet therapy (monotherapy or DAPT), endovascular procedures, and surgical interventions should be reported along with the treatment effectiveness results to determine the net benefit of therapies. Finally, although not a focus of this review, there was a lack of studies about the health care utilization and costs associated with the various therapies. Observational studies using administrative datasets, or RCTs and prospective studies collecting and reporting resource use data are needed to address this evidence gap.

Conclusions

The available evidence for treatment of patients with PAD is limited by the fact that few RCTs provide comparisons of meaningful treatment options. Several advances in care in both medical therapy and invasive therapy have not been rigorously tested. With respect to antiplatelet therapy for the prevention of cardiovascular events in patients with PAD, we found, from a limited number of studies, that it appears that aspirin has no benefit over placebo in asymptomatic PAD patients; clopidogrel monotherapy is more beneficial than or equivalent to aspirin; and DAPT is not significantly better than aspirin in reducing cardiovascular events in patients with PAD. For IC patients, exercise, medical therapy, and endovascular or surgical revascularization all had a positive effect on functional status and quality of life; the impact of these therapies on cardiovascular events is uncertain. Additionally, the potential additive effects of combined treatment strategies and the timing of these combined strategies are unknown. There do not appear to be significant differences in mortality or limb outcomes between endovascular and surgical revascularization in CLI patients. However, these data are derived from one RCT and many observational studies, and the presence of clinical heterogeneity in these results makes conclusions about clinical outcomes uncertain and provides an impetus for further research.

References

1. Hiatt WR, Goldstone J, Smith SC, Jr., et al. Atherosclerotic Peripheral Vascular Disease Symposium II: nomenclature for vascular diseases. Circulation. 2008;118(25):2826-9. PMID: 19106403.

2. Norgren L, Hiatt WR, Dormandy JA, et al. Inter-Society Consensus for the Management of Peripheral Arterial Disease (TASC II). Eur J Vasc Endovasc Surg. 2007;33 Suppl 1:S1-75. PMID: 17140820.

3. Criqui MH, Ninomiya JK, Wingard DL, et al. Progression of peripheral arterial disease predicts cardiovascular disease morbidity and mortality. J Am Coll Cardiol. 2008;52(21):1736-42. PMID: 19007695.

4. Criqui MH, Langer RD, Fronek A, et al. Mortality over a period of 10 years in patients with peripheral arterial disease. N Engl J Med. 1992;326(6):381-6. PMID: 1729621.

5. Remes L, Isoaho R, Vahlberg T, et al. Quality of life among lower extremity peripheral arterial disease patients who have undergone endovascular or surgical revascularization: a case-control study. Eur J Vasc Endovasc Surg. 2010;40(5):618-25. PMID: 20418121.

6. Nehler MR, McDermott MM, Treat-Jacobson D, et al. Functional outcomes and quality of life in peripheral arterial disease: current status. Vasc Med. 2003;8(2):115-26. PMID: 14518614.

7. Kannel WB. Risk factors for atherosclerotic cardiovascular outcomes in different arterial territories. J Cardiovasc Risk. 1994;1(4):333-9. PMID: 7621317.

8. Rooke TW, Hirsch AT, Misra S, et al. 2011 ACCF/AHA focused update of the guideline for the management of patients with peripheral artery disease (updating the 2005 guideline): a report of the American College of Cardiology Foundation/American Heart Association Task Force on Practice Guidelines: developed in collaboration with the Society for Cardiovascular Angiography and Interventions, Society of Interventional Radiology, Society for Vascular Medicine, and Society for Vascular Surgery. J Vasc Surg. 2011;54(5):e32-58. PMID: 21958560.

9. Dawson DL, Cutler BS, Hiatt WR, et al. A comparison of cilostazol and pentoxifylline for treating intermittent claudication. Am J Med. 2000;109(7):523-30. PMID: 11063952.

10. Schmieder FA, Comerota AJ. Intermittent claudication: magnitude of the problem, patient evaluation, and therapeutic strategies. Am J Cardiol. 2001;87(12A):3D-13D. PMID: 11434894.

11. Hirsch AT, Haskal ZJ, Hertzer NR, et al. ACC/AHA 2005 Practice Guidelines for the management of patients with peripheral arterial disease (lower extremity, renal, mesenteric, and abdominal aortic): a collaborative report from the American Association for Vascular Surgery/Sety for Vascular Surgery, Society for Cardiovascular Angiography and Interventions, Society for Vascular Medicine and Biology, Society of Interventional Radiology, and the ACC/AHA Task Force on Practice Guidelines (Writing Committee to Develop Guidelines for the Management of Patients With Peripheral Arterial Disease): endorsed by the American Association of Cardiovascular and Pulmonary Rehabilitation; National Heart, Lung, and Blood Institute; Society for Vascular Nursing; TransAtlantic Inter-Society Consensus; and Vascular Disease Foundation. Circulation. 2006;113(11):e463-654. PMID: 16549646.

12. Jaff MR, Cahill KE, Yu AP, et al. Clinical outcomes and medical care costs among medicare beneficiaries receiving therapy for peripheral arterial disease. Ann Vasc Surg. 2010;24(5):577-87. PMID: 20579582.

13. Agency for Healthcare Research and Quality. Methods Guide for Effectiveness and Comparative Effectiveness Reviews. Rockville, MD: Agency for Healthcare Research and Quality. www.effectivehealthcare.ahrq.gov/index.cfm/search-for-guides-reviews-and-reports/?pageaction=displayproduct&productid=318. Accessed March 16, 2012.

14. Evidence-based Practice Center Systematic Review Protocol. Project Title: Treatment Strategies for Patients With Peripheral Artery Disease. January 31, 2012. http://effectivehealthcare.ahrq.gov/index.cfm/search-for-guides-reviews-and-reports/?productid=948&pageaction=displayproduct. Accessed November 19, 2012.

15. Cohen J. Statistical Power Analysis for the Behavioral Sciences. 2nd ed Hillsdale, NJ: L. Erlbaum Associates; 1988.

16. Owens DK, Lohr KN, Atkins D, et al. AHRQ series paper 5: grading the strength of a body of evidence when comparing medical interventions--Agency for Healthcare Research and Quality and the Effective Health-Care Program. J Clin Epidemiol. 2010;63(5):513-23. PMID: 19595577.

17. Agency for Healthcare Research and Quality. Horizon Scan of Invasive Interventions for Lower Extremity Peripheral Artery Disease and Systematic Review of Studies Comparing Stent Placement to Other Interventions. Technology Assessment. October 2008. http://www.cms.gov/Medicare/Coverage/DeterminationProcess/downloads//id63TA.pdf. Accessed May 22, 2012.

18. Atkins D, Chang SM, Gartlehner G, et al. Assessing applicability when comparing medical interventions: AHRQ and the Effective Health Care Program. J Clin Epidemiol. 2011;64(11):1198-207. PMID: 21463926.

19. Belch J, MacCuish A, Campbell I, et al. The prevention of progression of arterial disease and diabetes (POPADAD) trial: factorial randomised placebo controlled trial of aspirin and antioxidants in patients with diabetes and asymptomatic peripheral arterial disease. BMJ. 2008;337:a1840. PMID: 18927173.

20. Catalano M, Born G, Peto R. Prevention of serious vascular events by aspirin amongst patients with peripheral arterial disease: randomized, double-blind trial. J Intern Med. 2007;261(3):276-84. PMID: 17305650.

21. Fowkes FG, Price JF, Stewart MC, et al. Aspirin for prevention of cardiovascular events in a general population screened for a low ankle brachial index: a randomized controlled trial. JAMA. 2010;303(9):841-8. PMID: 20197530.

22. Berger JS, Krantz MJ, Kittelson JM, et al. Aspirin for the prevention of cardiovascular events in patients with peripheral artery disease: a meta-analysis of randomized trials. JAMA. 2009;301(18):1909-19. PMID: 19436018.

23. Cacoub PP, Bhatt DL, Steg PG, et al. Patients with peripheral arterial disease in the CHARISMA trial. Eur Heart J. 2009;30(2):192-201. PMID: 19136484.

24. Belch JJ, Dormandy J, Biasi GM, et al. Results of the randomized, placebo-controlled clopidogrel and acetylsalicylic acid in bypass surgery for peripheral arterial disease (CASPAR) trial. J Vasc Surg. 2010;52(4):825-33, 833 e1-2. PMID: 20678878.

25. Tepe G, Bantleon R, Brechtel K, et al. Management of peripheral arterial interventions with mono or dual antiplatelet therapy-the MIRROR study: a randomised and double-blinded clinical trial. Eur Radiol. 2012;22(9):1998-2006. PMID: 22569995.

26. Wong Peng F, Chong Lee Y, Mikhailidis Dimitris P, et al. Antiplatelet agents for intermittent claudication. Cochrane Database of Systematic Reviews. 2011(11):CD001272. Epub 2011 Nov 9.

27. Frans FA, Bipat S, Reekers JA, et al. Systematic review of exercise training or percutaneous transluminal angioplasty for intermittent claudication. Br J Surg. 2011. PMID: 21928409.

28. Murphy TP, Cutlip DE, Regensteiner JG, et al. Supervised exercise versus primary stenting for claudication resulting from aortoiliac peripheral artery disease: six-month outcomes from the claudication: exercise versus endoluminal revascularization (CLEVER) study. Circulation. 2012;125(1):130-9. PMID: 22090168.

29. Leng GC, Fowler B, Ernst E. Exercise for intermittent claudication. Cochrane Database Syst Rev. 2000(2):CD000990. PMID: 10796572.

30. Watson L, Ellis B, Leng GC. Exercise for intermittent claudication. Cochrane Database Syst Rev. 2008(4):CD000990. PMID: 18843614.

31. National Institute for Health and Clinical Excellence. Lower limb peripheral arterial disease: diagnosis and management. NICE Clinical Guideline [draft]. March 2012. http://www.nice.org.uk/guidance/index.jsp?action=folder&o=58406. Accessed May 22, 2012.

32. Leng GC, Davis M, Baker D. Bypass surgery for chronic lower limb ischaemia. Cochrane Database Syst Rev. 2000(3):CD002000. PMID: 10908520.

33. Bradbury AW, Adam DJ, Bell J, et al. Bypass versus Angioplasty in Severe Ischaemia of the Leg (BASIL) trial: An intention-to-treat analysis of amputation-free and overall survival in patients randomized to a bypass surgery-first or a balloon angioplasty-first revascularization strategy. J Vasc Surg. 2010;51(5 Suppl):5S-17S. PMID: 20435258.

34. Robinson KA, Saldanha IJ, Mckoy NA. Frameworks for Determining Research Gaps During Systematic Reviews. Methods Future Research Needs Report No. 2. (Prepared by the Johns Hopkins University Evidence-based Practice Center under Contract No. HHSA 290-2007-10061-I.) AHRQ Publication No. 11-EHC043-EF. Rockville, MD: Agency for Healthcare Research and Quality; June 2011. www.effectivehealthcare.ahrq.gov/reports/final.cfm. Accessed May 22, 2012.

Glossary

ABI	ankle-brachial index
ACD	absolute claudication distance
ACC	American College of Cardiology
ACE	angiotensin-converting enzyme
AHA	American Heart Association

AHRQ	Agency for Healthcare Research and Quality
CI	confidence interval
CLI	critical limb ischemia
DAPT	dual antiplatelet therapy
HR	hazard ratio
IC	intermittent claudication
ICD	initial claudication distance
KQ	Key Question
LDL	low-density lipoprotein
MWD	maximal walking distance
MI	myocardial infarction
OR	odds ratio
PAD	peripheral artery disease
PFWD	pain-free walking distance
RCT	randomized controlled trial
SF-36®	Short-form (36) health survey
SOE	strength of evidence
TEP	Technical Expert Panel

Introduction

Background

Epidemiology of Peripheral Artery Disease (PAD)

Peripheral artery disease (PAD) is the preferred clinical term describing stenosis or occlusion of upper or lower extremity arteries due to atherosclerotic or thromboembolic disease.[1] In practice, however, the term PAD generally refers to chronic narrowing or blockage (also referred to as atherosclerotic disease) of the arteries of the *lower* extremities. Thus the focus of this systematic review is chronic atherosclerotic disease of the lower extremities.

PAD represents a spectrum of disease severity, encompassing both asymptomatic and symptomatic disease. Roughly 20 to 50 percent of patients diagnosed with PAD (diagnosis made by abnormal results of an ankle-brachial index (ABI) test, discussed in the next section) are asymptomatic, though they usually have functional impairment when tested.[2] If the disease progresses and blood vessels narrow, arterial flow into the lower extremities worsens and symptoms may manifest either as classic intermittent claudication (IC) or as atypical claudication or leg discomfort. IC is defined as leg muscle discomfort provoked by exertion that is relieved with rest, while atypical claudication (also called atypical leg discomfort) is defined as lower extremity discomfort that is exertional but does not consistently resolve with rest. Roughly 10 to 35 percent of all PAD patients report symptoms of classic IC, and 40 to 50 percent of patients present with the atypical form. If the disease worsens, patients often develop more severe claudication, with reduced walking distance and eventually with pain at rest. In 5 to 10 percent of cases, claudication progresses to a worsened severity of the disease, called critical limb ischemia (CLI)—defined as ischemic rest pain for more than 14 days, ulceration, or tissue loss/gangrene. CLI is the initial presentation in roughly 1 to 2 percent of all patients with PAD, and patients with CLI have 25 percent mortality at 1 year.[2]

The prevalence of PAD increases with age, such that roughly 20 percent of patients over age 65 have PAD (including symptomatic and asymptomatic disease).[3,4] Given the nearly 40 million Americans over age 65, this represents roughly 8 million Americans with the disease. The prevalence of PAD is lower among younger patients, such that estimates of asymptomatic or symptomatic PAD among patients 45 to 64 years of age is roughly 3 percent.[5] Given that PAD represents a more systemic atherosclerotic process that is similar to atherosclerotic disease of the coronary vessels, it is not surprising that PAD shares similar risk factors: male gender, age, diabetes, smoking, hypertension, high cholesterol, and renal insufficiency.[6] Furthermore, PAD is known to be associated with a reduction in functional capacity; quality of life; and an increased risk for myocardial infarction (MI), stroke, and death. PAD is also a major cause of limb amputation.[7-11] Therefore, PAD is prevalent and is associated with significant morbidity and mortality. Although the goals of cardiovascular protection, relief of symptoms, preservation of walking and functional status, and prevention of amputation are general goals of treatment for IC and CLI, the optimal treatment for patients with specific emphasis on the comparative effectiveness of treatment options is not known.[12]

Diagnostic Tests

Several tests are available to diagnose PAD. The initial test of choice includes the simple ABI measurement. Patients with an ABI of 0.41 to 0.90 are considered to have mild to moderate PAD, and patients with an ABI less than or equal to 0.40 are considered to have severe PAD. Similarly, an ABI greater than 1.30 is associated with noncompressible vessels and is nondiagnostic and requires further testing. Data have shown an inverse relationship between baseline ABI and the risk of ischemic events (MI, stroke, or cardiovascular death), such that as the ABI decreases, the risk of ischemic events increases.[13,14] Similarly, mortality increases with an ABI greater than 1.30. If an ABI measurement at rest or at exercise is suggestive of PAD, further noninvasive testing is usually performed to characterize the anatomic location and severity of the disease; such testing includes segmental pressure measurements, pulse-volume recordings, exercise ABI, duplex ultrasonography, computed tomography angiography, and magnetic resonance angiography.

Classification Schemes

While ABI measurements may quantify PAD severity, the ABI represents a numerical value that does not provide clinicians a full picture of the clinical severity of the disease. There are two classification systems, Rutherford and Fontaine,[2] generally used by clinicians to grade the severity of the clinical symptoms of patients. While these classification systems are frequently used, a large degree of heterogeneity exists in the spectrum of PAD. Tables 1 and 2 highlight these classification systems and show that patients with a higher stage of the disease have more advanced/severe PAD.

Table 1. Fontaine classification

Stage I	No symptoms
Stage IIa	IC >200m of walking distance (mild)
Stage IIb	IC <200m of walking distance (moderate to severe)
Stage 3	Rest pain
Stage 4	Necrosis/gangrene

Abbreviation: IC=intermittent claudication.

Table 2. Rutherford classification

Stage 0	Asymptomatic
Stage 1	Mild claudication
Stage 2	Moderate claudication
Stage 3	Severe claudication
Stage 4	Rest pain
Stage 5	Ischemic ulceration not exceeding ulcer of the digits of the foot
Stage 6	Severe ischemic ulcers or frank gangrene

The mapping of these classification schemes to the categories of PAD disease severity is as follows:
- Asymptomatic: Fontaine stage I, Rutherford stage 0
- Symptomatic (atypical leg symptoms, IC): Fontaine stages IIa and IIb; Rutherford stages 1, 2, and 3
- CLI: Fontaine stages 3 and 4; Rutherford stages 4, 5 and 6

Outcome Measures for PAD

This report examines several clinical outcomes of importance in the PAD population, including cardiovascular events, functional capacity, quality of life, pain, repeat revascularization, amputation, and vessel patency.

Cardiovascular Events

Measuring and preventing cardiovascular events such as MI, stroke, cardiovascular and all-cause mortality is important in patients with PAD because they are considered a population with a high risk of ischemia.

Functional Capacity

Functional capacity is often assessed by serial treadmill testing as an objective measure of assessing changes in performance in patients with IC. The most common measures reported in clinical studies to evaluate maximal walking performance are maximal walking distance (MWD), absolute claudication distance (ACD), and peak walking time (PWT). For measuring claudication-free walking time or distance, the measures commonly reported in clinical studies include pain-free walking distance (PFWD), pain-free walking time (PFWT), and claudication onset time (COT).

Quality of Life

Quality of life (QOL) of patients with PAD can be assessed by general and disease-specific measures. General measures include the Medical Outcomes Study Short Form-36 (SF-36®)[15] questionnaire and the EuroQOL-5D. The SF-36 evaluates the physical and mental functioning of patients along eight health dimensions—general health, change in health during the past year, physical functioning, social functioning, role limitations due to physical problems, role limitations due to emotional problems, mental health, and bodily pain.[16] The EuroQOL-5D[17] is a multiple attribute health utility instrument that assesses QOL from a societal perspective and classifies patients into various health states. Disease-specific measures include the Vascular Quality of Life (VascuQOL)[18] questionnaire, Walking Impairment Questionnaire (WIQ),[19] and Peripheral Artery Questionnaire (PAQ),[20] which were developed for PAD patients and are responsive to smaller treatment effects than the general QOL measures. The VascuQOL is a 35-item survey that measures 5 dimensions (activity, symptom, pain, emotion and social functioning). The WIQ measures the ability of PAD patients to walk defined distances and speeds, plus climb stairs, thus evaluating claudication severity and nonclaudication symptoms that limit walking ability. The PAQ is a 20-item questionnaire that quantifies patients' physical limitations, symptoms, social function, treatment satisfaction, and quality of life.

Limb Outcomes

Limb outcomes include repeat revascularization, amputation, and vessel patency. Vessel patency (open blood vessel) can be further characterized into primary patency, primary assisted patency and secondary patency. Primary patency is defined as uninterrupted patency following the revascularization procedure being evaluated. Primary assisted patency occurs when a revision of the revascularization method is performed to prevent progression of stenosis or an impending stenosis. Secondary patency refers to patency of the initially treated vessel following a reintervention to restore patency after occlusion.

Therapies for PAD

The backbone of treatment for PAD is smoking cessation, risk factor modification, dietary modification, and increased physical activity. The goals of therapy for PAD depend on the severity of the disease. For all patients with PAD, both symptomatic and asymptomatic, reducing the risk of cardiovascular morbidity and mortality is a primary concern. For patients with IC, improving functional status is an additional goal. Finally, for patients with CLI, preventing leg amputation, restoring mobility, and reducing mortality are of paramount concern. Depending on the population and the goal, different treatment choices are available. The following sections focus on the different options for achieving each goal.

Reducing Cardiovascular Morbidity and Mortality in All Patients With PAD

The goal of medical therapy in patients with PAD is to reduce the risk of future cardiovascular morbidity and mortality in patients with high ischemic risk, and/or to improve walking distance and functional status in patients with IC. Secondary prevention includes the use of antiplatelet agents and angiotensin-converting enzyme (ACE) inhibitors and the management of other risk factors such as tobacco use, diabetes, LDL levels, and hypertension. Some small studies have suggested that ACE inhibitors and statins may improve functional capacity or reduce the decline in lower extremity performance.[21-24] With respect to antiplatelet therapy, there is clinical uncertainty. It is not clear which antiplatelet strategy (aspirin versus clopidogrel, monotherapy versus dual antiplatelet therapy) is of most benefit. Further, the role of these agents in patients with asymptomatic PAD also is unclear. Therefore this review focused on the comparative effectiveness of antiplatelet therapy including aspirin and other antiplatelet agents in reducing the risk of adverse cardiovascular events, functional capacity, and quality of life.

Improving Functional Status in Patients With IC

There are three main treatment options for improving functional status and other clinical outcomes in patients with IC: (1) medical therapy, (2) exercise training, and (3) revascularization. Questions about comparative effectiveness include whether one approach is better than the others and whether certain combinations of them are most effective.

Medical Therapy

Selected medications, such as cilostazol and pentoxifylline, have been shown to improve walking distance in patients with PAD. Cilostazol has been shown to significantly improve MWD[25] and is, therefore, considered a Class I therapy in the 2005 ACC/AHA practice guidelines.[2] Cilostazol increases blood flow to the limbs both by preventing blood clots and by widening the blood vessels. Common side effects of this medication include headache and diarrhea, though its use is contraindicated in patients with congestive heart failure. An alternative medication to cilostazol is pentoxifylline, which rarely has side effects although occasionally patients complain of nausea and diarrhea. However, a prior study comparing cilostazol, pentoxifylline, and placebo found cilostazol to be superior by improving MWD by 24 weeks while pentoxifylline was not different than placebo.[25] The relative effect of medical therapy with regard to exercise therapy and invasive therapies is unknown and central to this review.

Exercise Training

Over the past 30 years, research efforts within PAD have focused on the potential benefits of noninvasive therapies, including exercise therapy. More recent work has refined the mechanism of proposed benefit in exercise therapy to (1) improved endothelial function, (2) reduced systemic inflammation, and (3) improved mitochondrial function and skeletal muscle metabolism.[26-35] Most studies have investigated differences in supervised exercise training when compared with home exercise training. More recently, supervised exercise training has also been compared with endovascular revascularization.

Revascularization

Historically, patients with IC have been treated conservatively for their leg symptoms with medical therapy, lifestyle modification, and exercise programs because of the low overall risk of limb-threatening ischemia.[36] Strategies for revascularization include surgical or endovascular procedures. Surgical procedures include vessel bypass with venous or prosthetic grafts or endarterectomy. The method of bypass surgery depends on the size and location of the affected artery (e.g., aortobifemoral, femoropopliteal, or femoral-tibial bypass). Endarterectomy is less common and typically performed on the femoral artery. Endovascular procedures include (1) angioplasty (cryoplasty, cutting, and standard angioplasty balloons are available for use in peripheral arteries and drug-coated balloons are being tested in clinical trials), (2) stenting (self-expanding and balloon-expandable stents are available, but drug-eluting stents are not currently approved for treating peripheral arteries in the United States), and (3) atherectomy (laser, directional, orbital, and rotational atherectomy devices are approved for use in the United States). With improvements in endovascular techniques and equipment, the use of balloon angioplasty, stenting, and atherectomy has led to applying endovascular revascularization to a wider range of patients over the past decade, both among those with more severe symptoms and those with less severe symptoms.[37] Large clinical studies have been performed that aim to determine the best revascularization strategy; however, many questions remain as newer endovascular therapies are applied to a broader population of patients.

Goals for treating IC with invasive therapies are to improve leg pain, walking distance, and quality of life. Decisions about whether to revascularize and how to revascularize patients with PAD depend on a number of factors, including patient-specific characteristics, anatomic location, severity of symptoms, need for possible repeat revascularization in the future, and patient and physician preferences.[2] Clinical guidelines remain vague regarding the absolute indications for and appropriate use of revascularization strategies in patients with PAD.[2] Clinical uncertainty exists around whether strategies of optimal medical therapy and exercise training with or without revascularization are better. Once clinicians have decided on a revascularization strategy, further uncertainty exists around the type of revascularization strategy to employ (i.e., endovascular versus surgical).

Patient characteristics such as advanced age, concomitant coronary artery disease or heart failure, and ongoing tobacco use often influence clinical decisionmaking and can make surgical revascularization unfavorable in patients for whom general anesthesia is risky. Endovascular revascularization offers multiple distinct advantages over surgical procedures. These advantages include the use of local anesthesia rather than general anesthesia, short recovery times, and reduced short-term morbidity and mortality. Critics of endovascular intervention cite the shorter duration of improvement and the need for/cost of repeat revascularization procedures as disadvantages. The introduction of hybrid revascularization techniques (endovascular and surgical revascularization performed in the same setting or with a staged approach) presents the potential advantage of combining the durability of surgical revascularization with the lower procedural risk of endovascular therapies.[38]

Anatomic location may help determine the preferable revascularization strategy (endovascular versus surgical); however, this topic remains controversial. The Trans-Atlantic Inter-Society Consensus Document on Management of Peripheral Arterial Disease[6] provides some guidance for the revascularization strategy based on anatomic location and severity. In general, in patients with stenosis of the aortoiliac segments, balloon angioplasty and stenting compare favorably with surgical patency rates while dramatically lowering the periprocedural mortality risk. However, there is still uncertainty about the most effective revascularization strategy in patients with femoropopliteal stenosis. Multiple studies are currently comparing exercise therapy, angioplasty with or without stenting, and surgical revascularization. While improved clinical outcomes have been reported with angioplasty and stenting when compared with medical therapy, the longevity of results in the femoropopliteal segment remains a concern. Tibioperoneal, or below-knee, endovascular interventions are typically reserved for patients with limb-threatening ischemia; however, multiple reports describe the adoption of tibioperoneal intervention for severe claudication.

In an effort to improve the patency rates and longevity seen with angioplasty and stenting, atherectomy devices have gained favor as tools to debulk atherosclerotic plaque. However, randomized comparisons between balloon angioplasty (with or without stenting) and atherectomy are lacking. Additional devices designed to reduce restenosis (cryoplasty balloons, cutting balloons, drug-coated balloons, and drug-eluting stents) are currently being evaluated in RCTs.

Improving Functional Status and Reducing Leg Amputation in Patients With CLI

CLI is the most severe manifestation of PAD, and it includes patients with lower extremity rest pain, ulceration, and gangrene.[2] There are currently no approved medical therapies for the treatment of CLI. At 1 year, CLI is associated with a 20-percent mortality rate and a 50-percent risk of major amputation in patients who do not undergo revascularization.[2] Medical treatment for CLI is often limited to local wound therapy because there are few available disease-modifying medical treatments. Consequently, revascularization is often attempted to restore blood flow, improve wound healing, and prevent amputation in patients with CLI. The decision to attempt revascularization in patients with CLI is based on a combination of factors, including patient characteristics, severity of symptoms, anatomic considerations, and patient and physician preferences. Few RCTs of revascularization for CLI have been performed, and the clinical endpoints have varied significantly.[39,40] Recently, objective performance goals have been established to standardize consensus metrics for clinical outcomes and assist in optimal clinical trial design in investigating peripheral revascularization for patients with CLI.[41] Amputation-free survival is defined as the time to first amputation or death from any cause, whichever occurs first, and is generally considered the best limb and patient outcome for revascularization in patients with CLI.[40]

CLI is a heterogeneous condition that makes the decision to revascularize extremely complex. Patient-specific characteristics such as age, inability to ambulate, and comorbid conditions (especially the presence of diabetes mellitus and coronary heart disease) often influence the decision to perform endovascular or surgical revascularization.[42] The presence and severity of tissue loss plays an important role in revascularization decisions and may impact the large degree of variation in amputation rates across geographic regions.[43] Finally, the higher prevalence of multilevel disease, involvement of smaller caliber vessels, and longer occlusions often make revascularization in patients with CLI more challenging than in patients with IC. Given these issues, the choice of revascularization strategy (endovascular versus surgical) is often made on an individual basis; however, more definitive data are needed to aid clinicians in decisionmaking. This review attempts to summarize the available comparative data on endovascular versus surgical revascularization strategies.

Scope and Key Questions (KQs)

Scope of the Review

This comparative effectiveness review was funded by the Agency for Healthcare Research and Quality (AHRQ). The review was designed to evaluate the effectiveness of available strategies—medications, exercise, revascularization—used to treat patients with PAD.

Although hundreds of RCTs have been published on the management of patients with PAD, notable uncertainties remain about several key components because of conflicting results, differences in outcomes measured, and differences in revascularization techniques. The following briefly summarizes the current controversies:

- Is aspirin effective for PAD, and if so, what is the optimal dose of aspirin to prevent cardiovascular events in patients with PAD?[44] Is there a differential effect of aspirin in patients who are symptomatic versus those who are asymptomatic?
- When patients with PAD are treated with thienopyridines for additional indications, what is the optimal dose of aspirin to prevent cardiovascular events?
- Should the decision to treat patients with PAD with aspirin and other antiplatelet agents be based on their comorbid conditions or symptomatic status?
- With increasing use of endovascular revascularization procedures in patients with IC, is there long-term benefit in functional status and quality of life when compared with medical therapy or exercise training?
- In patients with IC, what is the comparative effectiveness of balloon angioplasty, stenting, and atherectomy in patients treated with an endovascular approach in improving functional capacity and quality of life?
- In patients with CLI, what is the comparative effectiveness of endovascular revascularization techniques (balloon angioplasty, stenting, and atherectomy) and surgical revascularization techniques for outcomes such as vessel patency, revascularization, wound healing, pain, cardiovascular events, amputation, and mortality?

KQs

With input from our Technical Expert Panel (TEP), we constructed KQs using the general approach of specifying the population of interest, the interventions, comparators, outcomes, timing of outcomes, and settings (PICOTS; see the section on "Inclusion and Exclusion Criteria" in the Methods section for details). The KQs considered in this comparative effectiveness review were:

- **KQ 1.** In adults with peripheral artery disease (PAD), including asymptomatic patients and symptomatic patients with atypical leg symptoms, intermittent claudication (IC), or critical limb ischemia (CLI):
  a. What is the comparative effectiveness of aspirin and other antiplatelet agents in reducing the risk of adverse cardiovascular events (e.g., all-cause mortality, myocardial infarction, stroke, cardiovascular death), functional capacity, and quality of life?
  b. Does the effectiveness of treatments vary according to the patient's PAD classification or by subgroup (age, sex, race, risk factors, or comorbidities)?
  c. What are the significant safety concerns associated with each treatment strategy (e.g., adverse drug reactions, bleeding)? Do the safety concerns vary by subgroup (age, sex, race, risk factors, comorbidities, or PAD classification)?
- **KQ 2.** In adults with symptomatic PAD (atypical leg symptoms or IC):
  a. What is the comparative effectiveness of exercise training, medications (cilostazol, pentoxifylline), endovascular intervention (percutaneous transluminal angioplasty, atherectomy, or stents), and/or surgical revascularization (endarterectomy, bypass surgery) on outcomes including cardiovascular events (e.g., all-cause mortality, myocardial infarction, stroke, cardiovascular death), amputation, quality of life, wound healing, analog pain scale score, functional capacity, repeat revascularization, and vessel patency?
  b. Does the effectiveness of treatments vary by use of exercise and medical therapy prior to invasive management or by subgroup (age, sex, race, risk factors, comorbidities, or anatomic location of disease)?
  c. What are the significant safety concerns associated with each treatment strategy (e.g., adverse drug reactions, bleeding, contrast nephropathy, radiation, infection, exercise-related harms, and periprocedural complications causing acute limb ischemia)? Do the safety concerns vary by subgroup (age, sex, race, risk factors, comorbidities, anatomic location of disease)?
- **KQ 3.** In adults with CLI due to PAD:
  a. What is the comparative effectiveness of endovascular intervention (percutaneous transluminal angioplasty, atherectomy, or stents) and surgical revascularization (endarterectomy, bypass surgery) for outcomes including cardiovascular events (e.g., all-cause mortality, myocardial infarction, stroke, cardiovascular death), amputation, quality of life, wound healing, analog pain scale score, functional capacity, repeat revascularization, and vessel patency?
  b. Does the effectiveness of treatments vary by subgroup (age, sex, race, risk factors, comorbidities, or anatomic location of disease)?
  c. What are the significant safety concerns associated with each treatment strategy (e.g., adverse drug reactions, bleeding, contrast nephropathy, radiation, infection, and periprocedural complications causing acute limb ischemia)? Do the safety concerns vary by subgroup (age, sex, race, risk factors, comorbidities, or anatomic location of disease)?

Analytic Framework

Figure 1 shows the analytic framework for this comparative effectiveness review.

Figure 1. Analytic framework

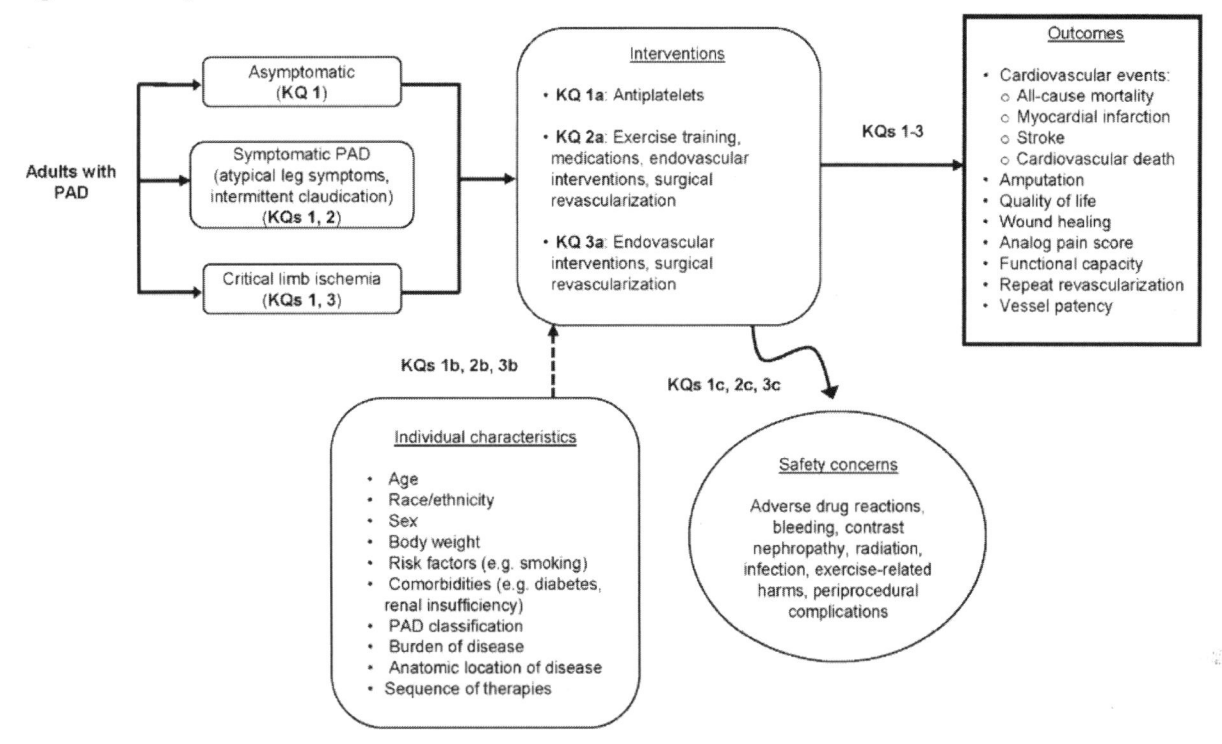

Abbreviations: KQ=Key Question; PAD=peripheral artery disease.

The analytic framework depicts the KQs within the context of the PICOTS described above. In general, the figure shows that the population of interest is adults with PAD, including asymptomatic patients and patients with IC or CLI. KQ 1 considers the comparative effectiveness of aspirin and other antiplatelet agents in reducing the risk of adverse cardiovascular events (e.g., MI, stroke, cardiovascular death) and whether the effectiveness of treatments varies according to the patient's symptomatic status or by subgroup (age, sex, race, comorbidities).

For patients with IC due to PAD, KQ 2 considers the comparative effectiveness of exercise training, medications (cilostazol, pentoxifylline), endovascular intervention (percutaneous transluminal angioplasty, atherectomy, or stents), and/or surgical revascularization (endarterectomy, bypass surgery) on improving functional capacity and quality of life as well as whether the effectiveness of treatments varies by subgroup (age, sex, race, comorbidities, anatomic location of disease).

For patients with CLI, KQ 3 considers the comparative effectiveness of endovascular intervention and surgical revascularization for outcomes including vessel patency, revascularization, wound healing, analog pain scale, cardiovascular events, amputation, and mortality (including amputation-free survival) and whether the effectiveness of treatments varies by subgroup (age, sex, race, comorbidities, anatomic location of disease). All three KQs consider the significant safety concerns associated with each treatment strategy (e.g., adverse drug reactions, contrast nephropathy, radiation, infection, bleeding, exercise-related harms, and periprocedural complications causing acute limb ischemia) as well as whether the risks vary by subgroup (age, sex, race, comorbidities, anatomic location of disease).

Methods

The methods for this comparative effectiveness review follow those suggested in the AHRQ "Methods Guide for Effectiveness and Comparative Effectiveness Reviews" (www.effectivehealthcare.ahrq.gov/methodsguide.cfm; hereafter referred to as the Methods Guide).[45] The main sections in this chapter reflect the elements of the protocol established for the systematic review; certain methods map to the PRISMA checklist.[46] All methods and analyses were determined a priori. Figure 2 depicts the steps undertaken for this systematic review.

Figure 2. Steps of a systematic review

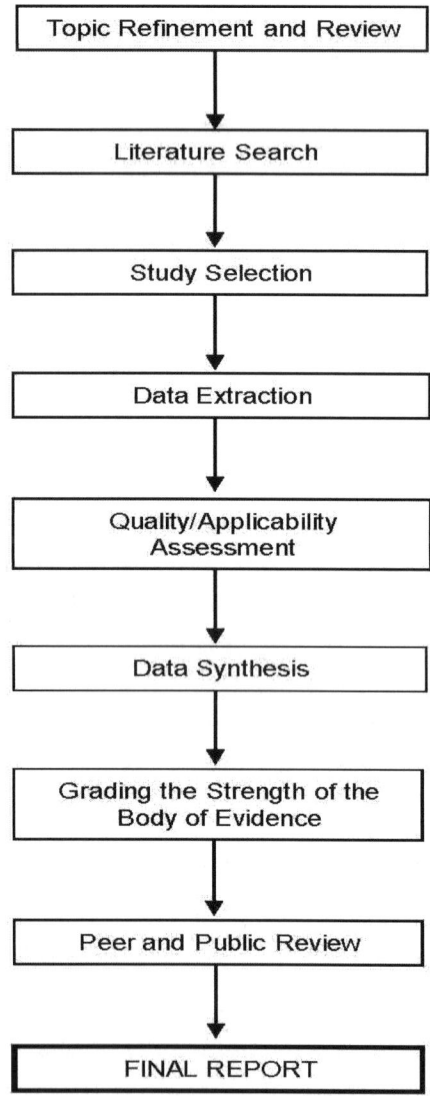

Topic Refinement and Review → Literature Search → Study Selection → Data Extraction → Quality/Applicability Assessment → Data Synthesis → Grading the Strength of the Body of Evidence → Peer and Public Review → FINAL REPORT

Topic Refinement and Review Protocol

During the topic refinement stage, we solicited input from KIs representing clinicians (cardiology, radiology, vascular surgery, general medicine, and nursing), patients, scientific experts, and Federal agencies, to help define the KQs. The KQs were then posted for public comment for 30 days, and the comments received were considered in the development of the research protocol. We next convened a TEP comprising clinical, content, and methodological experts to provide input in defining populations, interventions, comparisons, or outcomes as well as identifying particular studies or databases to search. The KIs and members of the TEP were required to disclose any financial conflicts of interest greater than $10,000 and any other relevant business or professional conflicts of interest. Any potential conflicts of interest were balanced or mitigated. Of the 10 TEP members, four held positions on scientific advisory boards representing 14 entities, of which two members overlapped on two entities; thus there was not majority interest in any particular company or institute. Neither KIs nor members of the TEP did analysis of any kind and did not contribute to the writing of the report. Members of the TEP were invited to provide feedback on an initial draft of the review protocol, which was then refined based on their input, reviewed by AHRQ, and posted for public access at the AHRQ Effective Health Care Web site.[47]

Literature Search Strategy

Sources Searched

Our search strategy used the National Library of Medicine's medical subject headings (MeSH) keyword nomenclature developed for MEDLINE® and adapted for use in other databases. In consultation with our research librarians, we searched PubMed®, Embase®, and the Cochrane Database of Systematic Reviews from January 1, 1995, to August 13, 2012. During peer and public review of this draft report, we updated the database searches and included any eligible studies identified either through that search or through suggestions from peer and public reviewers. Our search strategy for PubMed is included in Appendix A; this strategy was adapted as necessary for use in the other databases. We date-limited our search to articles published since January 1995, corresponding with the time period when contemporary studies on antiplatelet therapy, exercise training, endovascular interventions and surgical revascularization were published. We supplemented the electronic searches with a manual search of references from 132 systematic review articles, of which 10 articles were included. The reference list for identified pivotal articles was hand-searched and cross-referenced against our library, and 19 additional manuscripts were retrieved. All citations were imported into an electronic database (EndNote® X4; Thomson Reuters, Philadelphia, PA).

We also searched the gray literature of study registries and conference abstracts for relevant articles from completed studies and identified nine peer-reviewed articles for full-text screening. Gray literature databases included ClinicalTrials.gov; metaRegister of Controlled Trials; WHO International Clinical Trials Registry Platform Search Portal; and ProQuest COS Conference Papers Index. Scientific information packets were requested from the manufacturers of medications and devices and seven packets were received. These were reviewed for relevant articles from completed studies not previously identified in the literature searches, and no new publications were found (all suggested citations had been previously identified).

Inclusion and Exclusion Criteria

The PICOTS criteria used to screen articles for inclusion/exclusion at both the title-and-abstract and full-text screening stages are detailed in Table 3. Note that because study data in patients with PAD are limited—and because the indications for statin and angiotensin-converting enzyme inhibitor (ACE-I) therapy are based on baseline lipid levels, diabetic status, and blood pressure (all risk factors for PAD)—we did not include studies of these drugs in this review. These drugs are often covered and evaluated for those specific primary conditions. The management of risk factors (i.e., tobacco use, diabetes, LDL levels, and hypertension) is considered standard therapy for all patients with or without PAD regardless of PAD classification and was therefore considered concurrent therapy with the medical and revascularization strategies examined in this review.

Table 3. Inclusion and exclusion criteria

Study Characteristic	Inclusion Criteria	Exclusion Criteria
Population	Adult patients (≥18 years of age) with lower extremity PAD (e.g., ABI <0.9) who are asymptomatic or symptomatic (atypical leg symptoms, IC, or CLI)	• Patients with PAD, but results are not reported separately for the subgroup with lower extremity PAD • All patients are <18 years of age, or some patients are <18 years of age, but results are not broken down by age

Interventions and comparators	• KQ 1: Two or more antiplatelet agents (aspirin or clopidogrel)
	• KQ 2:
	  ○ Exercise training vs. medications (cilostazol, pentoxifylline)
	  ○ Exercise training vs. endovascular intervention (percutaneous transluminal arterial angioplasty, atherectomy, stenting)
	  ○ Exercise training vs. surgical revascularization (endarterectomy, bypass surgery)
	  ○ Medications vs. endovascular intervention
	  ○ Medications vs. surgical revascularization
	  ○ Usual care vs. another treatment modality (exercise training, medications, endovascular intervention, or surgical revascularization)
	• KQ 3:
	  ○ Endovascular intervention (percutaneous transluminal arterial angioplasty, atherectomy, stenting) vs. surgical revascularization (endarterectomy, bypass surgery)
	  ○ Usual care vs. endovascular intervention
	  ○ Usual care vs. surgical revascularization
		• Interventions not listed in KQs 1–3 (e.g., studies of tobacco cessation, statins, and were excluded since treatment of cardiovascular risk factors is considered standard therapy across the treatment strategies assessed in this report)
		• KQ 1: No active comparator (but placebo-controlled trials and studies comparing one antiplatelet agent with another antiplatelet agent are included); also excluded:
		  ○ Studies of ticlopidine (no longer prescribed due to hematologic side effects)
		  ○ Studies comparing anticoagulants (warfarin, low molecular weight heparin) with antiplatelet agents to prevent postrevascularization thrombosis
		• KQ 2 and KQ 3: No active comparator (but studies comparing usual care or placebo with another treatment are included), or comparisons of two treatments of the same type (i.e., one type of exercise vs. another type of exercise; endovascular approach vs. another endovascular approach; surgical approach vs. another surgical approach)

Table 3. Inclusion and exclusion criteria (continued)

Study Characteristic	Inclusion Criteria	Exclusion Criteria
Outcomes	KQs 1–3: • Functional capacity (e.g., PWT, MWD or PFWD, COT, and initial or ACD) • Quality of life (e.g., Short-Form 36, EuroQOL-5D, Walking Impairment Questionnaire, Peripheral Artery Questionnaire) • Vessel patency (primary, primary assisted, or secondary) • Repeat revascularization • Amputation • Wound healing • Analog pain scale score • Cardiovascular events (e.g., all-cause mortality, MI, stroke, cardiovascular death)	No primary or secondary outcomes of interest are reported
Outcomes (safety)	KQs 1–3: Intervention-related safety and adverse effects including adverse drug reactions, bleeding, contrast nephropathy, radiation, infection, exercise-related harms, and periprocedural complications causing acute limb ischemia	None
Timing	Short term (30 days), intermediate term (31 days to 1 year), and long term (>1 year)	Treatment or followup of <30 days
Setting	Inpatient and outpatient	None
Study design	• Randomized controlled trial, prospective or retrospective observational cohort study • Relevant systematic review or meta-analysis (used for background only) • Original data (or related methodology paper of an included article) for interventions listed in KQs 1–3 • All sample sizes	Not a clinical study (e.g., editorial, non–systematic review, letter to the editor, case series)
Publications	• English-language only • Peer-reviewed article • Published January 1, 1995, to present	Given the high volume of literature available in English-language publications (including the majority of known important studies), non-English articles were excluded

Abbreviations: ABI=ankle-brachial index; ACD=absolute claudication distance; COT=claudication onset time; KQ=Key Question; PAD=peripheral artery disease; PWT=peak walking time; PFWD=pain-free walking distance.

Study Selection

Using the prespecified inclusion and exclusion criteria, titles and abstracts were examined independently by two reviewers for potential relevance to the KQs. Articles included by any reviewer underwent full-text screening. At the full-text screening stage, two independent reviewers read each article to determine if it met eligibility criteria. At the full-text review stage, paired researchers independently reviewed the articles and indicated a decision to "include" or "exclude" the article for data abstraction. When the paired reviewers arrived at different decisions about whether to include or exclude an article, we reconciled the difference through a third-party arbitrator. Articles meeting our eligibility criteria were included for data abstraction. Relevant systematic review articles, meta-analyses, and methods articles were flagged for hand-searching and cross-referencing against the library of citations identified through electronic database searching.

Data Extraction

The investigative team created data abstraction forms and evidence table templates for abstracting data for the KQs. Based on clinical and methodological expertise, two investigators were assigned to the research questions to abstract data from the eligible articles. One investigator abstracted the data, and the second overread the article and the accompanying abstraction to check for accuracy and completeness. Disagreements were resolved by consensus or by obtaining a third reviewer's opinion if consensus was not reached between the first two investigators.

To aid in both reproducibility and standardization of data collection, investigators received data abstraction instructions directly on each form created specifically for this project with the DistillerSR data synthesis software program (Evidence Partners Inc., Manotick, ON, Canada). Data reported only in graphs were estimated quantitatively using Engauge Digitizer version 4.1 software (www.digitizer.sourceforge.net).

We designed the data abstraction forms for this project to collect data required to evaluate the specified eligibility criteria for inclusion in this review, as well as demographic and other data needed for determining outcomes (intermediate outcomes, health outcomes, and safety outcomes). Variables collected include:

- *Demographic factors* such as age, sex, and race
- *Vascular disease risk factors* such as diabetes, tobacco use, chronic kidney disease, hyperlipidemia, or other comorbid disease
- *Intervention-specific factors* such as dose of aspirin monotherapy, use of DAPT, type of exercise training, duration of exercise training, type of endovascular revascularization procedure (angioplasty, stenting, atherectomy), or type of surgical revascularization procedure (endarterectomy, surgical bypass)
- *Anatomy-specific factors* such as location of stenosis, pattern of stenosis, burden of disease, degree of calcification, or number of below-knee vessel runoff
- *Patient-specific factors* such as asymptomatic state, presence of atypical leg symptoms, IC or CLI
- *Hospital characteristics* such as hospital patient volume, setting, guideline-based treatment protocols

Safety outcomes were framed to help identify adverse events, including adverse drug reactions, contrast nephropathy, radiation exposure, infection, bleeding, exercise-related harms, and periprocedural complications causing acute limb ischemia

Data necessary for assessing quality and applicability, as described in the Methods Guide,[45] were also abstracted. Before they were used, abstraction form templates were pilot tested with a sample of included articles to ensure that all relevant data elements were captured and that there was consistency and reproducibility between abstractors. During the early phase of abstraction, forms were revised when relevant data elements were found in the published literature and needed to be captured in the database before full abstraction of all included articles. Appendix B lists the data elements used in the data abstraction forms.

Quality Assessment of Individual Studies

We evaluated the quality of individual studies using the approach described in the Methods Guide.[45] To assess quality, we used the strategy to (1) classify the study design, (2) apply predefined criteria for quality and critical appraisal, and (3) arrive at a summary judgment of the study's quality. To evaluate methodological quality, we applied criteria for each study type derived from the core elements described in the Methods Guide. For RCTs, criteria included adequacy of randomization and allocation concealment; the comparability of groups at baseline; blinding; the completeness of followup and differential loss to followup; whether incomplete data were addressed appropriately; the validity of outcome measures; and conflict of interest.

For observational studies, we assessed the following study-specific issues that may affect the internal validity of our systematic review: potential for selection bias (i.e., degree of similarity between intervention and control patients); performance bias (i.e., differences in care provided to intervention and control patients not related to the study intervention); attribution and detection bias (i.e., whether outcomes were differentially detected between intervention and control groups); and magnitude of reported intervention effects (see the section on "Selecting Observational Studies for Comparing Medical Interventions" in the Methods Guide).

To indicate the summary judgment of the quality of the individual studies, we used the summary ratings of good, fair, or poor based on their adherence to well-accepted standard methodologies and adequate reporting (Table 4).

Table 4. Definitions of overall quality ratings

Quality Rating	Description
Good	A study with the least bias; results are considered valid. A good study has a clear description of the population, setting, interventions, and comparison groups; uses a valid approach to allocate patients to alternative treatments; has a low dropout rate; and uses appropriate means to prevent bias, measure outcomes, and analyze and report results.
Fair	A study that is susceptible to some bias but probably not enough to invalidate the results. The study may be missing information, making it difficult to assess limitations and potential problems. As the fair-quality category is broad, studies with this rating vary in their strengths and weaknesses. The results of some fair-quality studies are possibly valid, while others are probably valid.
Poor	A study with significant bias that may invalidate the results. These studies have serious errors in design, analysis, or reporting; have large amounts of missing information; or have discrepancies in reporting. The results of a poor-quality study are at least as likely to reflect flaws in the study design as to indicate true differences between the compared interventions.

Included meta-analyses were appraised according to criteria adapted from the PRISMA Statement.[46] Grading was outcome specific; thus, a given study may have been graded of different quality for two individual outcomes reported within that study. Study design also was considered when grading quality. RCTs were graded as good, fair, or poor. Observational studies were graded separately, also as good (low risk of bias), fair (moderate risk of bias), or poor (high risk of bias). Appendix C summarizes our assessment of the quality and applicability for each included study.

Data Synthesis

We summarized the primary literature by abstracting relevant continuous (e.g., age, event rates) and categorical (e.g., race, presence of coronary disease risk factors) data. Continuous variable outcomes were summarized using what was reported by the authors. This included means, medians, standard deviations, interquartile ranges, ranges, and associated p-values. Dichotomous variables were summarized by proportions and associated p-values. We then determined the feasibility of completing a quantitative synthesis (i.e., meta-analysis). Feasibility depended on the volume of relevant literature, conceptual homogeneity of the studies, and completeness of the reporting of results. We considered meta-analysis for comparisons where at least three studies reported the same outcome at similar followup intervals.

Meta-analyses were based on the nature of the outcome variable, but random-effects models were used for all outcomes because of the heterogeneity of the studies. Continuous outcome measures comparing two treatments that used a similar scale were combined without transformation using a random-effects model as implemented in Comprehensive Meta-Analysis Version 2 (Biostat; Englewood, NJ). Continuous outcome measures comparing two treatments made on different scales (such as quality of life measures) were combined using a random-effects model on the effect sizes as implemented in Comprehensive Meta-Analysis. Dichotomous outcome measures comparing two treatments were combined and odds ratios were computed using a random-effects model as implemented in Comprehensive Meta-Analysis. When applicable, we grouped studies by PAD population and study design to show the summary estimates for each grouping. For studies with heterogeneous populations and study designs, we removed the overall summary estimate from the figure; however, the summary estimates for subgroups are still present due to the software configuration. Any subgroup summary estimate with fewer than three studies should be interpreted with caution.

For KQ 2, because several of the studies reported results from multiple treatment arms and used different measures for a similar outcome, we constructed an effect size for each relevant arm of each study and employed the methods of indirect comparative meta-analysis. We used a random-effects model that was a generalization of the standard random-effects model used in the meta-analysis of effect sizes. We assumed that each effect size for each arm, ES_{ij}, could be described by the following model:

$$ES_{ij} = \alpha_i + \sum_{j=1}^{5} x_{ij} \beta_j,$$

where i denotes the study and j denotes the specific treatment within a study. The αi represents the mean for placebo and assumed to be random and normal with variance ($SE_{ij}2 + \sigma2$). SE_{ij} is the standard error of the jth effect size from the ith study. $\sigma2$ is the extra variation from the random effects model. The x_{ij} are "1" if the jth treatment is present, and "0" otherwise. The βj (j=1, ... , 6) are the treatment effects ratios to be estimated for each treatment.

The model was fitted using SAS PROC NLMIXED (SAS Institute Inc.; Cary, NC) with "subject" set to the particular study, i. Any studies without estimates of the treatment effects, or without estimates of the variation or exact p-values, were excluded. This type of analysis was used for the maximal walking, claudication onset, and quality of life measures.

Effect size interpretation is based on Cohen's *d*, whereby 0 equates to no effect, 0.2 equates to a small effect, 0.5 equates to a medium effect, 0.8 equates to a large effect, and effects larger than 1.0 equate to very large effects.[48] The p-value is an indication of the significance of the effect, which is also reflected by the confidence interval around the summary estimate. Factors influencing the significance of the effect (or p-value) include the number of studies contributing to the estimate, the standard error of each individual study, and the heterogeneity of the individual study results.

Table 5 shows an example of effect size data for the Short Form-36 Item (SF-36) physical function score reported in Beebe et al., 1999[49] (from Table 4 of the publication). This three-arm study reported results for the endpoint of percent change from baseline of the physical function score.

Table 5. Example effect size calculation[a]

Arm	Sample Size	Percent Change
Cilostazol, 100 mg	106	7.1
Cilostazol, 50 mg	108	8.0
Placebo	102	2.0

[a]From Beebe et al.[49]

The authors reported a p-value of 0.02 for the three-way comparison. From this we used the inverse incomplete beta function to back-calculate the F-value, assuming 2 and 313 degrees of freedom. The corresponding F value is 3.961. Knowing the F value, we can calculate the mean square error. This value is 274.46. The square root of this value, 16.57, is the estimate of the pooled standard deviation. In order to calculate the effect size for cilostazol 100 mg versus placebo, we subtract 2.0 from 7.1 and divide by 16.57. This gives an effect size value of 0.31, which translates into a small effect of cilostazol when compared with placebo. The standard error of this value is the square root of the sum of the reciprocals of the samples sizes: $\sqrt{(1/106 + 1/102)} = 0.14$.

For the mortality outcome in KQ 2, the challenge of combining evidence from studies with several different treatment arms goes beyond standard meta-analysis techniques. The solution to the problem requires that we define parameters that describe the possible interventions. We made the same assumption that is used in standard meta-analyses, that is, we assumed that the odds ratio (or any other effect measure) comparing two treatments remains constant across studies. Because there are several different treatments, we assumed that all of the odds ratios between the various treatments remained constant. Thus the model made the same general assumptions as the Mantel-Haenszel method, one of the standard methods for combining odds ratios.

Because our outcome measures are dichotomous, they can be fitted using multiple logistic regression analysis. Dummy variables (α_j's) are used for study differences and treatment variables (β_k's) are used for various treatment effects. As is often done in meta-analyses, we used a random effects analysis. The random effects model is the same as that used for the fixed effects analysis, except that the model includes a coefficient, θ, times an error term:

$$Ln\left[\frac{p_i(x)}{1-p_i(x)}\right] = \sum_{j=1}^{m} \alpha_j x_{ij} + \sum_{k=1}^{m} \beta_k x_{kj} + \theta \varepsilon_i$$

where $p_i(x)$ is the probability of an event in the ith arm, ε_i is a standard normal random variable. This model can be fitted using the EGRET software (Cytel Software Corporation; Cambridge, MA) that estimates both fixed and random effects parameters and automatically generates the dummy variables (α's) for each study (Logistic-Normal Regression Model option). Hasselblad[50] described the application of this methodology to meta-regression problems. In order to minimize the impact that study populations and disease severity may have on clinical outcomes, we reviewed the PAD definition for study inclusion and the baseline population characteristics and found similar eligibility criteria and mean ABIs at study enrollment (within one standard deviation of each other). Therefore we did not perform statistical adjustment for the baseline severity of PAD. All studies were RCTs, most of which were good quality, and so randomization would have controlled for any selection and population bias in each treatment arm. Additionally, we performed a sensitivity analysis without one study[51] since it was a combination of cilostazol with percutaneous transluminal angioplasty versus placebo with percutaneous transluminal angioplasty, and there was minimal impact on the summary estimate for the cilostazol studies.

Given the heterogeneity of study design and patient population in KQ 3, we grouped the studies by study design (observational or RCT) and by population (CLI or mixed IC-CLI population) to evaluate the summary estimates for each study design-population combination separately and its contribution to the overall summary estimate.

We tested for statistical heterogeneity between studies (Q and I^2 statistics) while recognizing that the power to detect such heterogeneity may be limited. Potential heterogeneity between studies was reflected through the confidence intervals of the summary statistics obtained from a random-effects approach. We present summary estimates, standard errors, and confidence intervals in our data synthesis.

Strength of the Body of Evidence

The strength of evidence (SOE) for each KQ was assessed using the approach described in the Methods Guide.[52] The evidence was evaluated using the four required domains: risk of bias, consistency, directness, and precision (Table 6).

Table 6. SOE required domains

Domain	Rating	How Assessed
Risk of bias	Low Medium High	Assessed primarily through study design (randomized controlled trial versus observational study) and aggregate study quality
Consistency	Consistent Inconsistent Unknown/not applicable	Assessed primarily through whether effect sizes are generally on the same side of "no effect" and the overall range of effect sizes
Directness	Direct Indirect	Assessed by whether the evidence involves direct comparisons or indirect comparisons through use of surrogate outcomes or use of separate bodies of evidence
Precision	Precise Imprecise Unknown/not applicable	Based primarily on the size of the confidence intervals of effect estimates

Additionally, when appropriate, the studies were evaluated for dose-response association, the presence of confounders that would diminish an observed effect, strength of association (magnitude of effect), and publication bias. These domains were considered qualitatively, and a summary rating of high, moderate, or low SOE was assigned after discussion by two reviewers. In some cases, high, moderate, or low ratings were impossible or imprudent to make; for example, when no evidence was available or when evidence on the outcome was too weak, sparse, or inconsistent to permit any conclusion to be drawn. In these situations, a grade of insufficient was assigned. This four-level rating scale consists of the following definitions:

- **High**—High confidence that the evidence reflects the true effect. Further research is very unlikely to change our confidence in the estimate of effect.
- **Moderate**—Moderate confidence that the evidence reflects the true effect. Further research may change our confidence in the estimate of effect and may change the estimate.
- **Low**—Low confidence that the evidence reflects the true effect. Further research is likely to change the confidence in the estimate of effect and is likely to change the estimate.
- **Insufficient**—Evidence either is unavailable or does not permit estimation of an effect.

Applicability

We assessed applicability across our KQs using the method described in the Methods Guide.[45,53] In brief, the latter methods use the PICOTS format as a way to organize information relevant to applicability. We used these data to evaluate the applicability to clinical practice, paying special attention to study eligibility criteria, demographic features of the enrolled population (such as age, ethnicity, and sex) in comparison with the target population, version or characteristics of the intervention used in comparison with therapies currently in use (such as specific components of treatments considered to be "optimal medical therapy," plus advancements in endovascular and surgical revascularization techniques that have changed over time), and clinical relevance and timing of the outcome measures. We used a checklist to guide our assessment and summarized issues of applicability qualitatively (Appendix B).

Peer Review and Public Commentary

The peer review process is our principal external quality-monitoring device. Nominations for peer reviewers were solicited from several sources, including the TEP and interested Federal agencies. Experts in cardiology, radiology, vascular surgery, general medicine, and nursing, along with individuals representing stakeholder and user communities, were invited to provide external peer review of the draft report; AHRQ and an associate editor also provided comments. The draft report was posted on the AHRQ Web site for 4 weeks, from October 3 to November 7, 2012. We have addressed reviewer comments, revising the report as appropriate, and have documented our responses in a disposition of comments report available on the AHRQ Web site. A list of peer reviewers is given in the preface of this report.

Results

In this chapter, we describe the results of our literature searches followed by detailed results organized by KQ. For each KQ, we list the key points of the findings and provide a brief description of the included studies, followed by a detailed synthesis of the evidence. Across all KQs we present any relevant subgroup or harms data. (Tables C-1, C-2, and C-3 in Appendix C provide details and quality ratings for the included studies by population and comparison for each KQ.) We conducted quantitative syntheses where possible, as described in the Methods chapter. A list of abbreviations and acronyms used in this chapter is provided at the end of the report.

Results of Literature Searches

In Figure 3, we depict the flow of articles through the literature search and screening process for the review. Searches of PubMed,® Embase,® and the Cochrane Database of Systematic Reviews from January 1995 to August 2012 yielded 5908 citations, 1082 of which were duplicates. Manual searching and contacts to drug manufacturers identified 47 additional citations, for a total of 4873. After applying inclusion/exclusion criteria at the title-and-abstract level, 626 full-text articles were retrieved and screened. Of these, 521 were excluded at the full-text screening stage, leaving 105 articles (representing 83 unique studies) for data abstraction. Appendix D provides a detailed listing of included articles. Appendix E provides a complete list of articles excluded at the full-text screening stage, with reasons for exclusion.

As described in the Methods chapter, we searched ClinicalTrials.gov to identify completed but unpublished studies as a mechanism for ascertaining publication bias. Our search yielded 436 study records, 240 of which were completed at least 1 year prior to our search of the database and review of the published literature. A single reviewer identified 16 of these records as potentially relevant. We identified and screened publications for all 16 study records. Since we did not find any relevant study records without publications, we do not believe that there is significant publication bias in the evidence base that would impact our overall findings.

Figure 3. Literature flow diagram

```
┌─────────────────────────┐
│ 5908 citations          │
│ identified by           │──────► 1082 duplicates
│ literature search:      │
│  MEDLINE: 3573          │
│  Embase: 1460           │
│  Cochrane: 875          │
└─────────────────────────┘
            │
            │◄──── Manual searching: 47
            ▼
┌─────────────────────────┐
│ 4873 citations          │
│ identified              │──────► 4247 abstracts excluded
└─────────────────────────┘
            │
            ▼
┌─────────────────────────┐      ┌──────────────────────────────────────────────┐
│ 626                     │      │ 521 articles excluded:                        │
│ passed abstract         │─────►│  - Non-English: 26                            │
│ screening               │      │  - Not a full publication, not original data, │
└─────────────────────────┘      │    not peer-reviewed literature, or not grey  │
            │                    │    literature meeting specified criteria: 73  │
            │                    │  - Did not include a study population of      │
            │                    │    interest: 37                               │
            │                    │  - Did not include interventions or           │
            │                    │    comparators of interest: 165               │
            │                    │  - Did not include primary or secondary       │
            │                    │    outcomes of interest: 23                   │
            │                    │  - Single treatment strategy comparison: 196  │
            │                    │  - No outcomes of interest ≥30 days: 1        │
            ▼                    └──────────────────────────────────────────────┘
┌─────────────────────────┐
│ 105 articles            │
│ representing 83 studies │
│ passed full-text        │
│ screening               │
└─────────────────────────┘
            │
            ▼
┌─────────────────────────────────────────────────────────┐
│ 105 articles abstracted:                                │
│ KQ 1: 14 articles (11 studies; 10 RCT, 1 observational) │
│ KQ 2: 44 articles (35 studies; 27 RCT, 8 observational) │
│ KQ 3: 47 articles (37 studies; 3 RCT, 34 observational) │
└─────────────────────────────────────────────────────────┘
```

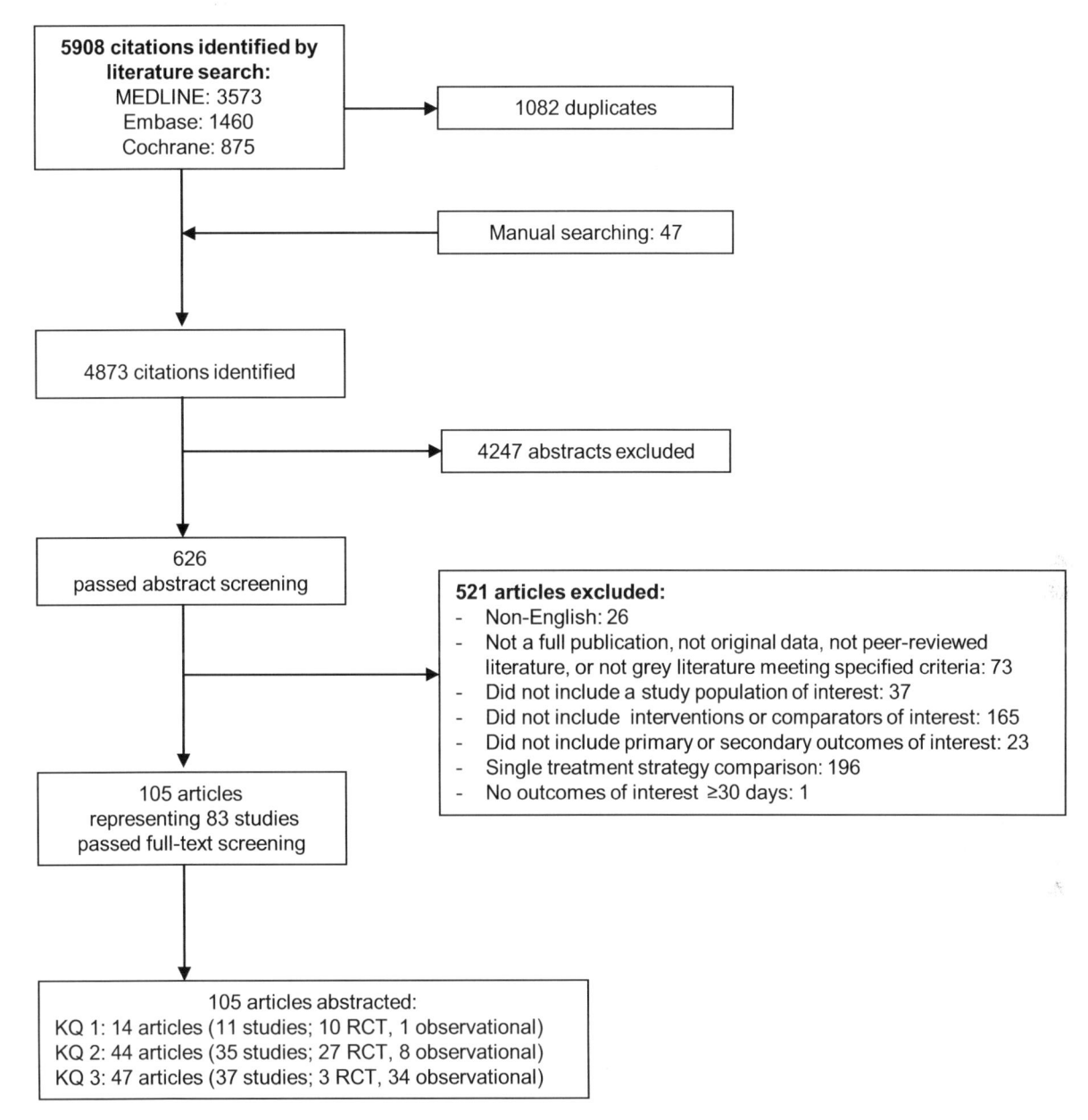

Abbreviations: KQ=Key Question; RCT=randomized controlled trial.

KQ 1. Comparative Effectiveness and Safety of Antiplatelet Therapy in Adults With PAD

KQ 1. In adults with peripheral artery disease (PAD), including asymptomatic patients and symptomatic patients with atypical leg symptoms, intermittent claudication (IC), or critical limb ischemia (CLI):

   a. What is the comparative effectiveness of aspirin and other antiplatelet agents in reducing the risk of adverse cardiovascular events (e.g., all-

cause mortality, myocardial infarction, stroke, cardiovascular death), functional capacity, and quality of life?
b. Does the effectiveness of treatments vary according to the patient's PAD classification or by subgroup (age, sex, race, risk factors, or comorbidities)?
c. What are the significant safety concerns associated with each treatment strategy (e.g., adverse drug reactions, bleeding)? Do the safety concerns vary by subgroup (age, sex, race, risk factors, comorbidities, or PAD classification)?

Key Points

Effectiveness of Interventions

- For asymptomatic PAD patients, there appears to be no benefit of aspirin over placebo for all-cause mortality, cardiovascular mortality, MI, or stroke (high SOE for all outcomes except cardiovascular mortality, which was rated moderate based on two good-quality RCTs).
- For IC patients, one small fair-quality RCT suggests with low SOE that aspirin compared with placebo may reduce MI (fatal and nonfatal) and composite vascular events (MI/stroke/pulmonary embolus), but there was insufficient SOE for all other outcomes due to study quality and imprecision.
- For IC patients, the PAD subgroup analysis of the CAPRIE RCT suggests that clopidogrel is more effective than aspirin for reducing cardiovascular mortality, nonfatal MI, and composite vascular events (moderate SOE for all outcomes). Clopidogrel and aspirin appear to be equivalent for prevention of nonfatal stroke, but the confidence interval was wide, making this conclusion less certain (low SOE).
- In patients with symptomatic or asymptomatic PAD, the PAD subgroup analysis of the CHARISMA RCT showed no difference between aspirin and dual therapy (clopidogrel plus aspirin) for outcomes of all-cause mortality (moderate SOE), nonfatal stroke (low SOE), cardiovascular mortality (low SOE), or composite vascular events (moderate SOE). There was a statistically significant benefit favoring dual therapy compared with aspirin for reducing nonfatal MI (low SOE).
- In patients with IC or CLI after unilateral bypass, the CASPAR RCT showed that DAPT resulted in no difference in nonfatal stroke and composite vascular events (low SOE), but there was insufficient SOE for other outcomes.
- In patients with IC or CLI after endovascular procedure, the MIRROR RCT showed no difference between dual therapy and aspirin in cardiovascular events or mortality at 6 months but was insufficiently powered for those outcomes (insufficient SOE).

Modifiers of Effectiveness

- Four RCTs reported subgroup analyses of demographic or clinical factors that modify the effect of antiplatelet agents in PAD and involved 5053 patients. Two of these RCTs included asymptomatic or high-risk patients and two included patients with either IC or CLI. Subgroups analyzed included diabetes (one RCT), age (one RCT), sex (two RCTs),

and PAD characteristics (two RCTs assessing ABI or type of bypass graft). The small number of and variation in subgroup analyses precluded the calculation of any overall estimate.
- One RCT of patients with IC or CLI showed a benefit of clopidogrel plus aspirin for reducing composite vascular events in patients with a prosthetic bypass graft compared with those with a venous bypass graft. Clinical outcomes were similar in men and women treated with antiplatelet agents. Given the heterogeneity of the subgroups, interventions, and clinical outcomes, the SOE for modifiers of effectiveness was insufficient.

Safety Concerns
- Seven RCTs reported safety concerns from antiplatelet treatment in the PAD population and involved 8297 patients. All seven RCTs reported bleeding as a harm. In general, use of antiplatelet agents was associated with higher rates of minor and moderate bleeding compared with placebo, ranging from 2 to 4 percent with aspirin, 2 percent with dual antiplatelet (no procedure), and 2.5 to 16.7 percent with dual antiplatelet (after percutaneous transluminal angioplasty or bypass grafting). Some RCTs reported adverse events such as rash and wound leak. The SOE for safety concerns is insufficient.

Description of Included Studies

We identified 11 unique studies (10 RCTs, 1 observational) that evaluated the comparative effectiveness of aspirin and antiplatelet agents in 15,150 patients with PAD.[54-64] Of these studies, seven were rated good quality, three fair, and one poor. (Characteristics for each study are presented in Table C-1 in Appendix C.) The following comparisons were assessed in the included studies and are detailed in this analysis:
1. Aspirin versus placebo or no antiplatelet (3 RCTs, 1 observational study)[54-57]
2. Clopidogrel/aspirin comparisons: clopidogrel with aspirin (dual antiplatelet) versus aspirin (4 RCTs)[60,61,63,64] and clopidogrel versus aspirin (1 RCT)[59]
3. Other antiplatelet comparisons: aspirin or iloprost versus no antiplatelet (1 RCT)[62] and high-dose aspirin versus low-dose aspirin (1 RCT)[58]

Detailed Synthesis

Effectiveness of Interventions

1. Aspirin Versus Placebo or No Antiplatelet
Two studies (both RCTs and rated good quality) compared aspirin with placebo, with no aspirin, or with no antiplatelet agent in asymptomatic patients.[54,56] These studies involved 3986 patients. One RCT (rated fair quality) compared aspirin with placebo in 181 patients with IC.[55] One observational study (retrospective cohort, rated poor quality) compared aspirin with no aspirin in 113 patients with CLI.[57] Sample sizes for individual studies ranged from 113 to 3350 patients. Study durations ranged from 2 to 10 years.

The mean age of study participants ranged from 60 to 72 years of age. The proportion of female patients ranged from 22 to 72 percent. None of the studies reported the racial and ethnic demographics of study participants. Few studies reported functional status or quality of life. Few studies reported the use of concomitant medications such as aspirin, antihypertensive medications, and HMG-CoA reductase medications.

All studies were conducted in Europe. Funding source was reported in three studies (75%), with two studies funded by a combination of government and industry funding[54,56] and one study funded by industry.[55]

Table 7 summarizes the clinical outcomes reported by the authors for each study as well as the calculated hazard ratio used in the meta-analyses. Meta-analyses of the hazard ratios were performed using Comprehensive Meta-Analysis Version 2.0.

Table 7. Calculated hazard ratios for aspirin versus placebo or no antiplatelet

Study Population	Type of Study N Analyzed[a] Comparison Quality	Length of Followup	Results Reported by Authors	Calculated HR (95% CI)[b]
Belch, 2008[54] POPADAD Study Patients with diabetes mellitus and asymptomatic PAD	RCT N: 636 ASA vs. placebo Good	6.7 yr	Nonfatal MI: ASA 34, no ASA 28 Nonfatal stroke: ASA 11, no ASA 22 CV mortality: ASA 20, no ASA 11 Composite vascular events: ASA 58, no ASA 57	Nonfatal MI: 0.98 (0.68 to 1.42) Nonfatal stroke: 0.71 (0.44 to 1.14) CV mortality: 1.23 (0.79 to 1.92) Composite vascular events: 0.98 (0.76 to 1.26)
Catalano, 2007[55] CLIPS Study Patients with IC	RCT N: 181 ASA vs. placebo Fair	2 yr	Nonfatal MI: ASA 0, placebo 2 Nonfatal stroke: ASA 0, placebo 5 CV mortality: ASA 2, placebo 3 Composite vascular events: ASA 1, placebo 10	Nonfatal MI: 0.18 (0.04 to 0.82) Nonfatal stroke: 0.54 (0.16 to 1.84) CV mortality: 1.21 (0.32 to 4.55) Composite vascular events: 0.35 (0.15 to 0.82)
Fowkes, 2010[56] Patients with asymptomatic PAD and no previous cardiovascular disease	RCT N: 3350 ASA vs. placebo Good	10 yr	Nonfatal MI: ASA 3.7%, placebo 4.1% Nonfatal stroke: ASA 0.4%, placebo 0.7% CV mortality: ASA 1.7%, placebo 1.1% Composite vascular events: ASA 10.8%, placebo 10.5%	Nonfatal MI: 0.91 (0.65 to 1.29) Nonfatal stroke: 0.97 (0.59 to 1.12) CV mortality: 0.95 (0.77 to 1.7) Composite vascular events: 1.00 (0.85 to 1.17)
Mahmood, 2003[57] Patients with CLI after infrainguinal bypass surgery	Retrospective cohort N: 113 ASA vs. no ASA Poor	2 yr	Nonfatal MI: ASA 1, no ASA 2 Nonfatal stroke: ASA 2, no ASA 3 CV mortality: ASA 26, no ASA 9 Composite vascular events: none reported	Nonfatal MI: ASA 1.2%, no ASA 5.9% Nonfatal stroke: ASA 2.5%, no ASA 8.8% CV mortality: ASA 33%, no ASA 26%

[a]Number of patients in the study arms of interest.
[b]Applies to studies used in the meta-analysis.
Abbreviations: ASA=acetylsalicylic acid (aspirin); CI=confidence interval; CV=cardiovascular; HR=hazard ratio; MI=myocardial infarction; RCT=randomized controlled trial; yr=year/years.

Effect on All-Cause Mortality

Two good-quality RCTs reported an all-cause mortality outcome in asymptomatic patients.[54,56] In the POPADAD study,[54] the total mortality rate was 11.9 percent in the aspirin group and 13.2 percent in the placebo group after a median followup time of 6.7 years. In the Fowkes study,[56] the total mortality rate was 12.8 percent in the aspirin group and 13.5 percent in the placebo group after 10 years (HR 0.95; 95% CI, 0.77 to 1.16). Results in both studies were not statistically significant. Given the consistent results from two good-quality RCTs on a direct outcome, the SOE was rated as high.

Effect on Nonfatal MI

Four studies reported nonfatal MI outcomes.[54-57] Three of these studies were RCTs and reported a nonfatal MI outcome in patients with PAD who were either asymptomatic or symptomatic without a recent procedure[54-56] with a median duration of 6.7 years. The fourth study[57] was excluded because of cohort study design (retrospective cohort) and patient population (postbypass patients with CLI).

Figure 4 shows the forest plot of the hazard ratios for the three RCTs that reported nonfatal MI events. Aspirin compared with placebo had no statistically significant effect on nonfatal MI. The confidence interval for the study by Catalano et al.[55] is wider since it is a smaller study, and the hazard ratio strongly favored aspirin and is likely due to the symptomatic (IC) population. The observational study[57] reported one nonfatal MI (1.2%) in the aspirin treatment arm and two nonfatal MIs (5.9%) in the no-aspirin treatment arm 2 years after infrainguinal bypass for CLI. The overall SOE was rated high for the asymptomatic population and low for the IC-CLI population and insufficient for the CLI population.

Figure 4. Forest plot for RCTs of aspirin versus placebo: nonfatal MI at 2 or more years

Study name	Population	Total N	Hazard ratio	Lower limit	Upper limit	p-Value
Belch, 2008 (POPADAD)	Asym PAD	636	0.98	0.68	1.42	0.92
Fowkes, 2010	Asym PAD	3350	0.91	0.65	1.29	0.60
Catalano, 2007 (CLIPS)	IC	181	0.18	0.04	0.82	0.03

Favors Aspirin   Favors Placebo

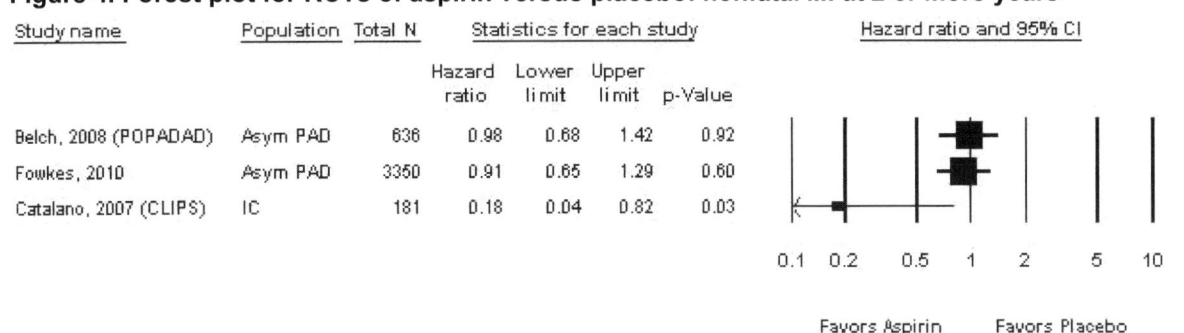

Abbreviations: CI=confidence interval; IC=intermittent claudication; PAD=peripheral artery disease.

Effect on Nonfatal Stroke

Four studies reported nonfatal stroke outcomes.[54-57] Three of these were RCTs and reported a stroke outcome in patients with PAD who were either asymptomatic or symptomatic without a recent procedure[54-56] with a median duration of 6.7 years. The fourth study[57] was a retrospective cohort study of patients with CLI receiving infrainguinal bypass surgery and was excluded because of study design and patient population.

Figure 5 shows the forest plot of the hazard ratios for the three RCTs that reported nonfatal stroke events. Aspirin compared with placebo had no statistically significant effect on nonfatal stroke. The summary estimate for Catalano et al. has a wider confidence interval since it is a smaller study and the hazard ratio appears to favor aspirin more than the Belch and Fowkes studies which is likely due to the symptomatic (IC) population, which can be assumed to have a higher degree of stenosis and CAD burden compared with the asymptomatic population. The findings from the Catalano study are inconclusive given the wide CI that crosses 1. The observational study[57] reported two strokes (2.5%) in patients receiving aspirin and three strokes (8.8%) in patients not receiving aspirin 2 years after infrainguinal bypass for CLI. The overall SOE was rated high for the asymptomatic population and insufficient for the IC-CLI and CLI populations.

Figure 5. Forest plot for RCTs of aspirin versus placebo: nonfatal stroke at 2 or more years

Study name	Population	Total N	Hazard ratio	Lower limit	Upper limit	p-Value
Belch, 2008 (POPADAD)	Asym PAD	636	0.71	0.44	1.14	0.16
Fowkes, 2010	Asym PAD	3350	0.97	0.62	1.53	0.91
Catalano, 2007 (CLIPS)	IC	181	0.54	0.16	1.84	0.32

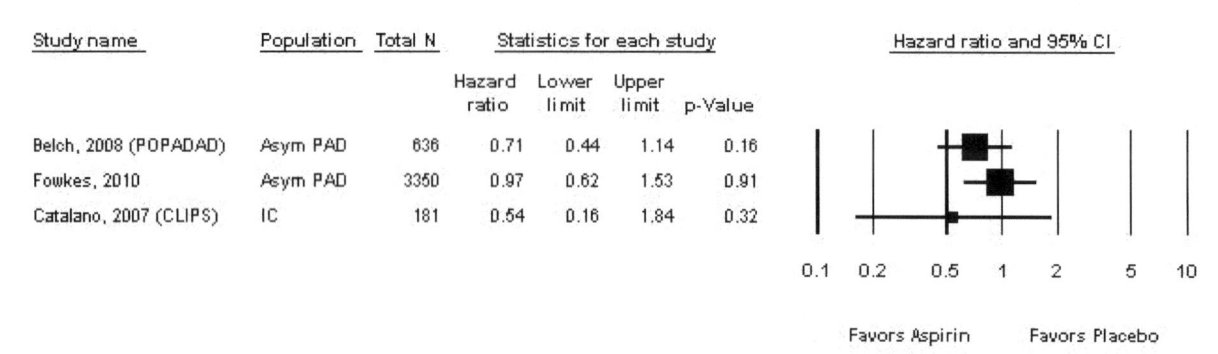

Abbreviations: CI=confidence interval; IC=intermittent claudication; PAD=peripheral artery disease.

Effect on Cardiovascular Mortality

Four studies reported cardiovascular mortality outcomes.[54-57] Three of these were RCTs and reported a cardiovascular mortality outcome in patients with PAD who were either asymptomatic or symptomatic without a recent procedure.[54-56] The fourth study[57] was a retrospective cohort study of patients with CLI receiving infrainguinal bypass surgery. Of the 79 patients in the treatment arm of that study, 47 received aspirin preoperatively and 32 received aspirin postoperatively; the comparison group (n=34) received no aspirin. Given the differences in study design (observational study) and patient population (postsurgical), this study was not included in the meta-analysis.

Figure 6 shows the forest plot of the hazard ratios for the three RCTs that reported cardiovascular mortality events. Aspirin compared with placebo had no statistically significant effect on cardiovascular mortality in either the asymptomatic PAD patients or the IC population. The observational study,[57] which was rated poor quality, reported a rate of vascular death in 33 percent of patients receiving aspirin and 26 percent in patients not receiving aspirin after 2 years after infrainguinal bypass for CLI (p=0.67). The overall SOE was rated moderate for the asymptomatic population and insufficient for the IC-CLI and CLI populations.

Figure 6. Forest plot for RCTs of aspirin versus placebo: cardiovascular mortality at 2 or more years

Study name	Population	Total N	Hazard ratio	Lower limit	Upper limit	p-Value
Belch, 2008 (POPADAD)	Asym PAD	636	1.23	0.79	1.92	0.36
Fowkes, 2010	Asym PAD	3350	0.95	0.77	1.17	0.62
Catalano, 2007 (CLIPS)	IC	181	1.21	0.32	4.55	0.78

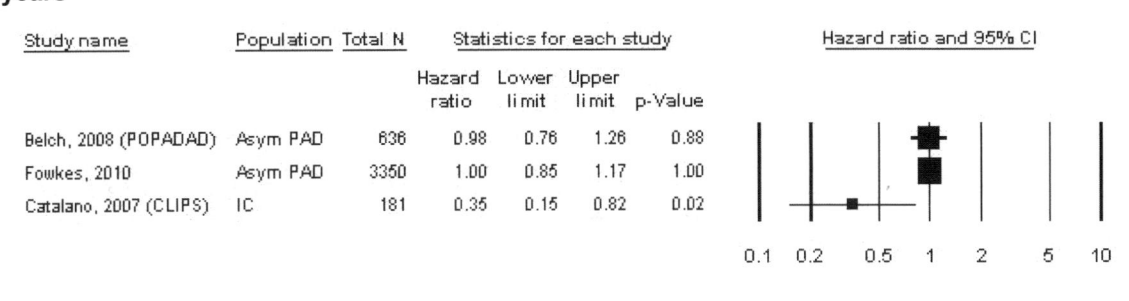

Abbreviations: Asym=asymptomatic; CI=confidence interval; IC=intermittent claudication; PAD=peripheral artery disease.

Effect on Composite Vascular Events

Three RCTs reported a composite of vascular event outcomes; namely, cardiovascular death, nonfatal stroke, and nonfatal MI in patients with PAD who were either asymptomatic or symptomatic at a median duration of 6.7 years.[54-56] Figure 7 shows the forest plot of the hazard ratios for these three RCTs. Similar to the analyses on the individual outcomes (cardiovascular mortality, nonfatal stroke, and nonfatal MI), aspirin compared with placebo had no statistically significant effect on vascular events. Again, the confidence interval for the study by Catalano et al.[55] is wider since it is a smaller study, and the hazard ratio strongly favored aspirin and is likely due to the symptomatic (IC) population. The overall SOE was rated high for the asymptomatic population and low for the IC population.

Figure 7. Forest plot for RCTs of aspirin versus placebo: composite vascular events at 2 or more years

Study name	Population	Total N	Hazard ratio	Lower limit	Upper limit	p-Value
Belch, 2008 (POPADAD)	Asym PAD	636	0.98	0.76	1.26	0.88
Fowkes, 2010	Asym PAD	3350	1.00	0.85	1.17	1.00
Catalano, 2007 (CLIPS)	IC	181	0.35	0.15	0.82	0.02

Abbreviations: Asym=asymptomatic; CI=confidence interval; IC=intermittent claudication; PAD=peripheral artery disease.

Effect on Other Outcomes

None of the studies comparing aspirin with placebo, with no aspirin, or with no antiplatelet drug reported functional outcomes such as MWD, PWT, or COT. The effect of aspirin on quality of life also was not reported. Therefore, SOE for the effect of aspirin on functional outcomes and quality of life is insufficient.

2. Clopidogrel/Aspirin Comparisons

Clopidogrel With or Without Aspirin Versus Aspirin Monotherapy

One good-quality RCT[59] compared clopidogrel monotherapy with aspirin monotherapy in a PAD subpopulation within a larger study of high-risk vascular populations (prior MI, cerebrovascular accident, PAD). This RCT was conducted internationally and involved 6452 PAD patients with a mean duration of follow up of 1.9 years.

Four studies (all RCTS and rated good quality) compared clopidogrel plus aspirin with aspirin monotherapy in patients with asymptomatic PAD (one RCT), IC (one RCT), and a mixed population of either IC or CLI (two RCTs) (Table 8).[60,61,63-65] These RCTs involved 4130 patients. Sample sizes for individual studies ranged from 80 to 3096 patients. Study durations ranged from 30 days to 28 months. Three RCTs were conducted internationally,[60,63-65] and one RCT was conducted at a single site in the United Kingdom.[61]

The mean age of study participants ranged from 64 to 70 years of age. The proportion of female patients ranged from 22 to 48 percent. None of the RCTs reported the racial and ethnic demographics of study participants. Few RCTs reported functional status or quality of life. Few RCTs reported the use of concomitant medications such as aspirin, antihypertensive medications, and HMG-CoA reductase medications. Industry funded the four international RCTs, and a mixture of nonprofit and industry funding sources was reported for the single-site study.[61]

Table 8. Calculated hazard ratio for clopidogrel with or without aspirin versus placebo with aspirin

Study Population	Type of Study N Analyzed[a] Comparison Quality	Length of Followup	Results Reported by Authors	Calculated HR (95% CI)[b]
Clopidogrel monotherapy vs. aspirin monotherapy				
Anonymous, 1996[59] CAPRIE Study Patients with IC or history of endovascular or bypass surgery	RCT N: 6452 Clopidogrel vs. ASA Good	2 yr	Nonfatal MI: Clopidogrel 50, ASA 81 Nonfatal stroke: Clopidogrel 70, ASA 74 CV mortality: Clopidogrel 66, ASA 87 Composite vascular events: Clopidogrel 215, ASA 277	Nonfatal MI: 0.62 (0.43 to 0.88) Nonfatal stroke: 0.95 (0.68 to 1.31) CV mortality: 0.76 (0.64 to 0.91) Composite vascular events: 0.78 (0.65 to 0.93)

Table 8. Calculated hazard ratio for clopidogrel with or without aspirin versus placebo with aspirin (continued)

Study Population	Type of Study N Analyzed[a] Comparison Quality	Length of Followup	Results Reported by Authors	Calculated HR (95% CI)[b]
Clopidogrel plus aspirin (dual antiplatelet) vs. aspirin monotherapy				
Belch, 2010[63] CASPAR Study Patients with IC or CLI status post unilateral bypass graft	RCT N: 851 Clopidogrel/ASA vs. ASA Good	2 yr	Nonfatal MI: HR 0.81 (0.32 to 2.06) Nonfatal stroke: HR 1.02 (0.41 to 2.57) CV mortality: HR 1.44 (0.77 to 2.68) Composite vascular events: HR 1.09 (0.65 to 1.82) Note: Actual event rates not reported	Nonfatal MI: 0.81 (0.32 to 2.06) Nonfatal stroke: 1.02 (0.41 to 2.56) CV mortality: 1.44 (0.77 to 2.69) Composite vascular events: 1.09 (0.65 to 1.82)
Cacoub, 2009[60] Bhatt, 2007[65] CHARISMA Study Patients with PAD (92% symptomatic [IC], 8% asymptomatic)	RCT N: 3096 Clopidogrel/ASA vs. ASA Good	28 mo	Nonfatal MI: Clopidogrel/ASA 2.3%, ASA 3.7% Nonfatal stroke: Clopidogrel/ASA 2.3%, ASA 3.0% CV mortality: Clopidogrel/ASA 4.2% ASA. 4.6% Composite vascular events: Clopidogrel 7.6%, ASA 8.9%	Nonfatal MI: 0.63 (0.42 to 0.96) Nonfatal stroke: 0.79 (0.0.51 to 1.21) CV mortality: 0.92 (0.65 to 1.28) Composite vascular events: 0.85 (0.66 to 1.08)
Cassar, 2005[61] Patients with IC	RCT N: 103 Clopidogrel/ASA vs. ASA Good	30 days	Only reports adverse drug reactions and platelet reactivity	Not estimated
Tepe, 2012[64] MIRROR Study Patients with IC or CLI status post endovascular procedure	RCT N: 80 Clopidogrel/ASA vs. ASA Good	6 mo	Mortality: Clopidogrel 0%, ASA 2.5% Composite vascular events: Clopidogrel 30%, ASA 37.5%	Mortality: OR 0.33 (0.01 to 8.22) Composite vascular events: OR 0.71 (0.28 to 1.81)

[a] Number of patients in the study arms of interest.
[b] Applies to studies used in the meta-analysis.
Abbreviations: ASA=acetylsalicylic acid (aspirin); CI=confidence interval; CLI=critical limb ischemia; CV=cardiovascular; HR=hazard ratio; IC=intermittent claudication; MI=myocardial infarction; mo=month/months; OR=odds ratio; RCT=randomized controlled trial; yr=year/years.

Clopidogrel Monotherapy Versus Aspirin Monotherapy

In the PAD subgroup of the CAPRIE RCT,[59] there was a statistically significant benefit of clopidogrel monotherapy over aspirin monotherapy, hazard ratio 0.76 (95% CI, 0.64 to 0.91, p=0.003), in regard to cardiovascular mortality. The overall SOE is moderate given the results of one large RCT on a direct outcome and narrow confidence interval. There was no difference in the rates of nonfatal stroke hazard ratio 0.95 (CI, 0.68 to 1.31, p=0.74). The overall SOE is low given the results of one large RCT on a direct outcome and wide confidence interval. CAPRIE also showed a statistically significant reduction in the rate of nonfatal MI, hazard ratio 0.62 (CI, 0.43 to 0.88, p=0.01). The overall SOE is moderate given the results of one large RCT on a direct outcome and narrow confidence interval. For composite vascular events (cardiovascular mortality, nonfatal stroke, and nonfatal MI), there was a statistically significant reduction, hazard ratio 0.78 (CI, 0.65 to 0.93, p=0.01). The overall SOE is moderate given the results of one large RCT on a direct outcome and narrow confidence interval. Overall, there is moderate evidence that clopidogrel monotherapy is superior to aspirin monotherapy in the reduction of cardiovascular mortality, nonfatal MI, and composite vascular events but low evidence that it affects nonfatal stroke in the PAD population (Figure 8). This study did not evaluate outcomes for all-cause mortality, functional outcomes, quality of life, modifiers of effectiveness, or safety concerns.

Figure 8. Clopidogrel versus aspirin for all outcomes in PAD subgroup of CAPRIE RCT

CAPRIE study outcome	Hazard ratio	Lower limit	Upper limit	p-Value
CV mortality	0.76	0.64	0.91	0.00
Nonfatal stroke	0.95	0.68	1.31	0.74
Nonfatal MI	0.62	0.43	0.88	0.01
Composite CV events	0.78	0.65	0.93	0.01

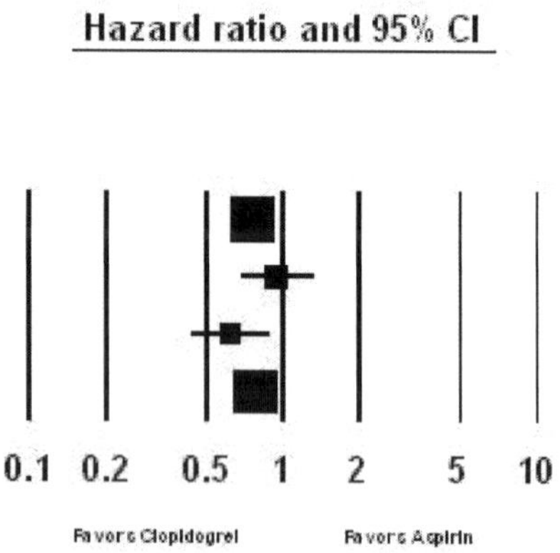

Abbreviations: CI=confidence interval; CV=cardiovascular; MI=myocardial infarction.

Clopidogrel Plus Aspirin (Dual Antiplatelet) Versus Aspirin Monotherapy

Four RCTs compared clopidogrel plus aspirin (DAPT) with aspirin monotherapy. The CHARISMA RCT[60] reported results for the PAD subpopulation (92% IC, 8% asymptomatic) within a larger study of high-risk vascular populations (prior MI, cerebrovascular accidents, and PAD). The CASPAR RCT[63] assessed a PAD population (33% IC, 67% CLI) who received unilateral below-the-knee (infrageniculate) bypass surgery. The MIRROR RCT[64] assessed a PAD population (66% IC, 44% CLI) that underwent percutaneous transluminal angioplasty. The RCT by Cassar et al.[61] reported adverse drug outcomes up to 30 days after an endovascular procedure for IC (see Safety Concerns section); the main finding was greater platelet function inhibition with dual therapy.

Effect on All-Cause Mortality

Three good-quality RCTs reported an all-cause mortality outcome.[60,63,64] In the CHARISMA RCT,[60] the all-cause mortality hazard ratio was 0.89 (0.68 to 1.16) in the clopidogrel plus aspirin group compared with the aspirin group after 28 months of followup. In the CASPAR RCT,[63] the all-cause mortality hazard ratio was 1.44 (95% CI, 0.77 to 2.69) in the clopidogrel plus aspirin group compared with the aspirin group after a followup time of 2 years. In the MIRROR RCT,[64] the all-cause mortality odds ratio was 0.33 (CI, 0.01 to 8.22) in the clopidogrel plus aspirin group compared with the aspirin group after a followup time of 6 months. In all three RCTs, the results were not statistically significant. Differences in these results among the RCTs may be due to the patient population (IC-asymptomatic vs. IC-CLI). The overall SOE was rated moderate for the IC-asymptomatic population and insufficient for the IC-CLI populations.

Effect on Nonfatal MI

Two RCTs reported nonfatal MI outcomes with a median duration of treatment of 2 years.[60,63,65] Clopidogrel plus aspirin reduced the rate of nonfatal MI compared with aspirin alone which was statistically significant in the CHARISMA RCT, hazard ratio 0.63 (95% CI, 0.42 to 0.95, p=0.03) and nonsignificant in the CASPAR RCT, hazard ratio 0.81 (CI, 0.32 to 2.06, p=0.66). The overall SOE was rated low for the IC-Asymptomatic population and insufficient for the IC-CLI postbypass population.

Effect on Nonfatal Stroke

Two RCTs reported nonfatal stroke outcomes with a median duration of 2 years.[60,63,65] The CHARISMA RCT showed a nonsignificant benefit of DAPT over aspirin monotherapy, hazard ratio 0.79 (95% CI, 0.51 to 1.22, p=0.28), but the CASPAR RCT showed no significant difference, hazard ratio 1.02 (CI, 0.41 to 2.55, p=0.97). The overall SOE was rated low for both the IC-Asymptomatic population and the IC-CLI postbypass population.

Effect on Cardiovascular Mortality

Two RCTs reported cardiovascular mortality outcomes with a median duration of 2 years.[60,63,65] In these RCTs (CHARISMA and CASPAR), DAPT had a no significant difference in the CHARISMA PAD subgroup, hazard ratio 0.92 (95% CI, 0.66 to 1.29, p=0.63), and was inconclusive in the CASPAR postbypass surgery population, hazard ratio 1.44 (CI, 0.77 to 2.69, p=0.25). The overall SOE was rated low for the IC-Asymptomatic population and insufficient for the IC-CLI postbypass population.

Effect on Composite Vascular Events

Three RCTs reported composite vascular event outcomes; namely, cardiovascular mortality, nonfatal stroke, and nonfatal MI, at around 6 months[64] or 2 years of followup.[60,63,65] Clopidogrel plus aspirin did not impact the rate of composite vascular events compared with aspirin alone: CHARISMA RCT, hazard ratio 0.85 (0.66 to 1.09, p=0.20), CASPAR RCT, hazard ratio 1.09 (0.65 to 1.82, p=0.74) and MIRROR RCT, OR 0.71 (0.28 to 1.81, p=0.48). The overall SOE was rated moderate for the IC-Asymptomatic population, low for the IC-CLI postbypass population and insufficient for the IC-CLI post percutaneous transluminal angioplasty population.

Effect on Other Outcomes

None of the RCTs comparing clopidogrel plus aspirin to aspirin reported functional outcomes such as MWD, ACD, PWT, or COT. The effect of clopidogrel plus aspirin on quality of life also was not reported. Therefore SOE for the effect of clopidogrel plus aspirin on functional outcomes and quality of life is insufficient. Figure 9 shows the hazard ratios for each outcome measured in the CHARISMA and CASPAR RCT. Figure 10 shows the odds ratios for each outcome measured in the MIRROR RCT.

Figure 9. Dual antiplatelet versus aspirin outcomes in CHARISMA and CASPAR RCTs

Study name (Population)	Outcome	Hazard ratio	Lower limit	Upper limit	p-Value
CHARISMA, 2009 (IC/Asym)	All death	0.89	0.68	1.16	0.39
CHARISMA, 2009 (IC/Asym)	Composite	0.85	0.66	1.09	0.20
CHARISMA, 2009 (IC/Asym)	CV death	0.92	0.66	1.29	0.63
CHARISMA, 2009 (IC/Asym)	MI	0.63	0.42	0.95	0.03
CHARISMA, 2009 (IC/Asym)	Stroke	0.79	0.51	1.22	0.28
CASPAR, 2010 (IC/CLI)	All death	1.44	0.77	2.69	0.25
CASPAR, 2010 (IC/CLI)	Composite	1.09	0.65	1.82	0.74
CASPAR, 2010 (IC/CLI)	CV death	1.44	0.77	2.69	0.25
CASPAR, 2010 (IC/CLI)	MI	0.81	0.32	2.06	0.66
CASPAR, 2010 (IC/CLI)	Stroke	1.02	0.41	2.55	0.97

Abbreviations: Asym=asymptomatic; CI=confidence interval; CLI=critical limb ischemia; CV=cardiovascular; IC=intermittent claudication; MI-myocardial infarction.

Figure 10. Dual antiplatelet versus aspirin outcomes in MIRROR RCT

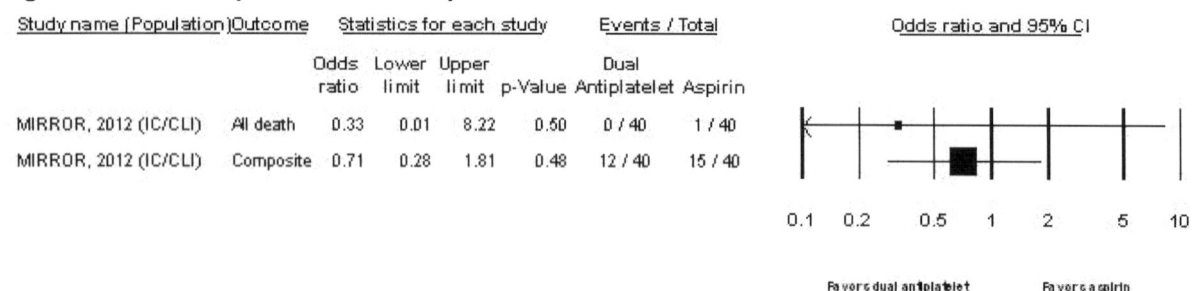

Study name (Population)	Outcome	Odds ratio	Lower limit	Upper limit	p-Value	Dual Antiplatelet	Aspirin
MIRROR, 2012 (IC/CLI)	All death	0.33	0.01	8.22	0.50	0 / 40	1 / 40
MIRROR, 2012 (IC/CLI)	Composite	0.71	0.28	1.81	0.48	12 / 40	15 / 40

Abbreviations: CI=confidence interval.

3. Other Antiplatelet Comparisons

Two studies (both RCTs and rated fair quality) assessed other antiplatelet comparisons in patients with IC or CLI.[58,62] The RCTs involved 254 patients and compared (1) aspirin or iloprost versus no antiplatelet agent in patients with IC or CLI after percutaneous transluminal angioplasty (PTA)[62] and (2) aspirin 1000 mg versus aspirin 100 mg in patients with IC or CLI after femoropopliteal PTA.[58] The smaller RCT included 38 patients while the larger RCT included 216 patients. Mean study duration was 1.5 years. The mean age of study participants was 66 to 68 years of age. The proportion of female patients ranged from 32 to 42 percent. Neither study reported the use of concomitant medications such as aspirin, antihypertensive medications, and HMG-CoA reductase medications. Both studies were conducted in Europe and neither reported funding source.

Results for various clinical outcomes are shown in Table 9. Due to the small number of studies and significant heterogeneity in the comparators, outcomes, and timing, a quantitative analysis was not possible. Neither RCT reported a composite outcome. Both RCTs assessed postprocedural outcomes and reported rates of vessel patency/restenosis/reocclusion. One RCT reported total mortality.[58] Neither RCT reported functional outcomes or quality of life. In both RCTs there were no significant differences found between the treatment groups for all outcomes measured.

Table 9. Results of other antiplatelet comparisons

Study	Type of Study N Analyzed[a] Comparison Quality	Outcome Length of Followup	Results Reported by Authors
Horrocks, 1997[62] Patients with IC or CLI	RCT (open label) N: 38 ASA or iloprost vs. no antiplatelet Fair	Restenosis Reocclusion 3 mo	Restenosis: ASA 5, iloprost 0, placebo 3 Reocclusion: ASA 0, iloprost 1, placebo 0
Minar, 1995[58] Patients with IC or CLI	RCT N: 216 ASA 1000 mg vs. ASA 100 mg Fair	Total mortality Primary vessel patency 2 yr	Total mortality: 1000 mg ASA 14; 100 mg ASA 13 Primary vessel patency: 1000 mg ASA 62.5% 100 mg ASA 62.6%

[a]Number of patients in the study arms of interest.
Abbreviations: ASA=acetylsalicylic acid (aspirin); CLI=critical limb ischemia; IC=intermittent claudication; LSM=least squares mean; mg=milligram; RCT=randomized controlled trial; yr=year/years.

Modifiers of Effectiveness

Four RCTs (three good quality, one fair) reported variations in treatment effectiveness by subgroup (Table 10).[54,56,58,63] Two RCTs compared aspirin with placebo in asymptomatic or high-risk patients,[54,56] one RCT compared 1000 mg of aspirin with 100 mg of aspirin in patients with IC or CLI,[58] and one RCT compared clopidogrel plus aspirin with aspirin alone in patients with IC or CLI undergoing unilateral below the knee bypass.[63]

Subgroups analyzed included diabetes (one study[54]), age (one RCT[56]), sex (two RCT[56,58]), type of bypass graft (one RCT[63]), and ABI (one RCT[56]). One RCT[63] showed a benefit of clopidogrel plus aspirin for reducing composite vascular events in patients with a prosthetic bypass graft compared to those with a venous bypass graft. Clinical outcomes were similar in men and women treated with antiplatelet agents. We found no studies reporting subgroup results by race or risk factors (e.g., tobacco use, presence of hyperlipidemia). Given the heterogeneity of the subgroups, interventions, and clinical outcomes, the SOE for modifiers of effectiveness was insufficient.

Table 10. Studies reporting subgroup results of antiplatelet therapy (modifiers of effectiveness)

Study Population	Type of Study N Analyzed[a] Comparison Quality	Subgroup	Results Reported by Authors
Belch, 2008[54] POPADAD Study Patients with diabetes mellitus and asymptomatic PAD	RCT N: 636 ASA vs. placebo Good	Diabetes	CV mortality: 21 ASA, 14 placebo Stroke: 0 ASA, 5 placebo
Belch, 2010[63] CASPAR Study Patients with IC or CLI	RCT N: 851 Clopidogrel/ASA vs. ASA Good	Type of bypass graft venous vs. prosthetic	Composite CV events: Venous: HR 1.25 (0.94 to 1.67) Prosthetic: HR 0.65 (0.45 to 0.95) Significant reduction in prosthetic graft patients receiving DAPT, but not in venous graft patients
Fowkes, 2010[56] Patients with asymptomatic PAD and no previous cardiovascular disease	RCT N: 3350 ASA vs. placebo Good	Age <62 yr vs. ≥62 yr Sex ABI ≤0.95, ≤0.90, ≤0.85, ≤0.80	Composite CV events: <62: HR 0.85 (0.65 to 1.20) ≥ 62: HR 1.13 (0.97 to 1.47) Composite CV events: Men: HR 1.15 (0.86 to 1.54) Women: HR 0.92 (0.68 to 1.23) Composite CV events: ≤0.95: HR 1.03 (0.84 to 1.27) ≤0.90: HR 1.02 (0.80 to 1.29) ≤0.85: HR 0.99 (0.73 to 1.35) ≤0.80: HR 1.06 (0.73 to 1.54)
Minar, 1995[58] Patients with IC or CLI	RCT N: 216 ASA 1000 mg vs. ASA 100 mg Fair	Sex	Vessel patency: Aspirin dosage had no influence on the cumulative patency in either sex

[a]Number of patients in the study arms of interest.
Abbreviations: ABI=ankle brachial index; ASA=acetylsalicylic acid (aspirin); CLI=critical limb ischemia; CV=cardiovascular; HR=hazard ratio; IC=intermittent claudication; RCT=randomized controlled trial.

Safety Concerns

Seven RCTs (six good quality, one fair) reported safety concerns associated with each treatment strategy (Table 11).[54-56,60,61,63,64] All seven RCTs reported bleeding, GI bleeding, or anemia as a harm: three RCTs comparing aspirin with placebo in asymptomatic patients[54,55] or patients with IC[56] and four RCTs comparing clopidogrel plus aspirin with aspirin alone in high-risk asymptomatic patients,[60] patients with IC,[61] and in a mixed population of patients with either IC or CLI.[63,64] A quantitative analysis of bleeding rates was not possible due to the low number of studies by treatment comparison, variation in the bleeding definition, and differences in measurement time points. In two aspirin versus placebo RCTs, the rates of major hemorrhage or bleeding were slightly higher in the aspirin groups; a third RCT showed lower rates of gastrointestinal bleeding in the aspirin group. In the dual antiplatelet groups, bleeding rates ranged from 2 to 3 percent (with one study showing a rate of 28 percent in the immediate postoperative period) compared with bleeding rates ranging from 0 to 6 percent in the placebo groups. There was no significant difference in bleeding except in the immediate postoperative period.

Two RCTs reported the adverse side effect of a rash (two studies[54,61]), which was higher in patients receiving aspirin compared with placebo and similar in patients receiving DAPT or aspirin. None of the RCTs reported on whether any harms varied by subgroup (age, sex, race, risk factors, comorbidities, anatomic location of disease). Therefore, the SOE for safety concerns is insufficient.

Table 11. Studies reporting harms of antiplatelet therapy

Study Population	Type of Study N Analyzed[a] Comparison Quality	Harm Length of Followup	Results Reported by Authors
Belch, 2008[54] POPADAD Study Patients with diabetes mellitus and asymptomatic PAD	RCT N: 636 ASA vs. placebo Good	1. GI bleed 2. GI symptoms 3. Arrhythmia 4. Rash 6.7 yr	1. GI bleed: ASA 13 (4%), placebo 18 (6%) 2. GI symptoms: ASA 40 (13%), placebo 58 (18%) 3. Arrhythmia: ASA 27 (9%), placebo 25 (8%) 4. Rash: ASA 38 (12%), placebo 30 (9%)
Belch, 2010[63] CASPAR Study Patients with IC or CLI status post unilateral bypass graft	RCT N: 851 Clopidogrel/ASA vs. ASA Good	Bleeding 2 yr	Bleeding: clopidogrel 71 (16.7%), placebo 30 (7.1%), p=0.001 Severe bleeding: clopidogrel 9 (2.1%); placebo 5 (1.2%), P=NS Moderate bleeding: clopidogrel 16 (3.8%); placebo 4 (0.9%), p=0.007 Mild bleeding: clopidogrel 46 (10.8%); placebo 21 (5%), p=0.002
Cacoub, 2009[60] CHARISMA Study PAD subgroup (92% CI, 8% asymptomatic)	RCT N: 3096 Clopidogrel/ASA vs. ASA Good	Bleeding 28 mo	Severe bleed: clopidogrel/ASA 1.7%, ASA 1.7%, p=0.90 Moderate bleed: clopidogrel/ASA 2.5%, ASA 1.9%, p=0.26 Minor bleed: clopidogrel/ASA 34.4%, ASA 20.8%, p<0.001
Cassar, 2005[61] Patients with IC status post-PTA	RCT N: 103 Clopidogrel/ASA vs. ASA Good	1. GI Bleed 2. Rash 3. Hematoma 4. Bruising 30 days	1. GI bleed: clopidogrel/ASA 1, ASA 0 2. Rash: clopidogrel/ASA 2, ASA 2 3. Hematoma: clopidogrel/ASA 2 peripheral and 1 retroperitoneal, ASA 2 4. Bruising: clopidogrel/ASA 25, ASA 16
Catalano, 2007[55] CLIPS Study Patients with IC	RCT N: 181 ASA vs. placebo Fair	Bleeding 2 yr	ASA 3%, placebo 0%

Table 11. Studies reporting harms of antiplatelet therapy (continued)

Study Population	Type of Study N Analyzed[a] Comparison Quality	Harm Length of Followup	Results Reported by Authors
Fowkes, 2010[56] Patients with asymptomatic PAD and no previous cardiovascular disease	RCT N: 3350 ASA vs. placebo Good	1. Major hemorrhage 2. GI ulcer 3. Retinal hemorrhage 4. Severe anemia 10 yr	1. Major hemorrhage: ASA 2.0%, placebo 1.2% 2. GI ulcer: ASA 0.8%, placebo 0.5% 3. Retinal hemorrhage: ASA 0.1%, placebo 0.2% 4. Severe anemia: ASA 25, placebo 16
Tepe, 2012[64] MIRROR study Patients with IC or CLI status post percutaneous transluminal angioplasty	RCT N: 80 Clopidogrel/ASA vs. ASA Good	Bleeding 6 mo	Bleeding: clopidogrel 1 (2.5%), placebo 2 (5%), p=0.559

[a]Number of patients in the study arms of interest.
Abbreviations: ASA=acetylsalicylic acid (aspirin); CI=confidence interval; CLI=critical limb ischemia; CV=cardiovascular; GI=gastrointestinal; HR=hazard ratio; IC=intermittent claudication; mo=month/months; NS=not significant; RCT=randomized controlled trial; SD=standard deviation; wk=week/weeks; yr=year/years.

SOE Ratings for KQ 1

Tables 12–14 summarize the SOE for the outcomes of cardiovascular mortality, nonfatal stroke, nonfatal MI, and composite vascular events. No studies reported results on functional outcomes or quality of life. Very few studies reported modifiers of effectiveness or safety outcomes.

Table 12. Detailed SOE for aspirin versus placebo in adults with asymptomatic or symptomatic PAD at 2+ years

Population Study Design Number of Studies (Total Patients)	Risk of Bias	Consistency	Directness	Precision	SOE and Magnitude of Effect Effect Estimate (95% CI)
All-cause mortality					
Asymptomatic RCT 2 (3986)	2 low risk	Consistent	Direct	Precise	HR 0.93 (0.71 to 1.24) HR 0.95 (0.77 to 1.16) No difference **High SOE**
Nonfatal MI					
Asymptomatic RCT 2 (3986)	2 low risk	Consistent	Direct	Precise	HR 0.98 (0.68 to 1.42) HR 0.91 (0.65 to 1.29) No difference **High SOE**
IC RCT 1 (181)	1 moderate risk	NA	Direct	Imprecise	HR 0.18 (0.04 to 0.82) Favors aspirin **Low SOE**
CLI Observational 1 (113)	1 high risk	NA	Direct	Unknown	No difference between aspirin (1.2%) and no-aspirin (5.9%) groups **Insufficient SOE**

Table 12. Detailed SOE for aspirin versus placebo in adults with asymptomatic or symptomatic PAD at 2+ years (continued)

Population Study Design Number of Studies (Total Patients)	Risk of Bias	Consistency	Directness	Precision	SOE and Magnitude of Effect Effect Estimate (95% CI)
Nonfatal stroke					
Asymptomatic RCT 2 (3986)	2 low risk	Consistent	Direct	Precise	HR 0.71 (0.44 to 1.14) HR 0.97 (0.62 to 1.53) No difference **High SOE**
IC RCT 1 (181)	1 moderate risk	NA	Direct	Imprecise	HR 0.54 (0.16 to 1.84) Inconclusive **Insufficient SOE**
CLI Observational 1 (113)	1 high risk	NA	Direct	Unknown	No difference between aspirin (2.5%) and no-aspirin (8.8%) groups **Insufficient SOE**
Cardiovascular mortality					
Asymptomatic RCT 2 (3986)	2 low risk	Consistent	Direct	Imprecise	HR 1.23 (0.79 to 1.92) HR 0.95 (0.77 to 1.17) No difference **Moderate SOE**
IC RCT 1 (181)	1 moderate risk	NA	Direct	Imprecise	HR 1.21 (0.32 to 4.55) Inconclusive **Insufficient SOE**
CLI Observational 1 (113)	1 high risk	NA	Direct	Unknown	No difference between aspirin (33%) and no-aspirin (26%) groups **Insufficient SOE**
Composite vascular events					
Asymptomatic RCT 2 (3986)	2 low risk	Consistent	Direct	Precise	HR 0.98 (0.76 to 1.26) HR 1.00 (0.85 to 1.17) No difference **High SOE**
IC RCT 1 (181)	1 moderate risk	NA	Direct	Imprecise	HR 0.35 (0.15 to 0.82) Favors aspirin **Low SOE**
Modifiers of effectiveness (subgroups)					
Asymptomatic IC-CLI RCT 3 (4202)	2 low risk, 1 moderate risk	NA	NA	NA	No differences in outcomes by age, sex, or baseline ABI in aspirin studies **Insufficient SOE**
Safety concerns					
Asymptomatic or IC RCT 3 (4167)	2 low risk, 1 moderate risk	NA	NA	NA	Bleeding rates slightly higher in aspirin group (2 to 4%) compared to placebo (0 to 6%) **Insufficient SOE**
Functional outcomes Quality of life Safety concerns (subgroups)					
0	NA	NA	NA	NA	**Insufficient SOE**

Abbreviations: ABI=ankle-brachial index; CI=confidence interval; CLI=critical limb ischemia; HR=hazard ratio; IC=intermittent claudication; NA=not applicable; Obs=observational; PTA=percutaneous transluminal angioplasty; RCT=randomized controlled trial; SOE=strength of evidence.

Table 13. Detailed SOE for clopidogrel versus aspirin in adults with IC at 2 years (CAPRIE)

Study Design Number of Studies (Total Patients)	Risk of Bias	Consistency	Directness	Precision	SOE and Magnitude of Effect Effect Estimate (95% CI)
Nonfatal MI					
IC RCT 1 (6452)	1 low risk	NA	Direct	Precise	HR 0.62 (0.43 to 0.88) Favors clopidogrel **Moderate SOE**
Nonfatal stroke					
IC RCT 1 (6452)	1 low risk	NA	Direct	Imprecise	HR 0.95 (0.68 to 1.31) No difference **Low SOE**
Cardiovascular mortality					
IC RCT 1 (6452)	1 low risk	NA	Direct	Precise	HR 0.76 (0.64 to 0.91) Favors clopidogrel **Moderate SOE**
Composite cardiovascular events					
IC RCT 1 (6452)	1 low risk	NA	Direct	Precise	HR 0.78 (0.65 to 0.93) Favors clopidogrel **Moderate SOE**
All-cause mortality Functional outcomes Quality of life Modifiers of effectiveness (subgroups) Safety concerns Safety concerns (subgroups)					
0	NA	NA	NA	NA	**Insufficient SOE**

Abbreviations: CI=confidence interval; HR=hazard ratio; NA=not applicable; RCT=randomized controlled trial; SOE=strength of evidence.

Table 14. Detailed SOE for clopidogrel plus aspirin versus aspirin monotherapy in adults with PAD at 2 years

Population Study Design Number of Studies (Total Patients)	Risk of Bias	Consistency	Directness	Precision	SOE and Magnitude of Effect Effect Estimate (95% CI)
All-cause mortality					
Symptomatic-asymptomatic RCT 1 (3096)	1 low risk	NA	Direct	Precise	HR 0.89 (0.68 to 1.16) No difference **Moderate SOE**
IC-CLI (postbypass) RCT 1 (851)	1 low risk	NA	Direct	Imprecise	HR 1.44 (0.77 to 2.69) Inconclusive **Insufficient SOE**
IC-CLI (post-PTA) RCT 1 (80)	1 low risk	NA	Direct	Imprecise	OR 0.33 (0.01 to 8.22) Inconclusive **Insufficient SOE**
Nonfatal MI					
Symptomatic-asymptomatic RCT 1 (3096)	1 low risk	NA	Direct	Precise	HR 0.63 (0.42 to 0.95) Favors dual antiplatelet **Low SOE**
IC-CLI (postbypass) RCT 1 (851)	1 low risk	NA	Direct	Imprecise	HR 0.81 (0.32 to 2.06) Inconclusive **Insufficient SOE**
Nonfatal stroke					
Symptomatic-asymptomatic RCT 1 (3096)	1 low risk	NA	Direct	Imprecise	HR 0.79 (0.51 to 1.22) No difference **Low SOE**
IC-CLI (postbypass) RCT 1 (851)	1 low risk	NA	Direct	Imprecise	HR 1.02 (0.41 to 2.55) No difference **Low SOE**
Cardiovascular mortality					
Symptomatic-asymptomatic RCT 1 (3096)	1 low risk	NA	Direct	Imprecise	HR 0.92 (0.66 to 1.29) No difference **Low SOE**
IC-CLI (postbypass) RCT 1 (851)	1 low risk	NA	Direct	Imprecise	HR 1.44 (0.77 to 2.69) Inconclusive **Insufficient SOE**

Table 14. Detailed SOE for clopidogrel plus aspirin versus aspirin monotherapy in adults with PAD at 2 years (continued)

Population Study Design Number of Studies (Total Patients)	Risk of Bias	Consistency	Directness	Precision	SOE and Magnitude of Effect Effect Estimate (95% CI)
Composite cardiovascular events					
Symptomatic-asymptomatic RCT 1 (3096)	1 low risk	NA	Direct	Precise	HR 0.85 (0.66 to 1.09) No difference **Moderate SOE**
IC-CLI (postbypass) RCT 1 (851)	1 low risk	NA	Direct	Imprecise	HR 1.09 (0.65 to 1.82) No difference **Low SOE**
IC-CLI (post-PTA) RCT 1 (80)	1 low risk	NA	Direct	Imprecise	OR 0.71 (0.28 to 1.81) Inconclusive **Insufficient SOE**
Modifiers of effectiveness (subgroups)					
IC-CLI (postbypass) RCT 1 (851)	1 low risk	NA	NA	NA	Patients with prosthetic graft had lower cardiovascular events on DAPT **Insufficient SOE**
Safety concerns					
All RCT 4 (4079)	4 low risk	NA	NA	NA	CASPAR study showed statistically significant higher rates of moderate and minor bleeding with DAPT; CHARISMA study showed statistically significant higher rate of minor bleeding with DAPT; Cassar study showed more bruising with DAPT but no significant difference in GI bleed or hematoma; MIRROR study showed no significant difference in bleeding **Insufficient SOE**
Functional outcomes Quality of life Safety concerns (subgroups)					
0	NA	NA	NA	NA	**Insufficient SOE**

Abbreviations: CI=confidence interval; CLI=critical limb ischemia; DAPT=dual antiplatelet therapy; GI=gastrointestinal; HR=hazard ratio; IC=intermittent claudication; MI=myocardial infarction; NA=not applicable; OR=odds ratio; RCT=randomized controlled trial; SOE=strength of evidence.

KQ 2. Comparative Effectiveness and Safety of Exercise, Medications, and Endovascular and Surgical Revascularization for IC

KQ 2. In adults with symptomatic PAD (atypical leg symptoms or IC):

a. What is the comparative effectiveness of exercise training, medications (cilostazol, pentoxifylline), endovascular intervention (percutaneous transluminal angioplasty, atherectomy, or stents), and/or surgical revascularization (endarterectomy, bypass surgery) on outcomes including cardiovascular events (e.g., all-cause mortality, myocardial infarction, stroke, cardiovascular death), amputation, quality of life, wound healing, analog pain scale score, functional capacity, repeat revascularization, and vessel patency?

b. Does the effectiveness of treatments vary by use of exercise and medical therapy prior to invasive management or by subgroup (age, sex, race, risk factors, comorbidities, or anatomic location of disease)?

c. What are the significant safety concerns associated with each treatment strategy (e.g., adverse drug reactions, bleeding, contrast nephropathy, radiation, infection, exercise-related harms, and periprocedural complications causing acute limb ischemia)? Do the safety concerns vary by subgroup (age, sex, race, risk factors, comorbidities, anatomic location of disease)?

Key Points

Effectiveness of Interventions
- In a random-effects network meta-analysis of 12 RCTs that assessed the effect of 6 comparisons on all-cause mortality, no specific treatment was found to have a statistically significant effect (low SOE for all comparisons).
- In a random-effects meta-analysis of 16 RCTs that compared the effect of multiple treatments on MWD or ACD, exercise training, pentoxifylline, and the combination of endovascular treatment with exercise were associated with large effects when compared with usual care. Cilostazol and endovascular intervention were associated with moderate effects when compared with usual care. None of the other treatments were found to have a statistically significant effect when compared against each other. A sensitivity analysis removing the pentoxifylline studies (due to inconsistency and imprecision) resulted in effect size estimates that are slightly increased for the remaining treatment modalities. We observed similar results in studies that were excluded due to measurement of peak walking time rather than distance. SOE was rated *moderate* for exercise; *low* for

cilostazol, endovascular treatment, and the combination of endovascular treatment with exercise; and *insufficient* for pentoxifylline.
- In a random-effects meta-analysis of 12 RCTs that compared the effect of multiple treatments on ICD or PFWD, cilostazol was associated with a statistically nonsignificant improvement when compared with usual care (effect size 0.63; 95% CI, -0.02 to 1.29, p=0.06); however, exercise training and endovascular revascularization were associated with moderate to large effects and a statistically significant improvement when compared with usual care (effect size 0.69; CI, 0.23 to 1.15, p=0.003; and effect size 0.79; CI, 0.29 to 1.29, p=0.002, respectively). When directly compared in head-to-head studies, there was no difference between the three treatments. Similar results were observed in studies excluded due to measurement of claudication onset time rather than distance. SOE was rated low across all comparisons.
- A random-effects meta-analysis of 10 RCTs examining the difference in the SF-36 measure of physical functioning assessed between 3 months and 6 months showed a significant improvement in quality of life from cilostazol, exercise training, endovascular intervention, and surgical revascularization ranging from moderate to large effects compared with usual care. However, the comparisons of all active treatments with each other showed that none of the treatments are significantly different from each other. SOE was rated low for all comparisons.
- Cardiovascular events (e.g. myocardial infarction, stroke, cardiovascular death), amputation, wound healing, analog pain scale score, repeat revascularization, and vessel patency were infrequently reported. SOE was rated insufficient for all comparisons.
- One observational study of surgical revascularization versus usual care reported mortality and vessel patency results at 5 years. SOE was rated insufficient.

Modifiers of Effectiveness
- Four RCTs and two observational studies reported variations in the treatment effectiveness by subgroup including severity of symptoms, functional limitations, anatomic location of disease, and success of revascularization. Despite limited data to draw definitive conclusions, one observational study reported improvements in quality of life measures and ABI in patients with successful endovascular revascularization when compared with patients without successful endovascular revascularization. Another study reported improvement in ABI in patients with successful surgical revascularization when compared with patients treated with exercise and medical therapy. One other RCT reported a statistically nonsignificant improvement in MWD favoring exercise training over endovascular revascularization in patients with superficial femoral artery (SFA) stenosis when compared with patients with iliac stenosis. Last, a single observational study reported variability in the patency of surgical revascularization based on anatomic location and graft type.
- We found no studies reporting results by the following subgroups: age, sex, race, presence of diabetes mellitus or renal disease, smoking status, use of exercise or medical therapy prior to invasive management, or prior revascularization. The SOE for modifiers of effectiveness was insufficient given the variation in subgroups that were studied and the outcomes reported.

Safety Concerns

Seventeen RCTs reported safety concerns. A single RCT of exercise therapy versus usual care did not identify side effects from exercise. RCTs of cilostazol had higher rates of headache (OR 3.00; 95% CI, 2.29 to 3.95; high SOE), diarrhea (OR 2.51; CI, 1.58 to 3.97; moderate SOE), and palpitation complications (OR 18.32; CI, 5.95 to 55.13; moderate SOE). RCTs of endovascular interventions reported more transfusions, arterial dissection/perforation, and hematomas compared to the usual care groups but the complication rates were low (1 to 2%). No studies were identified that measured contrast nephropathy, radiation, infection, or exercise-related harms. No studies reported on whether any of the harms vary by subgroup (age, sex, race, risk factors, comorbidities, anatomic location of disease). The SOE for safety concerns by subgroup was insufficient.

Description of Included Studies

We identified 35 unique studies that evaluated the comparative effectiveness of exercise training, medications, endovascular intervention, and/or surgical revascularization in 7475 patients who have PAD with IC.[16,25,49,51,66-96] Of these studies, 27 were RCTs (12 good quality, 13 fair, 2 poor) and 8 were observational (4 fair, 4 poor). (Characteristics for each study are presented in Table C-2 in Appendix C.)

The following comparisons were assessed in the included studies and are detailed in this analysis:

1. Medical therapy (cilostazol or pentoxifylline) versus usual care (10 RCTs; 4103 total patients)[25,49,51,73,85-90]
2. Exercise training versus usual care (10 RCTs, 2 observational; 754 total patients)[66,68-71,73-75,77-79,96]
3. Endovascular intervention versus usual care (5 RCTs, 4 observational; 1593 total patients)[70,72,74,77,91-95]
4. Surgical revascularization versus usual care (1 observational; 427 total patients)[76]
5. Endovascular intervention versus exercise training (9 RCTs; 1005 total patients)[16,70,74,77,80-84]
6. Surgical revascularization versus exercise training plus medical therapy (1 observational; 127 total patients)[67]
7. Endovascular intervention versus surgical revascularization (3 observational; 421 total patients)[91,92,94]

The literature search revealed many potential studies with the comparators of interest in the IC population; however, many of these studies used different measures for the same outcome. For example, peak performance or walking ability was measured by maximal walking distance (MWD), maximal walking time (MWT), absolute claudication distance (ACD), or peak walking time (PWT). Likewise, claudication onset was measured by initial claudication distance (ICD), pain-free walking distance (PFWD), claudication onset time (COT), or pain-free walking time (PFWT). Also, six studies had more than two treatment arms. Because several of the studies reported results from multiple treatment arms and used different measures for a similar outcome, we constructed an effect size for each relevant arm of each study. We used a random-effects model that was a generalization of the standard random-effects model used in the meta-analysis of effect sizes. Further details are outlined in the Methods section.

Detailed Synthesis

Description of Comparisons

1. Medical Therapy Versus Usual Care

Ten studies (all RCTs) compared medical therapy (cilostazol or pentoxifylline) with placebo in patients who have PAD with IC.[25,49,51,73,85-90] These studies included a total of 4103 patients. Of these studies, five were rated good quality and five fair quality. Sample sizes for individual studies ranged from 38 to 1439 patients. Study durations ranged from 12 weeks to 36 months, with a median of 6 months.

The mean age of study participants ranged from 55 to 71 years of age. The proportion of female patients ranged from 0 to 57.6 percent. Five studies[49,86,88-90,97] (50%) reported racial and ethnic demographics of the study participants. Few studies reported the treadmill exercise protocol used to measure maximal walking. Few studies reported the use of concomitant medications such as aspirin, antihypertensive medications, and HMG-CoA reductase medications.

Seven studies were conducted within the United States or Canada,[25,49,86,88-90,97] with the rest international. Funding source was reported in five studies[25,49,87,88,90,97,98] (50%), with four studies funded by the manufacturer of one of the study medications.

2. Exercise Training Versus Usual Care

Twelve studies (ten RCTs, two observational) compared exercise training with usual care in patients who have PAD with IC.[66,68-71,73-75,77-79,96] These studies included a total of 754 patients. Of the ten RCTs, four were rated good quality,[69,73,77,96] five fair quality,[66,68,70,71,74] and one poor quality.[79] The two observational studies were both rated poor quality.[75,78] Sample sizes for individual studies ranged from 21 to 264 patients. Study durations ranged from 12 weeks to 12 months, with a median of 6 months.

The mean age of study participants ranged from 63 to 76 years of age. The proportion of female patients ranged from 0 to 53 percent. Only two studies[69,96] (18%) reported the racial and ethnic demographics of study participants. Few studies reported the treadmill exercise protocol used to measure maximal walking. Few studies reported the use of concomitant medications such as aspirin, antihypertensive medications, and HMG-CoA reductase medications.

Four studies (27%) were conducted within the United States or Canada,[68,69,77,96] with the rest international. Funding source was reported in five studies (45%), with those studies funded by government sources or national societies.[68-70,77,96]

3. Endovascular Intervention Versus Usual Care

Nine studies (five RCTs, four observational studies) compared endovascular intervention with usual care in patients who have PAD with IC.[70,72,74,77,91-95] These studies included a total of 1593 patients. Of the RCTs, two were rated good quality[77,93] and three fair quality.[70,73,95] Three of the observational studies were rated fair quality[72,91,94] while one was rated poor.[92] Sample sizes for individual studies ranged from 32 to 526 patients. Study durations ranged from 6 months to 24 months.

The mean age of study participants was 62 to 69 years of age. The proportion of female patients ranged from 17.7 to 44.6 percent. Only one study reported the racial and ethnic demographics of the study participants. Few studies reported the treadmill exercise protocol used to measure maximal walking. Few studies reported the use of concomitant medications such as aspirin, antihypertensive medications, and HMG-CoA reductase medications.

Two studies (25%) were conducted within the United States or Canada,[77,91] with the rest international. Funding source was reported in all studies, with the majority of studies (six; 67%) funded by government agencies.

A majority of the endovascular procedures for this comparison and the following comparisons consisted of percutaneous transluminal angioplasty (PTA) with or without stent placement, and the type of stent was not specified.

4. Surgical Revascularization Versus Usual Care

One study compared surgical revascularization with usual care in patients who have PAD with IC.[76] This observational study included a total of 427 patients and was rated poor quality. The study duration was 5 years and the mean age of the participants was 65 years of age. The study did not report the proportion of female patients or the racial and ethnic demographics of the study participants. The study also failed to report the use of concomitant medications such as aspirin, antihypertensive medications, and HMG-CoA reductase medications. The study was conducted internationally and the funding source was not noted.

5. Endovascular Intervention Versus Exercise Training

Nine studies (all RCTs) compared endovascular intervention with exercise training in patients who have PAD with IC.[16,70,74,77,80-84] These studies included a total of 1005 patients. Of these studies, five were rated good quality and five fair quality. Sample sizes for individual studies ranged from 23 to 264 patients. Study durations ranged from 6 months to 72 months, with a median of 6 months.

The mean age of study participants ranged from 62 to 70 years of age. The proportion of female patients ranged from 25 to 45 percent. No study reported the racial and ethnic demographics of the study participants. Few studies reported the treadmill exercise protocol used to measure maximal walking. Few studies reported the use of concomitant medications such as aspirin, antihypertensive medications, and HMG-CoA reductase medications.

One study was conducted within the United States or Canada,[77] with the rest international. Funding source was reported in seven studies[70,73,77,80,82-84] (70%), with the majority of studies (50%) funded by government agencies.

6. Surgical Revascularization Versus Exercise Plus Medical Therapy

One study compared the use of surgical revascularization with exercise therapy plus pentoxifylline 600 mg twice daily in patients who have PAD with IC.[67] This observational study included a total of 127 patients and was rated fair quality. The study duration was 12 weeks and the mean age of the participants was 58 years of age. The study did not report the proportion of female patients or the racial and ethnic demographics of the study participants. The study did not report the treadmill exercise protocol used to measure maximal walking and did not report the use of concomitant medications such as aspirin, antihypertensive medications, and HMG-CoA reductase medications. The study was conducted internationally and the funding source was not noted.

7. Endovascular Intervention Versus Surgical Revascularization

Three studies compared the use of endovascular intervention with surgical revascularization in patients who have PAD with IC.[91,92,94] These studies included a total of 421 patients. Of these studies, all three were observational studies (two fair quality, one poor). Sample sizes for individual studies ranged from 153 to 526 patients. Study durations ranged from 6 months to 18 months, with a median of 12 months.

The mean age of study participants was 67 years of age. The proportion of female patients ranged from 20 to 38.8 percent. No studies reported the racial and ethnic demographics of the study participants. No studies reported the treadmill exercise protocol used to measure maximal walking. No studies reported the use of concomitant medications such as aspirin, antihypertensive medications, and HMG-CoA reductase medications. One study was conducted within the United States or Canada,[91] with the rest international. Funding source was reported in all three studies, with the majority (67%) funded by government agencies.

Effectiveness of Interventions

Effect on Cardiovascular Events (Mortality, MI, Stroke)

We identified 16 studies that assessed the effect of various treatments on cardiovascular events in patients with PAD.

Medical Therapy Versus Usual Care

Mortality was reported in four studies with a range of followup between 4 months and 3 years[49,51,88,89] with death occurring in equal proportions in the medical and usual care groups. Myocardial infarction was reported in two studies[49,51] with MI occurring in 8 of 385 patients treated with medical therapy and 2 of 209 patients treated with usual care. Stroke was reported in three studies[49,51,88] and occurred in equal proportions in patients treated with medical therapy (1.3%) versus usual care (1.4%).

Exercise Training Versus Usual Care

Mortality was reported in two studies[68,70] with death occurring in 5.3 percent (6/113 patients) in the control groups, 5.2 percent (6/116 patients) in the exercise groups, and 5.7 percent (5/87 patients) in the intervention group of the Gelin study. MI and stroke were reported in a single study[69] with MI occurring in one patient in the home-based exercise group and stroke occurring in one patient in the usual care and supervised exercise groups.

Endovascular Intervention Versus Usual Care

Mortality was reported in four studies,[70,72,93,94] with a range of followup between 1 and 3 years. One of these studies[94] did not report outcomes based on treatment assignment, and the other studies were mixed with one reporting that death occurred more frequently in patients treated with endovascular revascularization (5.2%) than with usual care (3.4%) and the other reporting the opposite (endovascular 2.3% vs. usual care 6.5%).[72] Stroke was reported in two studies[72,91] but outcomes were reported based on treatment assignment in only one (1.1% PTA vs. 1.4% usual care).[72] MI (3.0% PTA vs. 8.8% usual care), coronary artery bypass graft surgery (1.1% PTA vs. 2.3% usual care), coronary intervention (0.8% PTA vs. 2.3% usual care) and carotid intervention (0% vs. 0.9%) were reported in one study.[72]

Surgical Revascularization Versus Usual Care

Mortality was reported in a single observational study,[76] with death occurring in 10.4% (27/259) in the surgical revascularization group and 16.7% (28/168) of the usual care group. MI and stroke were not reported.

Endovascular Intervention Versus Exercise Training

Mortality was reported in five studies[16,70,80,83,84] with a range of followup between 1 and 6 years. All five studies showed either a reduction of mortality in the endovascular group or no difference between groups. MI and stroke were reported in a single study,[80] with no MIs occurring in either group, and one stroke occurring in each group throughout the study period.

Endovascular Intervention Versus Surgical Revascularization

Mortality was reported in two studies,[91,94] with a range of followup between 1 and 2 years, but the results were not presented by treatment group (3% in one study, 8% in the other). Stroke was reported in a single study[91] and MI was not reported in any study of endovascular intervention versus surgical revascularization.

Analysis of Mortality for All Treatment Comparisons

Table 15 describes the 12 RCTs and 3 observational studies we identified for the analysis of various treatments on mortality in patients with PAD, organized alphabetically. The observational study by Mori[76] was not included in the meta-analysis since it was the only study with a surgical revascularization arm and our indirect analysis required at least two studies for each intervention in the model. The study by Giugliano[72] also was not included in the meta-analysis since it was the only observational study assessing endovascular intervention compared with usual care. The study by Pell[94] was not included in the meta-analysis because it did not report outcomes based on treatment assignment. Therefore, this analysis is limited to the 12 RCTs only (Figure 11). Of note, the Greenhalgh findings are treated as two separate studies since the results for the femoropopliteal and aortoiliac populations are reported separately; i.e., randomization was stratified by anatomic location.[80]

Table 15. Mortality analysis for all treatment comparisons

Study	Type of Study N Enrolled or Observed[a] Quality	Outcome Length of Followup	Mortality Results Reported by Authors
Beebe, 1999[49]	RCT N: 516 Good	Mortality 6 mo	N Cilostazol=346 N death=3 N Placebo=170 N death=2
Gardner, 2002[68]	RCT N: 52 Fair	Mortality 18 mo	N Supervised exercise=28 N death=1 N Usual care=24 N death=2

Table 15. Mortality analysis for all treatment comparisons (continued)

Study	Type of Study N Enrolled or Observed[a] Quality	Outcome Length of Followup	Mortality Results Reported by Authors
Gelin, 2001[70]	RCT N: 264 Fair	Mortality 12 mo	N Endovascular=87 N death=5 N Exercise=88 N death=5 N Usual Care=89 N death=4
Giugliano 2012[72]	Observational N: 479 Fair	Cardiovascular death Median followup 21 mo IQR (12.0–29)	Endovascular group N =264 N death=6 N Usual care=215 N death=14
Greenhalgh, 2008[80] MIMIC Study	RCT N: 93 Fair	Mortality 3 mo	Femoropopliteal group N Endovascular=48 N death=2 N Exercise=45 N death=2
	RCT N: 34 Fair	Mortality 3 mo	Aortoiliac group N Endovascular=19 N death=1 N Exercise=15 N death=2
Hiatt, 2008[88] Stone, 2008[97] CASTLE Study	RCT N: 1435 Good	Mortality 36 mo	N Cilostazol=717 N death=49 N Placebo=718 N death=52
Money, 1998[89]	RCT N: 239 Fair	Mortality 4 mo	N Cilostazol=119 N death=1 N Placebo=120 N death=1
Mori, 2002[76]	Observational N: 427 Poor	Mortality 5 years	N Surgical revascularization=259 N death=27 N Usual care=168 N death=28
Nordanstig, 2011[83]	RCT N: 201 Good	Mortality 24 mo	N Endovascular=100 N death=1 N Usual care=101 N death=6
Nylaende, 2007[93] OBACT Study	RCT N: 56 Good	Mortality 24 mo	N Endovascular=28 N death=1 N Usual care=28 N death=0
Pell, 1997[94]	Observational N: 201 Fair	Mortality 6 mo	6 total deaths (number by treatment arm not reported)

Table 15. Mortality analysis for all treatment comparisons (continued)

Study	Type of Study N Enrolled or Observed[a] Quality	Outcome Length of Followup	Mortality Results Reported by Authors
Perkins, 1996[84]	RCT N: 56 Fair	Mortality 6 yr	N Endovascular=30 N death=4 N Exercise=26 N death=6
Soga, 2009[51]	RCT N: 78 Good	Mortality 24 mo	N Cilostazol=39 N death=1 N Placebo=39 N death=2
Spronk, 2009[16]	RCT N: 150 Fair	Mortality 12 mo	N Endovascular=75 N death=3 N Exercise=75 N death=5

[a] Number of patients in the study arms of interest.
Abbreviations: mo=month/months; RCT=randomized controlled trial; yr=year/years.

The random-effects network meta-analysis of the 12 RCTs[16,49,51,68-70,80,83,84,88,89,93] of mortality is shown in Figure 11 for each treatment comparison. No specific treatment was found to have a statistically significant effect. The wide confidence intervals make conclusions less certain, and therefore the SOE is rated low. The Soga et al. study compared cilostazol with placebo but included endovascular surgery in each arm. As a sensitivity analysis, we ran a random-effects meta-analysis without the Soga study, and the odds ratio for cilostazol versus control was essentially the same (OR 0.93; 95% CI, 0.63 to 1.38).

Figure 11. Network meta-analysis of treatment effects versus usual care and each other on mortality in IC patients

Treatment comparison	Odds ratio	Lower limit	Upper limit	p-Value
Cilostazol vs. Control	0.91	0.62	1.35	0.65
Exercise vs. Control	0.84	0.34	2.07	0.70
Exercise vs. Cilostazol	0.65	0.27	1.55	0.33
Endovascular vs. Control	0.91	0.34	2.45	0.86
Endovascular vs. Cilostazol	0.71	0.27	1.84	0.48
Endovascular vs. Exercise	0.77	0.39	1.54	0.47

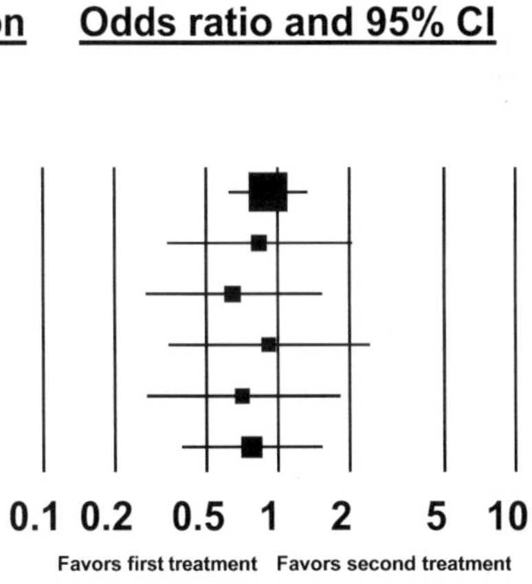

Favors first treatment   Favors second treatment

Abbreviation: CI=confidence interval.

Effect on Maximal Walking Measures

We identified 25 unique studies that reported the walking measures MWD, ACD, or PWT. Results by study comparison are listed in Table 16. There was significant heterogeneity in the study protocols and data reporting.

Medical Therapy Versus Usual Care

Maximal walking measures were reported in eight studies: cilostazol (five studies), pentoxifylline (two), and both (one). Seven of these studies reported MWD or ACD; no studies reported PWT. We included these seven studies (three good quality, four fair)[25,49,73,85,86,89,90] that reported MWD or ACD with median duration of treatment of 6 months in the random-effects meta-analysis (Figure 12). The one study not included in the analysis (De Sanctis et al.[87,98]) reported total walking distance at 12 months and reported a mean percentage change as 404% in the pentoxifylline group and 280% in the placebo group. We calculated an effect size (standard error) of 0.408 (0.175) for this comparison.

Exercise Training Versus Usual Care

Maximal walking measures were reported in 11 studies: MWD (3 studies), ACD (5), and PWT (3). We included five RCTs (two good quality, three fair quality)[68,71,73,74,96] in the random-effects meta-analysis (Figure 12). The Gelin study[70] was not included since it reported MWD results at 12 months; we calculated an effect size (standard error [SE]) of -0.08 (0.10) for this study, which essentially shows no difference in effect between the two treatments. The observational study by Sugimoto[78] reported ACD results at 6 months and the calculated effect size (SE) was 0.70 (0.13) showing a large effect of exercise training over usual care. We were unable to calculate an effect size for Lee et al. (2007)[75] since it did not report the standard deviation or exact p-value; that study found that the improvement in MWD (183 meters) was higher in the exercise group compared to usual care (33 meters) after 6 months. The three studies reporting PWT found improvements in the group that received supervised exercise compared to usual care.[69,77,79]

Endovascular Intervention Versus Usual Care

Maximal walking measures were reported in four studies: MWD (two studies), ACD (one), and PWT (one). Two of these studies (one good quality, one fair)[74,93] reporting MWD or ACD were included in the random-effects meta-analysis (Figure 12). The Gelin study[70] reported MWD results at 12 months; we calculated an effect size (SE) of 0.51 (0.13) for this study that showed a moderate effect of endovascular intervention compared to usual care. The study by Murphy et al. (2012)[77] reported an improvement in PWT in the endovascular group compared to usual care, calculated effect size (SE) of 5.66 (0.278).

Endovascular Intervention Versus Exercise Training

Maximal walking measures were reported in eight studies: MWD (five studies), ACD (two), and PWT (one). Five of these studies (one good quality, three fair)[16,74,82,84] were included in the random-effects meta-analysis (Figure 12). The Gelin study[70] reported MWD results at 12 months and showed a larger effect in the endovascular group compared to the exercise group. The Greenhalgh study[80] reported mean change in the MWD at 24 months with the group in the endovascular plus exercise group having a moderate effect compared to exercise alone in the femoropopliteal patients (ES=0.43) and a large effect in the aortofemoral patients (ES=0.70). In the Murphy study reporting PWT change at 6 months,[77] mean change in the endovascular group was 3.7 min (SD 4.9) and the exercise group was 5.8 min (SD 4.6), p=0.04. Our calculated effect size of endovascular intervention compared to exercise was -0.48 (SE 0.23), which means there was a moderate effect favoring exercise.

Surgical Revascularization Versus Exercise Plus Medical Therapy

One study reported MWT as a measure of maximal walking.[67] MWT (minutes) improved from 4.9 (SD 0.4) to 11.8 (SD 1.7) in the exercise plus medical therapy (pentoxifylline) arm and from 3.7 (SD 1.1) to >15 in the surgical revascularization arm. We were unable to compute an effect size since the 12-week result in the surgical arm was a categorical (nonexact) value and the authors did not report an exact p-value.

Endovascular Intervention Versus Surgical Revascularization

No study reported measures of MWD for this comparison.

Analysis of Walking Measures

Table 16 presents the 25 studies that reported walking measures MWD, ACD, or PWT, organized alphabetically by study comparison. Of these studies, 16 studies were included in the random-effects network meta-analysis (Figure 12).

Table 16. Calculated effect size: maximal walking measures

Study	Type of Study N Analyzed[a] Quality	Outcome Length of Followup	Results Reported by Authors	Calculated Effect Size[b]
Medical therapy vs. usual care				
Beebe, 1999[49]	RCT N: 316 Good	MWD (m) 6 mo	Cilostazol 100 mg Mean geometric % change: 1.51 Placebo: 1.15	**ES: 0.46 EffSE: 0.10**
Belcaro, 2002[85]	RCT N: 53 Fair	MWD (m) 6 mo	Mean MWD (SD) Pentoxifylline: baseline 56 (8) 3 mo 122 (10) Placebo: baseline 59 (12) 3 mo 99 (13)	**ES: 4.89 EffSE: 0.19**
Dawson, 1998[86]	RCT N: 66 Good	ACD (m) 12 wk	Mean change from baseline least square (SE) Cilostazol: 42.6 (8.2) Placebo: 3.5 (11.7)	**ES: 0.72 EffSE: 0.14**
Dawson, 2000[25]	RCT N: 643 Fair	MWD (m) 6 mo	Mean change in MWD (SD) Cilostazol 107 (158) Pentoxifylline 64 (127) Placebo 65 (135)	**ES (cilostazol): 0.91 EffSE: 0.07** ES (pentoxifylline): 0.55 EffSE: 0.07
De Sanctis, 2002[87,98]	RCT N: 101 Poor	TWD (m) 12 mo	Mean % change in TWD Pentoxifylline: 404% Placebo: 280%	ES: 0.41 EffSE: 0.18
Hobbs, 2007[73] INEXACT Study	RCT N: 18 Good	ACD (m) 6 mo	Ratio of 6 mo: baseline ACD (SD) Cilostazol: 1.69 (1.55) Usual care: 1.09 (0.34)	**ES: 1.69 EffSE: 0.33**
Money, 1998[89]	RCT N: 212 Fair	ACD (m) 4 mo	Mean ACD (SE) Cilostazol: baseline 236.9 (13.6) 4 mo 332.6 (20.0) Placebo: baseline 244.3 (13.7) 4 mo 281.1 (19.2)	**ES: 1.39 EffSE: 0.10**
Strandness, 2002[90]	RCT N: 377 Fair	MWD (m) 6 mo	Cilostazol 100 mg Estimated treatment effect: 1.21 (1.09 to 1.35)	**ES: 0.46 EffSE: 0.90**

51

Table 16. Calculated effect size: maximal walking measures (continued)

Study	Type of Study N Analyzed[a] Quality	Outcome Length of Followup	Results Reported by Authors	Calculated Effect Size[b]
Exercise training vs. usual care				
Treat-Jacobson, 2009[96]	RCT N: 15 Good	MWD (m) 24 wk	Mean change in MWD (SD) Exercise: 294.4 (162.2) Usual care: 73.3 (65.6)	**ES: 2.38** **EffSE: 0.44**
Gardner, 2002[68]	RCT N: 31 Fair	ACD (m) 18 months	Percent change in ACD Exercise: 80% Control: 0%	**ES: 1.13** **EffSE: 0.24**
Gardner, 2011[69]	RCT N: 63 Good	PWT (sec) 12 wk	Mean change in PWT (SD) Exercise: 215 (207) Usual care: -10 (176)	ES: 1.19 EffSE: 0.27
Gelin, 2001[70]	RCT N: 149 Fair	MWD (m) 12 mo	Mean MWD (SD) Exercise: baseline 258 (142) 1 yr 247 (111) Control: baseline 272 (153) 1 yr 261 (131)	ES: -0.08 EffSE: 0.10
Gibellini, 2000[71]	RCT N: 37 Fair	ACD (m) 6 mo	ACD (SD) Exercise: baseline 203 (66.1) 6 mo 393.6 (208.8) Control: baseline 230.1 (109.8) 6 mo 276.4 (191.2)	**ES: 0.98** **EffSE: 0.44**
Hobbs, 2006[74] EXACT Study	RCT N: 14 Fair	ACD (m) 6 mo	Ratio of 6 mo: baseline ACD (SD) Exercise: 1.45 (0.80) Usual care: 1.09 (0.34)	**ES: 1.20** **EffSE: 0.33**
Hobbs, 2007[73] INEXACT Study	RCT N: 18 Good	ACD (m) 6 mo	Overall effect at 6 mo (ACD) Exercise: 1.33 Best medical therapy: 1.0	**ES: 0.59** **EffSE: 0.48**
Lee, 2007[75]	Observational N: 70 Poor	MWD (m) 6 mo	Median MWD (IQR) Exercise: baseline 117.6 (73.5 to 205.8) 6 mo 300 (143.8 to 300) Usual care: baseline 152.2 (76.7 to 279.3) 6 mo 185 (102.0 to 300)	Unable to compute (no SD or p-value)
Murphy, 2012[77] CLEVER Study	RCT N: 58 Good	PWT (min) 6 mo	Mean change in PWT (SD) Exercise: 5.8 (4.6) Usual care: 1.2 (2.6)	ES: 1.04 EffSE: 0.29
Sugimoto, 2010[78]	Observational N: 100 Poor	ACD (m) 6 mo	Mean ACD (SD) Exercise: baseline 143 (90) 6 mo 257 (161) Usual care: baseline 249 (177) 6 mo 317 (168)	ES: 0.70 EffSE: 0.13
Tsai, 2002[79]	RCT N: 53 Poor	PWT (min) 3 mo	Mean PWT (SD) Exercise: baseline 7.4 (3.9) 3 mo 12.5 (3.7) Control: baseline 7.2 (3.2) 3 mo 7.6 (3.8)	ES: 1.25 EffSE: 0.30

Table 16. Calculated effect size: maximal walking measures (continued)

Study	Type of Study N Analyzed[a] Quality	Outcome Length of Followup	Results Reported by Authors	Calculated Effect Size[b]
Endovascular intervention vs. usual care				
Gelin, 2001[70]	RCT N: 152 Fair	MWD (m) 12 mo	Mean MWD (SD) Baseline: Revascularization 274 (172), control 272 (153) 1 year: Revascularization 344 (169), control 261 (131)	ES: 0.51 EffSE: 0.13
Hobbs, 2006[74] EXACT Study	RCT N: 16 Fair	ACD (m) 6 mo	Median change in ACD (IQR) Endovascular: 513 (110 to 1000) Usual care: 61 (75 to 435)	**ES: 0.47** **EffSE: 0.51**
Murphy, 2012[77] CLEVER Study	RCT N: 61 Good	PWT (min) 6 mo	Mean change in PWT (SD) Endovascular: 3.7 (4.9) Usual care: 1.2 (2.6)	ES: 0.57 EffSE: 0.28
Nylaende, 2007[93] OBACT Study	RCT N: 56 Good	MWD (m) 24 mo	Mean MWD (SD) Baseline: Endovascular 323.9 (231.5), usual care 265.4 (173.5) 2 year: Endovascular 539.2 (144.3), usual care 319.5 (220.4)	**ES: 0.51** **EffSE: 0.19**
Endovascular intervention vs. exercise training				
Gelin, 2001[70]	RCT N: 149 Fair	MWD (m) 12 mo	Mean MWD (SD) Baseline: Revascularization (274 (172), exercise 258 (142), control 272 (153) 1 year: Revascularization 344 (169), exercise 247 (111), control 261 (131)	ES (endo): 0.51 EffSE: 0.13 ES (ex): -0.08 EffSE: 0.10
Greenhalgh, 2008[80] MIMIC Study	RCT N: 94 Fair	MWD (m) 24 mo	Mean change in MWD Femoropopliteal group Endovascular + exercise: 224 Exercise: 150 Aortoiliac group Endovascular + exercise: 354 Exercise: 168	ES (femor): 0.43 EffSE: 0.21 ES (aorto): 0.70 EffSE: 0.36
Hobbs, 2006[74] EXACT Study	RCT N: 16 Fair	ACD (m) 6 mo	Median Change in ACD (IQR) Endovascular: 513 (110 to 1000) Exercise: 13 (69 to 352)	**ES: 0.76** **EffSE: 0.52**
Kruidenier, 2011[81]	RCT N: 61 Good	ACD (m) 6 mo	Mean ACD (SD) Baseline: Endovascular 343.3 (247.9), endovascular + exercise 293.4 (189.6) 6 month: Endovascular 685.0 (313.5), endovascular + exercise 956.3 (490.4)	**ES: 0.63** **EffSE: 0.25**

Table 16. Calculated effect size: maximal walking measures (continued)

Study	Type of Study N Analyzed[a] Quality	Outcome Length of Followup	Results Reported by Authors	Calculated Effect Size[b]
Mazari, 2012[82]	RCT N: 109 Good	MWD (m) 6 mo	Median MWD (IQR) Baseline: Endovascular 77.62 (49.16 to 116.11), exercise 83.41 (58.32 to 141.65) 6 mo: Endovascular 146.15 (67.45 to 215.0), exercise 215.0 (104.97 to 215.0)	ES (endo): 0.78 EffSE: 0.12 ES (ex): 0.96 EffSE: 0.15 ES (endo+ex): 1.90 EffSE: 0.12
Murphy, 2012[77] CLEVER Study	RCT N: 79 Good	PWT (min) 6 mo	Mean change in PWT (SD) Endovascular 3.7 (4.9) Exercise 5.8 (4.6) Usual care 1.2 (2.6)	ES: -0.48 EffSE: 0.23
Perkins, 1996[84]	RCT N: 56 Fair	MWD (m) 6 yr	Median MWD (SE) Baseline: Endovascular 82.3735 (18.8482), exercise 104.014 (20.924) 70 mo: Endovascular 181.5 (53.8), exercise 124.3 (46.8)	ES (endo): 0.11 EffSE: 0.18 ES (ex): 0.4 EffSE: 0.20
Spronk, 2009[16]	RCT N: 150 Fair	MWD (m) 12 mo	Mean improvement score (99% CI) Endovascular : 826 (680 to 970) Exercise: 1034 (896 to 1170)	ES (endo): 3.56 EffSE: 0.13 ES (ex): 5.36 EffSE: 0.11
Surgical revascularization vs. exercise plus medical therapy (pentoxifylline)				
Drozdz 2001[67]	Prospective Cohort N: 127 Fair	MWT (min) 12 wk	Mean MWT (SD) Surgical revascularization 1. Baseline: 3.70 (1.10) 2. 12 wk: >15 Usual care 1. Baseline: 4.90 (0.40) 2. 12 wk: 11.8 (1.7)	Unable to compute (no exact p-value, categorical value for 12-wk surgical result)
Endovascular intervention vs. surgical revascularization				
No studies				

[a]Number of patients in the study arms of interest.
[b]Values used in meta-analysis appear in bold.
Abbreviations: ACD=absolute claudication distance; EffSE=standard error of effect; endo=endovascular; ES=effect size; ex=exercise; IQR=interquartile range; m=meters; min=minute/minutes; mo=month/months; MWD=maximal walking distance; MWT=maximal walking time; PWT=peak walking time; RCT=randomized controlled trial; SD=standard deviation; sec=second/seconds; TWD=total walking distance; wk=week/weeks.

We conducted a random-effects meta-analysis with 16 studies[16,25,49,68,71,73,74,82,84-86,89,90,93,96] to compare the multiple treatment arms on continuous measures (PROC NLMIXED). The results show summary effect sizes of 0.89 (95% CI, 0.06 to 1.71, p=0.04) for exercise training; 0.62 (CI, -0.21 to 1.45, p=0.14) for cilostazol; 1.70 (CI, 0.36 to 3.04 p=0.01) for pentoxifylline; 0.41 (CI,

-0.54 to 1.36, p=0.40) for endovascular intervention; and 1.08 (CI, -0.37 to 2.53, p=0.14) for the combination of endovascular intervention and exercise. These effects are all relative to usual care and are summarized in Figure 12.

Figure 12. Network meta-analysis of treatment effects versus usual care on walking distance in IC patients

Treatment	Std diff in means	Lower limit	Upper limit	p-Value
Exercise training	0.89	0.06	1.71	0.04
Cilostazol	0.62	-0.21	1.45	0.14
Pentoxifylline	1.70	0.36	3.04	0.01
Endovascular intervention	0.41	-0.54	1.36	0.40
Endovascular intervention & exercise	1.08	-0.37	2.53	0.14

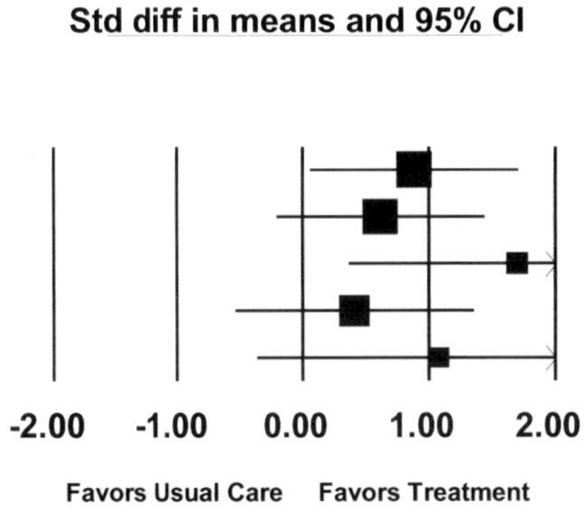

Abbreviation: CI=confidence interval.

Thus, large effects were seen with exercise training (moderate SOE; nine studies), pentoxifylline (insufficient SOE due to imprecision and inconsistency; two studies), and the combination of endovascular intervention and exercise (low SOE; 2 studies). Moderate effects were seen with endovascular intervention (moderate SOE; five studies) and cilostazol (low SOE; six studies). Clinically, this equates to an improvement in MWD or ACD of 135 meters for exercise training, 63 meters for endovascular intervention, and 166 for the combination of endovascular intervention and exercise. For the medical therapies, this equates to an improvement in MWD or ACD of 95 meters for cilostazol and 260 meters for pentoxifylline.

Since the level of evidence for pentoxifylline was insufficient due to inconsistency and imprecision, we ran a sensitivity analysis removing the pentoxifylline studies.[25,85] The results show summary effect sizes of 0.98 (95% CI, 0.23 to 1.74, p=0.01) for exercise training; 0.61 (CI, -0.20 to 1.42, p=0.14) for cilostazol; 0.51 (CI, -0.35 to 1.37, p=0.25) for endovascular intervention; and 1.20 (CI, -0.11 to 2.50, p=0.07) for the combination of endovascular intervention and exercise. These effects are all relative to usual care and are summarized in Figure 13.

Figure 13. Network sensitivity meta-analysis of treatment effects versus usual care on walking distance in IC patients

Treatment	Std diff in means	Lower limit	Upper limit	p-Value
Exercise training	0.98	0.23	1.74	0.01
Cilostazol	0.61	-0.20	1.42	0.14
Endovascular intervention	0.51	-0.35	1.37	0.25
Endovascular intervention & exercise	1.20	-0.11	2.50	0.07

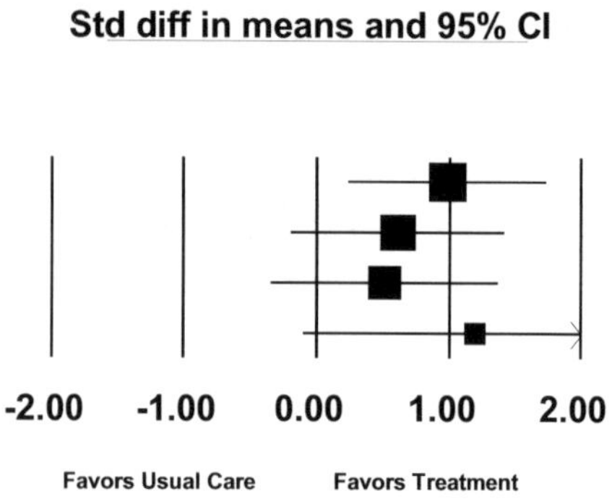

Abbreviation: CI=confidence interval.

Similar to the full analysis, large effects were seen with exercise training (moderate SOE; nine studies) and the combination of endovascular intervention plus exercise (low SOE; 2 studies). Moderate effects were seen with endovascular intervention (moderate SOE; five studies) and cilostazol (low SOE; six studies). Clinically, this equates to an improvement in MWD or ACD of 150 meters for exercise training, 93 meters for cilostazol, 78 meters for endovascular intervention, and 184 for the combination of endovascular intervention plus exercise.

When indirectly compared against each other, none of the treatment arms were found to be significantly different. This is summarized in Figure 14, with the effect sizes favoring the first treatment (negative values) on the left and the second treatment (positive values) on the right. There was a small effect between cilostazol and endovascular intervention (ES=-0.21, favoring cilostazol) and between exercise and cilostazol (ES=-0.27, favoring exercise). There were medium effects seen between exercise and endovascular interventions (ES=-0.47, favoring exercise), between cilostazol and the combination of endovascular intervention with exercise (ES=0.46, favoring the combination), between pentoxifylline and the combination of endovascular with exercise (ES=-0.62, favoring pentoxifylline), as well as between endovascular and the combination of endovascular with exercise (ES=0.67, favoring the combination). There were large effects seen between cilostazol and pentoxifylline (ES=1.08, favoring pentoxifylline), exercise and pentoxifylline (ES=0.82, favoring pentoxifylline), and between pentoxifylline and endovascular intervention (ES=-1.29, favoring pentoxifylline).

Figure 14. Network meta-analysis of treatment effects versus each other on walking distance in IC patients

Treatment comparison	Std diff in means	Lower limit	Upper limit	p-Value
Cilostazol vs Pentoxifylline	1.08	-0.35	2.52	0.14
Cilostazol vs Endovascular	-0.21	-1.33	0.92	0.72
Cilostazol vs Endovascular & exercise	0.46	-1.10	2.03	0.56
Pentoxifylline vs Endovascular	-1.29	-2.84	0.26	0.10
Pentoxifylline vs Endovascular & exercise	-0.62	-2.51	1.27	0.52
Exercise vs Cilostazol	-0.27	-1.29	0.76	0.61
Exercise vs Pentoxifylline	0.82	-0.67	2.30	0.28
Exercise vs Endovascular	-0.47	-1.40	0.46	0.32
Exercise vs Endovascular & exercise	0.20	-1.23	1.63	0.79
Endovascular vs Endovascular & exercise	0.67	-0.71	2.05	0.34

(Statistics for each comparison)

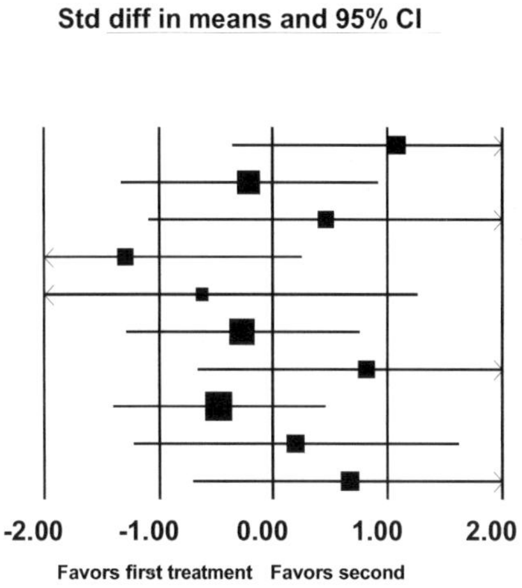

Abbreviation: CI=confidence interval.

Again, we ran a sensitivity analysis removing the pentoxifylline studies and had similar results to the full analysis (Figure 15). When indirectly compared against each other, none of the treatment arms were found to be significantly different, with effect sizes favoring the first treatment (negative values) on the left and the second treatment (positive values) on the right. There was a minimal effect between cilostazol and endovascular intervention (ES=-0.10, no difference). There was a small effect between exercise and the combination endovascular with exercise (ES=0.22, favoring the combination) and between exercise and cilostazol (ES=-0.37, favoring exercise). There were medium effects seen between exercise and endovascular interventions (ES=-0.47, favoring exercise), between cilostazol and the combination of endovascular with exercise (ES=0.58, favoring the combination), as well as between endovascular and the combination of endovascular with exercise (ES=0.68, favoring the combination).

Figure 15. Network sensitivity meta-analysis of treatment effects versus each other on walking distance in IC patients

Treatment comparison	Std diff in means	Lower limit	Upper limit	p-Value
Cilostazol vs Endovascular	-0.10	-1.16	0.96	0.85
Cilostazol vs Endovascular & exercise	0.58	-0.84	2.01	0.42
Exercise vs Cilostazol	-0.37	-1.34	0.60	0.45
Exercise vs Endovascular	-0.47	-1.31	0.36	0.27
Exercise vs Endovascular & exercise	0.22	-1.05	1.50	0.73
Endovascular vs Endovascular & exercise	0.68	-0.55	1.91	0.28

(Statistics for each comparison)

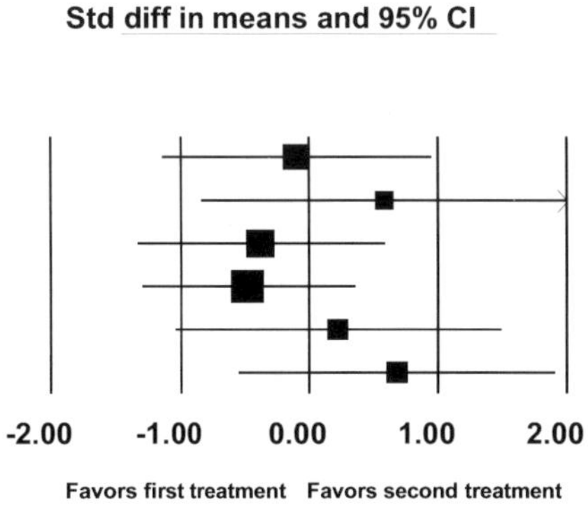

Abbreviation: CI=confidence interval.

We consider the network sensitivity meta-analyses without the pentoxifylline studies (Figures 13 and 15) to be the definitive analysis for the following reasons. First, there were few pentoxifylline studies published since 1995, with 6 studies excluded from the analysis because they were conducted prior to current clinical practice where secondary prevention of cardiovascular events includes treatment of hypertension, diabetes, hyperlipidemia, and tobacco use. Second, the studies that were included in the full analysis were inconsistent and imprecise (i.e., insufficient SOE), and therefore the effect sizes shown in Figure 14 comparing pentoxifylline with usual care and other treatments were also imprecise. Third, the ACC/AHA guidelines recommend pentoxifylline as an alternative therapy to cilostazol since the clinical effectiveness for IC is marginal and not well established.[2]

Effect on Claudication Onset Measures

Twenty-one unique studies reported claudication onset measures ICD, PFWD, PFWT, or COT. Results by study comparison are listed in Table 17. There was significant heterogeneity in the study protocols and data reporting.

Medical Therapy Versus Usual Care

Claudication onset measures were reported in five studies: ICD (three studies) and PFWD (two); no studies reported COT. Three of these studies (two good quality, one fair) were included in the random-effects meta-analysis (Figure 16).[25,73,86] For two studies,[49,89] we were unable to calculate an effect size since the results provided did not contain a standard deviation or exact p-value. Both studies showed mild increases in the PFWD and ICD on cilostazol compared to placebo.

Exercise Training Versus Usual Care

Claudication onset measures were reported in 10 studies: ICD (5 studies), PFWD (1), PFWT (1), and COT (3). Five of these studies (two good quality, three fair)[68,71,73,74,96] reporting ICD or PFWD were included in the random-effects meta-analysis. The effect size for Lee et al.[75] could not be calculated due to no reported SD or p-value. The five studies reporting timing measures showed an improvement with supervised exercise compared with usual care with moderate to large effect sizes (SE) ranging from 0.70 (0.28) to 1.06 (0.47).

Endovascular Intervention Versus Usual Care

Claudication onset measures were reported in five studies: ICD (two studies), PFWD (two), and COT (one). A random-effects meta-analysis included three of these studies (one good quality, two fair).[74,93,95] The effect size for the Koivunen et al. study[92] could not be calculated since the distribution of values in each study arm was unusual. The Murphy et al. (2012) study[77] reported mean change in COT (SD) of 3.6 (4.2) in the endovascular arm, and 0.7 (1.1) in the usual care arm. Our calculated effect size was 0.88 (SD 0.28), which means a large effect significantly favoring endovascular intervention over usual care.

Endovascular Intervention Versus Exercise Training

Claudication onset measures were reported in five studies: ICD (three studies), PFWD (one), and COT (one). A random-effects meta-analysis included four of these studies (one good quality, three fair)[16,74,80,82] reporting ICD or PFWD. In the study reporting COT change at 6 months,[77] mean change from baseline in the endovascular group was 3.6 sec (SD 4.2) and the exercise group was 3.0 sec (SD 2.9), p=NS. Our calculated effect size of endovascular intervention compared to exercise was 0.18 (SE 0.23), which means there was a small, nonsignificant effect favoring endovascular treatment.

Surgical Revascularization Versus Exercise Plus Medical Therapy

One study reported COT.[67] COT (minutes) improved from 2.8 (SD 0.3) to 7.3 (SD 0.9) in the exercise plus medical therapy (pentoxifylline) arm and from 1.4 (SD 0.5) to >10 in the surgical revascularization arm. We were unable to compute an effect size since the 12-week result in the surgical arm was a categorical (nonexact) value and the authors did not report an exact p-value.

Endovascular Intervention Versus Surgical Revascularization

No study reported measures of claudication onset distance for this comparison.

Analysis of Claudication Onset Measures

Table 17 presents the 21 studies that reported claudication onset measures ICD, PFWD, PFWT, or COT, organized alphabetically by study comparison. Of these studies, 12 were included in the random-effects network meta-analysis (Figure 16).

Table 17. Calculated effect size: claudication onset measures

Study	Type of Study N Analyzed[a] Quality	Outcome Length of Followup	Results Reported by Authors	Calculated Effect Size[b]
Medical therapy vs. usual care				
Beebe, 1999[49]	RCT N: 316 Good	PFWD (m) 6 mo	Mean geometric % change PFWD Cilostazol 100: 1.51 Cilostazol 50: 1.38 Placebo: 1.15	Unable to compute (no exact p-value, SD in wrong units)
Dawson, 1998[86]	RCT N: 66 Good	ICD (m) 12 wk	ICD (SE) Cilostazol: baseline 71.2 (6.0) 3 mo 112.5 (13.8) Placebo: 77.7 (8.4) 3 mo 84.6 (13.7)	**ES (cilostazol): 0.68 EffSE: 0.25**
Dawson, 2000[25]	RCT N: 643 Fair	PFWD (m) 6 mo	Mean % change in PFWD Pentoxifylline: 74 (106) Cilostazol: 94 (127) Placebo: 57 (93)	**ES (pentoxifylline): 0.17 EffSE: 0.10** **ES (cilostazol): 0.38** **EffSE: 0.10**
Hobbs, 2007[73] INEXACT Study	RCT N: 18 Good	ICD (m) 6 mo	Ratio of 6 mo: baseline ICD (SD) Cilostazol: 3.34 (4.23) Best medical therapy: 1.23 (0.73)	**ES (cilostazol): 0.72 EffSE: 0.49**
Money, 1998[89]	RCT N: 212 Fair	ICD (m) 4 mo	% change in ICD compared to placebo Cilostazol: 27%	Unable to compute (no exact p-value or SD)

59

Table 17. Calculated effect size: claudication onset measures (continued)

Study	Type of Study N Analyzed[a] Quality	Outcome Length of Followup	Results Reported by Authors	Calculated Effect Size[b]
Exercise training vs. usual care				
Treat-Jacobson, 2009[96]	RCT N: 31 Good	PFWD (m) 24 wk	Change in PFWD (SD) Walking: 155.1 (180.7) Usual care: 10.9 (27.4) Arm ergometry: 39.7 (97.2) Walking + arm ergometry: 21.6 (81.3)	**ES: 1.30** **EffSE: 0.51**
Crowther, 2008[66]	RCT N: 21 Fair	PFWT (sec) 12 mo	Mean PFWT in seconds (SD): Exercise: baseline 132.8 (61.1) 1 yr 360.0 (188.3) Control: 115.9 (99.5) 1 yr 166.3 (89.4)	ES: 1.06 EffSE: 0.47
Gardner, 2002[68]	RCT N: 31 Fair	ICD (m) 18 mo	Percent Change in ICD Exercise: 189% Control: 0%	**ES: 1.32** **EffSE: 0.24**
Gardner, 2011[69]	RCT N: 63 Good	COT (sec) 12 wk	COT change from baseline (SD) Supervised exercise: 165 (173) Control: -16 (125) Home exercise: 134 (197)	ES: 1.06 EffSE: 0.47
Gibellini, 2000[71]	RCT N: 37 Fair	ICD (m) 6 mo	Mean ICD (SD) Exercise: baseline 116.8 (48.2) 6 mo 351.4 (209.5) Control: 111.6 (64.6) 6 mo 114.5 (79.6)	**ES: 2.14** **EffSE: 0.79**
Hobbs, 2006[74] EXACT Study	RCT N: 14 Fair	ICD (m) 6 mo	Median ICD (IQR) Exercise: baseline 59 (35 to 63) 6 mo 92 (47 to169) Best medical therapy: baseline 47 (30 to 118) 6 mo 56 (45 to 325) Median ICD (range) Usual care: baseline 59 (48 to 72) 6 mo 64 (47 to 77) Usual care + exercise: baseline 60 (45 to 95) 6 mo 127 (62 to 180)	**ES: 0.01** **EffSE: 0.54**
Hobbs, 2007[73] INEXACT Study	RCT N: 18 Good	ICD (m) 6 mo	Overall effect at 6 mo (ICD) Exercise: 1.80 Best medical therapy: 1.0	**ES: 0.34** **EffSE: 0.48**
Lee, 2007[75]	Observational N: 70 Poor	ICD (m) 6 mo	Median ICD (range) Exercise: baseline 58.5 (39.2 to 112.7) 6 mo 107.5 (52.5 to 153.8) Usual care: baseline 78.4 (39.2 to 131.2) 6 mo 75 (45 to 180)	Unable to compute (no SD or p-value)
Murphy, 2012[77] CLEVER Study	RCT N: 58 Good	COT (sec) 6 mo	Mean change in COT from baseline (SD) Exercise: 3.0 (2.9) Usual care: 0.7 (1.1)	ES: 0.70 EffSE: 0.28
Tsai, 2002[79]	RCT N: 53 Poor	COT (min) 3 mo	Mean COT (SD) Exercise: baseline 3.3 (3.1) 3 mo 6.2 (2.7), Usual care: baseline 2.9 (2.6) 3 mo 3.2 (3.4)	ES: 0.74 EffSE: 0.28

Table 17. Calculated effect size: claudication onset measures (continued)

Study	Type of Study N Analyzed[a] Quality	Outcome Length of Followup	Results Reported by Authors	Calculated Effect Size[b]
Endovascular intervention vs. usual care				
Hobbs, 2006[74] EXACT Study	RCT N: 16 Fair	ICD (m) 6 mo	Median ICD (IQR) Baseline: Endovascular 84 (43 to 127), best medical therapy 47 (30 to 118) 6 mo: Endovascular 698 (147 to 1000), best medical therapy 56 (43 to 325)	ES: 0.74 EffSE: 0.52
Koivunen, 2008[92]	Observational N: 129 Poor	PFWD (m) 12 mo	Median PFWD (IQR) Baseline: Endovascular 100 (50 to 200), surgery 100 (50 to 200), usual care 200 (100 to 500) 12 mo: Endovascular 400 (100 to 10,000), surgery 2250 (2250 to 10,000), usual care 200 (100 to 1000)	Distribution of values are unusual therefore effect sizes cannot be computed
Murphy, 2012[77] CLEVER Study	RCT N: 61 Good	COT (sec) 6 mo	Mean change in COT (SD) Endovascular 3.6 (4.2) Usual Care 0.7 (1.1)	ES: 0.88 EffSE: 0.28
Nylaende, 2007[93] OBACT Study	RCT N: 56 Good	PFWD (m) 24 mo	Mean PFWD (SD) Baseline: Endovascular 93.5 (72.9) usual care 69.6 (54.2), 24 mo: Endovascular 435.0 (223.8), usual care: 174.9 (171.8)	ES: 1.28 EffSE: 0.27
Whyman, 1997[95]	RCT N: 19 Fair	ICD (m) 24 mo	Median ICD (IQR) Baseline: Endovascular 56 (33 to 133), usual care 78 (58 to 100) 24 mo: Endovascular 383 (85 to 667), usual care 333 (106 to 667)	ES: 0.25 EffSE: 0.18
Endovascular intervention vs. exercise training				
Greenhalgh, 2008[80] MIMIC Study	RCT N: 94 Fair	ICD (m) 24 mo	Adjusted HR (95% CI) Femoropopliteal group Endovascular: 3.11 (1.42 to 6.81) Exercise + optimal medical therapy 1.0 Aortoiliac group Endovascular: 3.6 (1.0 to 12.8) Exercise + optimal medical therapy 1.0	ES (femor): 0.61 EffSE: 0.21 ES (aorto): 0.70 EffSE: 0.36
Hobbs, 2006[74] EXACT Study	RCT N: 16 Fair	ICD (m) 6 mo	Median ICD (IQR) Baseline: Endovascular 84 (43 to 127), exercise 59 (35 to 63) 6 month: Endovascular 698 (147 to 1000), exercise 92 (47 to 169)	ES: 0.73 EffSE: 0.52

Table 17. Calculated effect size: claudication onset measures (continued)

Study	Type of Study N Analyzed[a] Quality	Outcome Length of Followup	Results Reported by Authors	Calculated Effect Size[b]
Mazari, 2012[82]	RCT N: 109 Good	ICD (m) 12 mo	Median ICD (IQR) Baseline: Endovascular 31.30 (20.70 to 63.13), exercise 42.71 (26.65 to 74.17) 12 mo: Endovascular 75.80 (46.07 to 209.82), exercise 103.15 (64.1 to 129.3)	**ES (endo): 0.58** **EffSE: 0.17** ES (ex): 0.61 EffSE: 0.06 ES (endo+ex): 0.49 EffSE: 0.16
Murphy, 2012[77] CLEVER Study	RCT N: 79 Good	COT (sec) 6 mo	Mean change in COT from baseline in seconds (SD) Endovascular 3.6 (4.2) Exercise 3.0 (2.9) Usual Care 0.7 (1.1)	ES: 0.18 EffSE: 0.23
Spronk, 2009[16]	RCT N: 150 Fair	PFWD (m) 12 mo	Mean improvement in PFWD (99% CI) Endovascular 806 (646 to 960) Exercise 943 (786 to 1099)	**ES (endo): 1.28** **EffSE: 0.12** ES (ex): 1.52 EffSE: 0.11
Surgical revascularization vs. exercise training plus medical therapy (pentoxifylline)				
Drozdz, 2001[67]	Prospective Cohort N: 127 Fair	COT (min) 12 wk	Mean COT (SD) Baseline: Usual care 2.8 (0.3), surgical revascularization 1.4 (0.5) 12 wk: Usual care 7.30 (0.9), surgical revascularization >10	Unable to compute (no exact p-value, categorical value for 12-wk surgical result)
Endovascular intervention vs. surgical revascularization				
No studies				

[a]Number of patients in the study arms of interest.
[b]Values used in meta-analysis appear in bold.
Abbreviations: COT=claudication onset time; EffSE=standard error of effect; ES=effect size; ICD=initial claudication distance; IQR=interquartile range; m=meters; min=minute/minutes; mo=month/months; PFWD=pain-free walking distance; PFWT=pain-free walking time; RCT=randomized controlled trial; SD=standard deviation; wk=week/weeks.

We conducted a random-effects network meta-analysis with 12 studies[16,25,68,71,73,74,80,82,86,93,95,96] to compare the multiple treatment arms on continuous measures (PROC NLMIXED). The results show summary effect sizes of 0.63 (95% CI, -0.02 to 1.29, p=0.059) for cilostazol; 0.69 (CI, 0.23 to 1.15, p=0.003) for exercise training; and 0.79 (CI, 0.29 to 1.29, p=0.002) for endovascular intervention compared with usual care. These effects are summarized in Figure 16. Note that the three treatments are not significantly different from each other, with effect sizes ranging from 0.06 to 0.16 (no effect to small effect).

Figure 16. Network meta-analysis of treatment effects versus usual care and each other on claudication distance in IC patients

Treatment comparison	Std diff in means	Lower limit	Upper limit	p-Value
Usual Care vs Cilostazol	0.631	-0.024	1.286	0.059
Usual Care vs Exercise training	0.691	0.230	1.152	0.003
Usual Care vs Endovascular intervention	0.789	0.292	1.286	0.002
Cilostazol vs Exercise training	0.059	-0.668	0.786	0.874
Cilostazol vs Endovascular intervention	0.158	-0.593	0.909	0.680
Exercise vs Endovascular intervention	0.098	-0.376	0.572	0.685

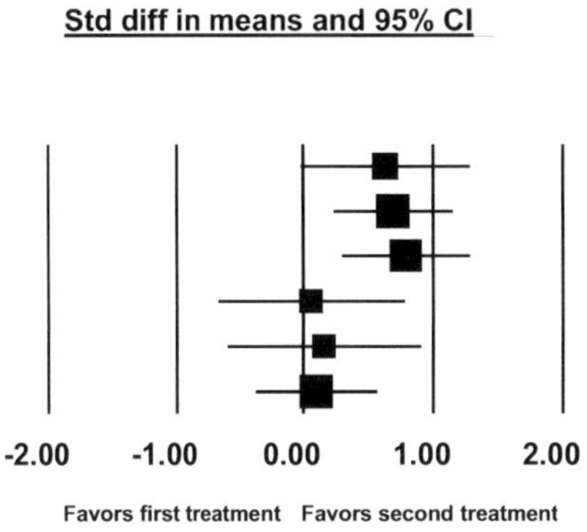

Abbreviation: CI=confidence interval.

Thus, cilostazol, exercise training, and endovascular interventions had a medium effect compared with usual care. Clinically, this equates to an improvement in ICD or PFWD of 35 meters for cilostazol, 39 meters for exercise training, and 44 meters for endovascular intervention. There was no effect seen between exercise training and cilostazol (ES=0.06) and small effects seen between endovascular intervention compared with cilostazol (ES=0.16) and exercise (ES=0.10), both favoring endovascular intervention. The overall SOE was rated low for all six comparisons.

Effect on Quality-of-Life Measures

We identified 13 unique studies that reported measures quality of life, such as the SF-36, WIQ, EQ-5D, VascuQOL, or PAQ. Results by study comparison are listed in Table 18. There was significant heterogeneity in the study protocols and data reporting.

Medical Therapy Versus Usual Care

Two studies (1 good quality, 1 fair) reported SF-36 as a measure of quality of life and were included in the random-effects meta-analysis.[49,89] None of these studies reported EQ-5D, VascuQOL, PAQ, or WIQ.

Exercise Training Versus Usual Care

Five studies (two good quality, one fair, two poor) reported SF-36 as a measure of quality of life, and three reported WIQ. A random-effects meta-analysis included all of these studies[68,69,75,77,79] examining the difference in SF-36 measure of physical functioning between exercise and usual care.

Endovascular Intervention Versus Usual Care

Five studies reported SF-36 as a measure of quality of life, and no studies reported EQ-5D, VascuQOL, PAQ, or WIQ. The random-effects meta-analysis included two RCTs (two good quality)[77,93] but not the two prospective observational studies (both fair)[91,94] reporting SF-36 physical functioning.

Endovascular Intervention Versus Exercise Training

Four studies reported SF-36 as a measure of quality of life, one reported EQ-5D, one reported VascuQOL, one reported PAQ, and one reported WIQ. The random-effects meta-analysis included all four studies (two good quality, two fair)[16,77,80,82] reporting SF-36 physical functioning scores.

Endovascular Intervention Versus Surgical Revascularization

Two studies included in the random-effects meta-analysis reported SF-36 as a measure of quality of life,[91,94] and no studies reported EQ-5D, VascuQOL, PAQ, or WIQ.

Analysis of Quality-of-Life Measures

Table 18 presents the 13 studies that reported measures of quality of life, organized alphabetically by study comparison. Of these studies, ten were included in the random-effects network meta-analyses (Figures 17 and 18).

Table 18. Calculated effect size: quality-of-life measures

Study	Type of Study N Analyzed[a] Quality	Outcome Length of Followup	Results Reported by Authors	Calculated Effect Size[b]
Medical therapy vs. usual care				
Beebe, 1999[49]	RCT N: 419 Good	Mean SF-36 improvement from baseline 1. Physical function 2. Role-physical 3. Bodily pain Mean WIQ change from baseline: 1. walking speed 2. walking distance 6 mo	SF-36: 1. Cilostazol 100 BID: 7.1 Cilostazol 50 BID: 8.0 Placebo: 2.0 2. Cilostazol 100 BID: 5.3 Cilostazol 50 BID: 4.4 Placebo: -2.8 3. Cilostazol 100 BID: 7.2 Cilostazol 50 BID: 4.6 Placebo: -1.8 WIQ: 1. Cilostazol 100 BID: 0.1 Cilostazol 50 BID: 0.2 Placebo: 0.1 2. Cilostazol 100 BID: 0.2 Cilostazol 50 BID: 0.2 Placebo: 0.1	ES (cilostazol 100): 0.31 EffSE: 0.14 ES (cilostazol 50): 0.36 EffSE: 0.14
Money, 1998[89]	RCT N: 212 Fair	SF-36 physical score 4 mo	Score Improvement: Cilostazol: 20% Placebo: 0%	ES (cilostazol): 0.36 EffSE: 0.13

Table 18. Calculated effect size: quality-of-life measures (continued)

Study	Type of Study N Analyzed[a] Quality	Outcome Length of Followup	Results Reported by Authors	Calculated Effect Size[b]
Exercise training vs. usual care				
Gardner, 2002[68]	RCT N at 6 mo: 40 N at 18 mo: 31 Fair	1. WIQ distance 2. WIQ speed 3. WIQ stair climbing 18 mo 4. SF36 QOL physical composite score 5. SF36 QOL mental health composite score 6 mo	Percent change in score 1. Supervised exercise 21%, usual care 3% 2. Supervised exercise 34%, usual care 6% 3. Supervised exercise 24%, usual care 15% Mean SF-36 QOL (SD) 4. Supervised exercise baseline: 41 (2) 6 mo: 41(2) Usual care baseline: 40 (3) 6 mo: 39 (2) 5. Supervised exercise baseline: 55 (3) 6 mo: 59 (2) Usual care baseline: 53(3) 6 mo: 53 (3)	**ES: 0.16** **EffSE: 0.32**
Gardner, 2011[69]	RCT N: 63 Good	1. SF-36 physical function 2. WIQ distance 3. WIQ speed 4. WIQ stair climbing 12 wk	Mean change score (SD) 1. Supervised exercise 9 (16), usual care -1 (17), home exercise 8 (15) 2. Supervised exercise 13 (28), usual care 8 (20), home exercise 10 (25) 3. Supervised exercise 9(15), usual care 4 (25), home exercise 11 (22) 4. Supervised exercise 12 (15), usual care 3 (25), home exercise 10 (22)	**ES: 0.60** **EffSE: 0.26**

Table 18. Calculated effect size: quality-of-life measures (continued)

Study	Type of Study N Analyzed[a] Quality	Outcome Length of Followup	Results Reported by Authors	Calculated Effect Size[b]
Lee, 2007[75]	Observational N: 70 Poor	SF-36 1. Physical function 2. Role limited 3. Bodily pain 4. General health 5. Vitality 6 mo	Median SF-36 score (IQR) 1. Exercise: baseline 45.0 (25 to 62.5) 6 mo 50 (35 to 67.5) Usual care: baseline 52.5 (45 to 70) 6 mo 37.5 (11.3 to 63.8) 2. Exercise: baseline 0 (0 to 75) 6 mo 25 (0 to 87.5) Usual care: baseline 25 (0 to 100) 6 mo 0 (0 to 100) 3. Exercise: baseline 52 (42 to 69) 6 mo 42 (31 to 52) Usual care: baseline 31 (22 to 60) 6 mo 32 (22 to 52) 4. Exercise: baseline 65 (52 to 72) 6 mo 60 (47 to 52.5) Usual care: baseline 52 (40 to 60) 6 mo 47.5 (31.2 to 67) 5. Exercise: baseline 55 (50 to 70) 6 mo 55 (50 to 60) Usual care: baseline 55 (40 to 62) 6 mo 45 (32.5 to 57.5)	ES: 0.08 EffSE: 0.24
Murphy, 2012[77] CLEVER Study	RCT N: 58 Good	1. SF12 physical 2 WIQ walking distance 3. WIQ pain severity 4. WIQ walking speed 5. WIQ stair climbing 6. PAQ summary 6 mo	Mean change from baseline (SD) 1. Exercise 5.9 (10.1) Usual care 1.2 (11.0) 2. Exercise 25.1 (27.6) Usual care 0.5 (26.0) 3. Exercise 26.3 (36.3) Usual care 16.3 (34.7) 4. Exercise 16.5 (19.7) Usual care 1.47 (15.69) 5. Exercise 24.0 (10.9) Usual care 10.2 (29.3) 6. Exercise 13.8 (17.0) Usual care -3.1 (18.6)	**ES: 0.61** **EffSE: 0.17**

Table 18. Calculated effect size: quality-of-life measures (continued)

Study	Type of Study N Analyzed[a] Quality	Outcome Length of Followup	Results Reported by Authors	Calculated Effect Size[b]
Tsai, 2002[79]	RCT N: 53 Poor	SF-36 1. Physical function 2. Role limitation 3. Bodily pain 3 mo	Mean SF-36 Score (SD) 1. Exercise: baseline 39.5 (11.0) 3 mo 58.0 (10.6) Control: baseline 49.2 (11.2) 3 mo 48.0 (9.6) 2. Exercise: baseline 22.5 (30.0) 3 mo 62.5 (31.7), Control: baseline 22.9 (19.8) 3 mo 33.3 (16.3) 3. Exercise: baseline 64.8 (15.9) 3 mo 81.5 (18.4) Control: baseline 71.1 (20.4) 3 mo 77.3 (17.8)	ES: 1.79 EffSE: 0.21
Endovascular intervention vs. usual care				
Feinglass, 2000[91]	Observational N: 321 Fair	1. WIQ walking distance 2. SF-36 bodily pain 18 mo	Effect Size 1. Endovascular 0.98, usual care -0.11 2. Endovascular 0.2, usual care -0.11	Not calculated
Murphy, 2012[77] CLEVER Study	RCT N: 61 Good	1. SF12 physical 2. WIQ walking distance 3. WIQ pain severity 4. WIQ walking speed 5. WIQ stair climbing 6. PAQ summary 6 mo	Mean change from baseline (SD) 1. Usual care 1.2 (11.0), Endovascular therapy 6.6 (8.5) 2. Usual care 0.5 (26.0), Endovascular therapy 43.8 (42.2) 3. Usual care 16.3 (34.7), endovascular therapy 40.4 (43.9) 4. Usual care 1.47 (15.69), Endovascular therapy 30.8 (31.0) 5. Usual care 10.2 (29.3), Endovascular therapy 29.3 (39.1) 6. Usual care -3.1 (18.6), Endovascular therapy 28.0 (26.4)	ES: 0.69 EffSE: 0.14
Nylaende, 2007[93] OBACT Study	RCT N: 56 Good	SF-36 physical function 24 mo	Mean change in SF-36 Physical Functioning Score (SD) Endovascular 0.11 (0.32), usual care -0.06 (0.26)	ES: 0.13 EffSE: 0.21

Table 18. Calculated effect size: quality-of-life measures (continued)

Study	Type of Study N Analyzed[a] Quality	Outcome Length of Followup	Results Reported by Authors	Calculated Effect Size[b]
Pell, 1997[94]	Observational N: 138 Fair	SF-36 1. Physical function 2. Role limited 3. Bodily pain 4. General Health 5. Vitality 6 mo	Mean change (SE) 1. Endovascular 10.8 (6), usual care -0.7 (2.2) 2. Endovascular 18.1 (10), usual care -10.7 (3.8) 3. Endovascular 12.3 (5.3), usual care -3.3 (2.1) 4. Endovascular -1.3 (5.3), usual care -8.2 (2.3) 5. Endovascular 0 (5.1), usual care -9.7 (2.4)	ES: 0.77 EffSE: 0.25
Endovascular intervention vs. exercise training				
Greenhalgh, 2008[80] MIMIC Study	RCT N: 94 Fair	SF-36 physical function score 24 mo	Mean score (SD) <u>Femoropopliteal group</u> Baseline: Exercise 39.7 (7.4), endovascular 38.9 (8.5) 24 mo: Exercise 39.2, endovascular 40.9 <u>Aortoiliac group</u> Baseline: Exercise 37.7 (8.2), endovascular 38.3 (9.0) 24 mo: Exercise 38.6, endovascular 46.4	**ES (femor): -0.02** **EffSE: 0.11** **ES (aortoiliac): 0.49** **EffSE: 0.20**

Table 18. Calculated effect size: quality-of-life measures (continued)

Study	Type of Study N Analyzed[a] Quality	Outcome Length of Followup	Results Reported by Authors	Calculated Effect Size[b]
Mazari, 2012[82]	RCT N: 109 Good	SF-36 1. Physical function 2. Role limited 3. Bodily pain 4. General health 5. Vitality VascuQOL 12 mo	Median score (IQR) 1. Baseline: Endovascular 35 (25 to 45), exercise 35 (20 to 53) 12 mo: Endovascular 47.5 (28.69 to 80), exercise 47.5 (28.75 to 76.25) 2. Baseline: Endovascular 0 (0 to 75), exercise 18.75 (0 to 50) 12 mo: Endovascular 25 (0 to 100), exercise 25 (0 to 100) 3. Baseline: Endovascular 41 (22 to 72), exercise 41 (31 to 68.5) 12 mo: Endovascular 57.5 (34.25 to 78.5), exercise 52 (41 to 72.5) 4. Baseline: Endovascular 57 (35 to 72), exercise 55 (37.75 to 64.25) 12 mo: Endovascular 55 (35 to 77), exercise 57 (37.5 to 72) 5. Baseline: Endovascular 45 (35, 65), exercise 47.5 (35 to 65) VascuQOL Baseline: Endovascular 3.88 (3.16 to 5.0), exercise 4.16 (3.02 to 5.12) 12 mo: 5.29 (3.82 to 6.46), exercise 5.14 (3.96 to 6.08)	ES (endo): **0.62** **EffSE: 0.14** ES (ex): **0.47** **EffSE: 0.12**

Table 18. Calculated effect size: quality-of-life measures (continued)

Study	Type of Study N Analyzed[a] Quality	Outcome Length of Followup	Results Reported by Authors	Calculated Effect Size[b]
Murphy, 2012[77] CLEVER Study	RCT N: 79 Good	1. SF12 physical 2. WIQ walking distance 3. WIQ pain severity 4. WIQ walking speed 5. WIQ stair climbing 6. PAQ summary 6 mo	Mean change from baseline (SD) 1. Exercise 5.9 (10.1), Usual care 1.2 (11.0), Endovascular therapy 6.6 (8.5) 2. Exercise 25.1 (27.6), Usual care 0.5 (26.0), Endovascular therapy 43.8 (42.2) 3. Exercise 26.3 (36.3), Usual care 16.3 (34.7), endovascular therapy 40.4 (43.9) 4. Exercise 16.5 (19.7), Usual care 1.47 (15.69), Endovascular therapy 30.8 (31.0) 5. Exercise 24.0 (10.9), Usual care 10.2 (29.3), Endovascular therapy 29.3 (39.1) 6. Exercise 13.8 (17.0), Usual care -3.1 (18.6), Endovascular therapy 28.0 (26.4)	**ES (endo): 0.69** **EffSE: 0.14** **ES (ex): 0.61** **EffSE: 0.17**
Spronk, 2009[16]	RCT N: 150 Fair	SF-36 1. Physical score 2. Role limitation 3. Bodily pain 4. General health VascuQOL EQ-5D 12 mo	Adjusted mean change (99% CI) 1. Endovascular 17 (12, 22), exercise 13 (8, 18) 2. Endovascular 21 (10, 32), exercise 6 (-4, 16) 3. Endovascular 11 (5, 17), exercise 10 (4, 16) 4. Endovascular 2 (-3, 7), exercise 5 (1,9) VascuQOL: endovascular 0.7 (0.3 to 1.1), exercise 0.6 (0.3, 0.9) EQ-5D score: endovascular 0.11 (0.04, 0.18), exercise 0.07 (0.02, 0.13)	**ES (endo): 1.01** **EffSE: 0.12** **ES (ex): 0.77** **EffSE: 0.12**

Table 18. Calculated effect size: quality-of-life measures (continued)

Study	Type of Study N Analyzed[a] Quality	Outcome Length of Followup	Results Reported by Authors	Calculated Effect Size[b]
Endovascular intervention vs. surgical revascularization				
Feinglass, 2000[91]	Observational N: 104 Fair	SF-36 18 mo	Mean change (SD) Medication -2 (19) Matched medication 3 (23) Surgical 17 (26) Endovascular 14 (21)	ES: 0.12 EffSE: 0.20
Pell, 1997[94]	Observational N: 138 Fair	SF-36 1. Physical functioning 2. Physical role 3. Bodily pain 4. General health 5. Vitality 6 mo	Mean (SD) 1. Conservative management 42.5 (2.1), endovascular 42.4 (5.3), surgical 32.9 (4.6) 2. Conservative management 39.9 (3.9), endovascular 44.4 (10.0), surgical 27.8 (9.9) 3. Conservative management 48.3 (2.1), endovascular 46.5 (4.8), surgical 43.3 (6.4) 4. Conservative management 57.1 (1.4), endovascular 56.7 (2.4), surgical 53.9 (3.4) 5. Conservative management 54.6 (1.9), endovascular 37.4 (5.6), surgical 51.3 (4.3)	ES: 0.14 EffSE: 0.33

[a] Number of patients in the study arms of interest.
[b] Values used in meta-analysis of RCTs appear in bold.
Abbreviations: BID=two times a day; EffSE=standard error of effect; ES=effect size; IQR=interquartile range; m=meters; min=minute/minutes; mo=month/months; RCT=randomized controlled trial; SD=standard deviation; SF-36=short-form (36) health survey; WIQ=walking impairment questionnaire; wk=week/weeks.

We conducted a random-effects meta-analysis with 10 studies[16,49,68,69,77,79,80,82,89,91,93,94] to compare the multiple treatment arms on continuous measures (PROC NLMIXED). Results showed summary effect sizes that were statistically significant compared to usual care for cilostazol (2 studies; p=0.0278), exercise training (7 studies; p=0.0003), endovascular intervention (6 studies; p=0.0001), and surgical revascularization (2 studies; p=0.0044). The results comparing active treatments with each other were not significantly different. These effects are summarized in Figures 17 and 18. We also ran a sensitivity analysis without the three observational studies,[75,91,94] and the summary effect sizes for cilostazol, exercise training, and endovascular interventions were similar and still significantly better than usual care. Note that removing the Feinglass and Pell observational studies also removes the surgical versus endovascular and surgical versus usual care indirect comparison. Therefore, the full analysis combining RCTs and observational studies is presented below.

Figure 17. Network meta-analysis of treatment effects versus usual care on quality of life in IC patients

Treatment Comparison	Statistics for each comparison			
	Std diff in means	Lower limit	Upper limit	p-Value
Cilostazol	0.4400	0.0479	0.8321	0.0278
Exercise	0.5630	0.2559	0.8701	0.0003
Endovascular	0.6120	0.2989	0.9251	0.0001
Surgical	0.8230	0.2560	1.3900	0.0044

Std diff in means and 95% CI

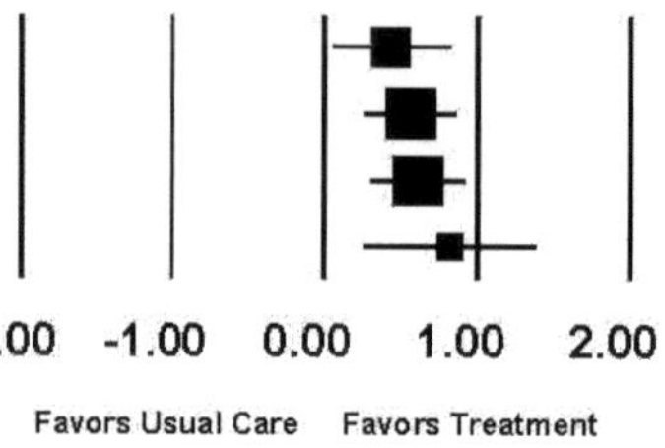

Abbreviation: CI=confidence interval.

Figure 18. Network meta-analysis of treatment effects versus each other on quality of life in IC patients

Treatment comparison	Statistics for each comparison		
	Std diff in means	Lower limit	Upper limit
Cilostazol vs exercise training	0.12	-0.32	0.56
Cilostazol vs endovascular	0.17	-0.27	0.62
Cilostazol vs surgical	0.38	-0.27	1.03
Exercise training vs endovascular	0.05	-0.24	0.34
Exercise training vs surgical	0.26	-0.31	0.83
Endovascular vs surgical	0.21	-0.34	0.76

Std diff in means and 95% CI

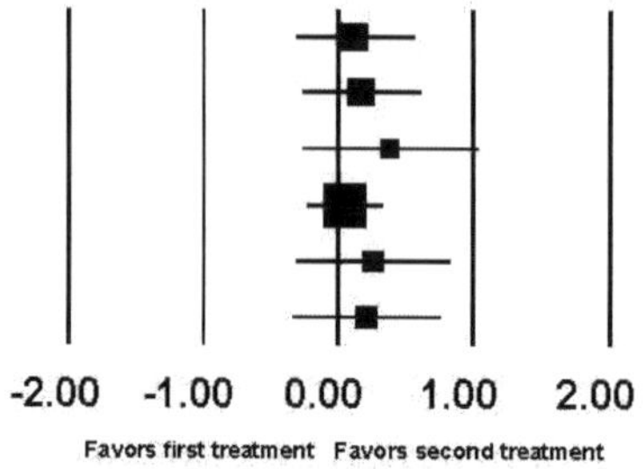

Abbreviation: CI=confidence interval.

Thus, when compared with usual care, cilostazol and exercise training had moderate effects on physical functioning, while endovascular and surgical interventions had large effects (Figure 17). Clinically, this equates to an improvement in SF-36 physical functioning domain score of 4.4 for cilostazol, 5.6 for exercise training, 6.1 for endovascular intervention, and 8.3 for surgical intervention. Figure 18 shows that the effect sizes comparing cilostazol, exercise training, endovascular intervention, and surgical intervention were negligible or small, ranging from 0.05 to 0.38. The overall SOE was rated low for all comparisons on the basis consistent results of an indirect analysis with a wide confidence interval.

Effect on Other Outcome Measures

We identified six studies that reported other outcome measures, such as amputation, repeat revascularization, vessel patency, wound healing, bleeding, and analog pain scale.

Medical Therapy Versus Usual Care

Amputation was measured in two studies[49,51] and occurred in only one patient (treated with usual care). Revascularization was measured in the same two studies and occurred more frequently in patients treated with usual care (10.5%) compared with medical therapy (3.6%). Vessel patency, wound healing and analog pain scale were not measured in any of the studies for this comparison.

Exercise Training Versus Usual Care

Amputation was measured in a single study[68] and occurred in only one patient (treated with exercise). Vessel patency was measured in a single study;[70] however, it was only measured in the endovascular and surgical revascularization groups (results reported under endovascular versus usual care section) and not in the exercise or control groups. Repeat revascularization, wound healing, analog pain scale, bleeding, and amputation were not measured in any of the studies for this comparison.

Endovascular Intervention Versus Usual Care

Amputation was measured in two studies with a range of followup between 1 and 2 years[70,91] with amputation occurring in similar proportions in patients treated with endovascular revascularization and usual care (Gelin study: 2% usual care, 1% endovascular; Feinglass study: two in medical therapy arm, three in endovascular arm). Vessel patency was reported in a single study,[70] and only patients receiving revascularization procedures had vessel patency outcomes reported (endovascular group 59%, surgical group 98%). Repeat revascularization, wound healing, analog pain scale, and bleeding were not measured in any of the studies for this comparison.

Surgical Revascularization Versus Usual Care

Vessel patency was measured in a single study;[76] however, it was measured only in the surgical revascularization group and not in the usual care group. Amputation, repeat revascularization, wound healing, analog pain scale, and bleeding were not measured in any of the studies for this comparison.

Endovascular Intervention Versus Exercise Training

Vessel patency and amputation were each measured in a single study.[70] Vessel patency was not reported in the exercise group. Amputation occurred in one patient in the endovascular group and in none of the patients in the exercise group. Repeat revascularization, wound healing, analog pain scale, and bleeding were not measured in any of the studies for this comparison.

Endovascular Intervention Versus Surgical Revascularization

Vessel patency, repeat revascularization, amputation, wound healing, analog pain scale, and bleeding were not measured in any of the studies for this comparison.

Modifiers of Effectiveness

Table 19 summarizes the six studies—four RCTs (two good quality, two fair) and two observational studies (one fair, one poor)—that reported variations in treatment effectiveness by subgroup, arranged alphabetically. Two studies compared medical therapy with usual care,[51,86] one study compared endovascular revascularization with exercise training,[84] and two studies compared endovascular revascularization or surgical revascularization and with usual care.[70,76,91] Despite limited data to draw definitive conclusions, one study reported improvements in quality-of-life measures and ABI in patients with successful endovascular revascularization when compared with patients without successful endovascular revascularization. One other study reported a statistically nonsignificant improvement in MWD favoring exercise training over endovascular revascularization in patients with SFA stenosis when compared with patients with iliac stenosis.

We found no studies reporting results by the following subgroups: age, sex, race, presence of diabetes mellitus or renal disease, smoking status, use of exercise or medical therapy prior to invasive management, or prior revascularization. The SOE for modifiers of effectiveness was insufficient given the variation in subgroups that were studied and the outcomes reported.

Table 19. Studies reporting subgroup results (modifiers of effectiveness) in the IC population

Study	Type of Study N Analyzed[a] Comparison Quality	Subgroup	Results Reported by Authors
Dawson, 1998[86]	RCT N: 81 Cilostazol vs. placebo Good	On treatment analysis (limited to those completing 12 wk of therapy)	Percent change in walking distances from baseline (geometric mean) Cilostazol (N=44): 31% Placebo (N=22): -4.6%
Feinglass, 2000[91]	Observational N: 526 Endovascular revascularization vs. medical therapy Fair	Success of revascularization technique only on the revascularization group	QOL Bypass grafting ABI change >0.1 (mean [SD]) (N=37) 1. SF-36 physical functioning score 28 (23) 2. WIQ walking distance score 0.43 (0.27) 3. SF36 bodily pain score 25 (24) 4. ABI 0.36 (0.15) Bypass grafting ABI change <0.1 (mean [SD]) (N=23) 1. SF36 physical functioning score -0.8 (18) 2. WIQ walking distance score 0.01 (0.23) 3. SF36 bodily pain score 5 (24) 4. ABI -0.01 (0.12) Angioplasty ABI change >0.1 (mean [SD]) (N=22) 1. SF-36 physical functioning score 20 (23) 2. WIQ walking distance score 0.35 (0.28) 3. SF36 bodily pain score 12 (24) 4. ABI 0.23 (0.11) Angioplasty ABI change <0.1 (mean [SD]) (N=22) 1. SF-36 physical functioning score 7 (17) 2. WIQ walking distance score 0.20 (0.26) 3. SF-36 bodily pain score 13 (18) 4. ABI -0.01 (0.01)
Gelin, 2001[70]	RCT N: 264 Supervised exercise vs. invasive therapy (surgical or endovascular) vs. control Fair	Suprainguinal vs. infrainguinal reconstructions	1-yr patency Suprainguinal 89% (24 of 27) Infrainguinal 76% (26 of 34) p-value not provided by author; our calculated p-value=0.21

Table 19. Studies reporting subgroup results (modifiers of effectiveness) in the IC population (continued)

Study	Type of Study N Analyzed[a] Comparison Quality	Subgroup	Results Reported by Authors
Mori, 2002[76]	Observational N: 427 Surgical revascularization vs. usual care Poor	Suprainguinal patency 1. Aortofemoral bypass 2. Axillofemoral bypass 3. Femorofemoral bypass Infrainguinal patency 1. Above knee femoropopliteal bypass 2. Below knee femoropopliteal bypass Above knee bypass 1. Synthetic graft 2. Auto vein graft Below knee bypass 1. Synthetic graft 2. Auto vein graft 5 yr	Suprainguinal patency 1. 95.1% 2. 95.5% 3. 83.3% Infrainguinal patency 1. 67.6% 2. 45.2% Above knee bypass 1. 64.2% 2. 85.7% Below knee bypass 1. 38.9% 2. 57.1%
Perkins, 1996[84]	RCT N: 56 Endovascular revascularization vs. supervised exercise Fair	Iliac stenosis vs. superficial femoral stenosis in exercise vs. PTA	Median MWD at 15 mo (SE) SFA stenosis: PTA (N=15) 161.43 (66), exercise (N=13) 723.8 (124.7) Iliac stenosis: PTA (N=15) 171.3 (125.8), exercise (N=13) 374.3 (96)
Soga, 2009[51]	RCT N: 78 Cilostazol vs. placebo Good	Occlusive vs. nonocclusive disease	Repeat revascularization Occlusive disease: Cilostazol 50% Placebo 36% Nonocclusive disease: Cilostazol 3.4% Placebo 39%

[a]Number of patients in the study arms of interest.
Abbreviations: ABI=ankle-brachial-index; ACD=absolute claudication distance; ICD=initial claudication distance; MWD=maximal walking distance; PTA=percutaneous transluminal angioplasty; QOL=quality of life; RCT=randomized controlled trial; SD=standard deviation; SE=standard error; SFA=superficial femoral artery; WIQ=Walking Impairment Questionnaire.

Safety Concerns

Table 20 describes the 17 RCTs (8 good, 8 fair, 1 poor) that reported safety concerns, arranged alphabetically. Ten RCTs measured harm in a comparison of medical therapy and usual care, three RCTs measured harm in a comparison of exercise training and usual care, three RCTs measured harm in a comparison of endovascular revascularization and usual care, and five RCTs measured harm in a comparison of endovascular revascularization and exercise training. Five RCTs reported both headache and diarrhea.[25,49,73,89,90] Five RCTs reported serious adverse events,[25,85,87,89,90] and three RCTs reported bleeding.[51,88,93]

Table 20. Studies reporting harms of therapies in the IC population

Study	Type of Study N Analyzed[a] Comparison Quality	Harm Length of Followup	Results Reported by Authors
Beebe, 1999[49]	RCT N: 419 Cilostazol 100 mg vs. cilostazol 50 mg vs. placebo Good	1. Headache 2. Abnormal stools 3. Diarrhea 4. Dizziness 5. Palpitations 24 wk	1. Headache: cilostazol 100 34.3%, cilostazol 50 23.4%, placebo 14.7% 2. Abnormal stool: cilostazol 100 14.9%, cilostazol 50 14.6%, placebo 3.5% 3. Diarrhea: cilostazol 100 12%, cilostazol 50 9.9%, placebo 8.7% 4. Dizziness: cilostazol 100 10.3%, cilostazol 50 8.8%, placebo 4.7% 5. Palpitations: cilostazol 100 11.4%, cilostazol 50 4.7%, placebo 0%
Belcaro, 2002[85]	RCT N: 53 Pentoxifylline vs. placebo Fair	Serious side effects 6 mo	Serious side effects: pentoxifylline 0, placebo 0
Dawson, 1998[86]	RCT N: 77 Cilostazol vs. placebo Good	1. Hospitalizations 2. pneumonia 12 wk	1. Cilostazol 6, placebo 0 2. Cilostazol 2, placebo 0
Dawson, 2000[25]	RCT N: 698 Cilostazol vs. pentoxifylline vs. placebo Good	1. Headache 2. Pain 3. Diarrhea 4. Pharyngitis 5. Peripheral vascular disorder 6. Abnormal stools 7. Palpitation 8. Serious adverse events 28 wk	1. Headache: cilostazol 28%, pentoxifylline 11%, placebo 12% 2. Pain: cilostazol 13%, pentoxifylline 16%, placebo 14% 3. Diarrhea: cilostazol 19%, pentoxifylline 8%, placebo 5% 4. Pharyngitis: cilostazol 10%, pentoxifylline 14%, placebo 7% 5. Peripheral vascular disorder: cilostazol 6%, pentoxifylline 10%, placebo 11% 6. Abnormal stools: cilostazol 15%, pentoxifylline 5%, placebo 3% 7. Palpitation: cilostazol 17%, pentoxifylline 2%, placebo 1% 8. Serious adverse events: cilostazol 12%, pentoxifylline 13%, placebo 13%
De Sanctis, 2002[98]	RCT N: 135 Pentoxifylline vs. placebo Fair	Side effects 12 mo	Side effects: pentoxifylline 0, placebo 0
De Sanctis, 2002[87]	RCT N: 101 Pentoxifylline vs. placebo Poor	Serious side effects	Serious Side Effects: pentoxifylline 0, placebo 0
Gardner, 2002[68]	RCT N: 31 Supervised exercise vs. control Fair	Side effects 18 mo	Supervised exercise: 0, usual care: 0

Table 20. Studies reporting harms of therapies in the IC population (continued)

Study	Type of Study N Analyzed[a] Comparison Quality	Harm Length of Followup	Results Reported by Authors
Greenhalgh, 2008[80]	RCT N: 106 Supervised exercise + best medical therapy vs. supervised exercise + best medical therapy + PTA Fair	1. Minor hematomas 2. Dissected artery 3. Sensory deficit 24 mo	1. Minor hematomas: supervised exercise + best medical therapy + PTA 8, supervised exercise + best medical therapy 0 2. Dissected artery: supervised exercise + best medical therapy + PTA 1, supervised exercise + best medical therapy 0 3. Sensory deficit: supervised exercise + best medical therapy + PTA 8, supervised exercise + best medical therapy 0
Hiatt, 2008[88]	RCT N: 1435 Cilostazol vs. placebo Good	1. Dyspnea 2. Serious bleeding 36 mo	1. Dyspnea: cilostazol 7 (1%), placebo 3 (0.4%) 2. Serious bleeding: cilostazol 18 (2.5%), placebo 22 (3.1%)
Hobbs, 2007[73]	RCT N: 34 Medical therapy + supervised exercise vs. medical therapy + cilostazol vs medical therapy + supervised exercise + cilostazol Good	1. Headache 2. Diarrhea 6 mo	1. Headache: patients taking cilostazol 2, medical therapy 0 2. Diarrhea: patients taking cilostazol 3, medical therapy 0
Money, 1998[89]	RCT N: 212 Cilostazol vs. placebo Fair	1. Headache 2. Abnormal stools 3. Diarrhea 4. Dizziness 5. Serious adverse events 16 wk	1. Headache: cilostazol 30.3%, placebo 9.2% 2. Abnormal stool: cilostazol 16%, placebo 5.0% 3. Diarrhea: cilostazol 12.6%, placebo 6.7% 4. Dizziness: cilostazol 12.6%, placebo 5.0% 5. Serious adverse events: cilostazol 11.8%, placebo 9.2%
Murphy, 2012[77]	RCT N: 99 Supervised exercise vs. primary stenting vs. optimal medical care for IC Good	1. Transfusion 2. Arterial dissection 3. Arterial perforation 6 mo	1. Transfusion: PTA 1, supervised exercise 0, optimal medical therapy 0 2. Arterial dissection: PTA 2, supervised exercise 0, optimal medical therapy 0 3. Arterial perforation PTA 1, supervised exercise 0, optimal medical therapy 0
Nylaende, 2007[93]	RCT N: 56 Optimal medical therapy vs. PTA + optimal medical therapy Good	1. Bleeding 2. Emboli 3. Local thrombosis 4. Arterial dissection / perforation 5. Hematoma requiring surgical management 24 mo	1. Bleeding: PTA + optimal medical therapy 0, optimal medical therapy 0 2. Emboli: PTA + optimal medical therapy 0, optimal medical therapy 0 3. Local thrombosis: PTA + optimal medical therapy 0, optimal medical therapy 0 4. Arterial dissection / perforation: PTA + optimal medical therapy 0, optimal medical therapy 0 5. Hematoma requiring surgical management: PTA + optimal medical therapy 0, optimal medical therapy 0
Perkins, 1996[84]	RCT N: 56 Exercise vs. PTA Fair	1. Contralateral angioplasty 2. Surgery 6 yr	1. Contralateral angioplasty: exercise 3/26, PTA 3/30 2. Surgery: exercise 2/26, PTA 2/30

Table 20. Studies reporting harms of therapies in the IC population (continued)

Study	Type of Study N Analyzed[a] Comparison Quality	Harm Length of Followup	Results Reported by Authors
Soga, 2009[51]	RCT N: 78 Cilostazol vs. control Good	1. Major bleeding 2. Palpitations 24 mo	1. Major bleeding: cilostazol 0/39, control 0/39 2. Palpitations: cilostazol 2/39, control 0/39
Spronk, 2009[16]	RCT N: 150 PTA vs. exercise Fair	1. Minor complications 2. Hematoma 3. Dissection 12 mo	1. Minor complications: PTA 7/75, exercise 0/75 2. Hematoma: PTA 6/75, exercise 0/75 3. Arterial dissection: PTA 1/75, exercise 0/75
Strandness, 2002[90]	RCT N: 394 Cilostazol vs. placebo Fair	1. Abnormal stools 2. Serious adverse event 3. Headache 4. Infection 5. Pain 6. Diarrhea 24 wk	1. Abnormal stools: cilostazol 100 19.5%, cilostazol 50 6.1%, placebo 5.4% 2. Serious adverse event: cilostazol 100 18.8%, cilostazol 50 16.7%, placebo 15.5% 3. Headache: cilostazol 100 40.6%, cilostazol 50 26.5%, placebo 12.4% 4. Infection: cilostazol 100 18%, cilostazol 50 17.4%, placebo 12.4% 5. Pain: cilostazol 100 11.3%, cilostazol 50 19.7%, placebo 14.0% 6. Diarrhea: cilostazol 100 16.5%, cilostazol 50 10.6%, placebo 6.2%

[a] Number of patients in the study arms of interest.
Abbreviations: ABI=ankle-brachial-index; ACD=absolute claudication distance; ICD=initial claudication distance; mo=month/months; PTA=percutaneous transluminal angioplasty; RCT=randomized controlled trial; SFA=superficial femoral artery; wk=week/weeks.

Figure 19 shows the forest plot for the random-effects meta-analysis of the five RCTs comparing cilostazol with placebo and reporting headache as a side effect. The result is an estimated odds ratio of 3.00 (95% CI, 2.29 to 3.95) favoring placebo. There was no evidence of heterogeneity, with a Q-value of 2.46 for 4 degrees of freedom, p=0.65; I^2=0.00.

Figure 19. Forest plot for meta-analysis of cilostazol versus placebo on headache complications in the IC population

Study name	Odds ratio	Lower limit	Upper limit	p-Value
Money, 1998	4.2905	2.0632	8.9224	0.0001
Beebe, 1999	2.3598	1.4544	3.8288	0.0005
Dawson, 2000	2.8519	1.7542	4.6363	0.0000
Strandness, 2002	3.5716	1.9950	6.3941	0.0000
Hobbs, 2007 (INEXACT)	6.3327	0.2624	152.8497	0.2558
	3.0036	2.2860	3.9465	0.0000

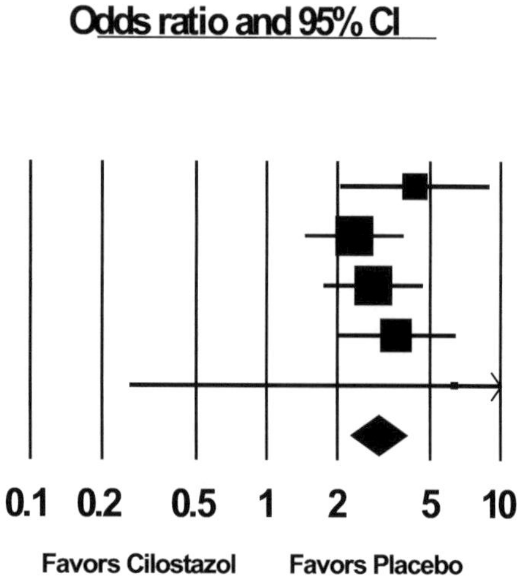

Favors Cilostazol   Favors Placebo

Abbreviation: CI=confidence interval.

Figure 20 shows the forest plot for the random-effects meta-analysis of the five RCTs comparing cilostazol with placebo and reporting diarrhea as a side effect. The result is an estimated odds ratio of 2.51 (95% CI, 1.58 to 3.97) favoring placebo. There was no evidence of heterogeneity, with a Q-value of 5.85 for 4 degrees of freedom, p=0.21; I^2=31.61.

Figure 20. Forest plot for meta-analysis of cilostazol vs. placebo on diarrhea complications in the IC population

Study name	Statistics for each study			
	Odds ratio	Lower limit	Upper limit	p-Value
Money, 1998	2.0075	0.8184	4.9247	0.1280
Beebe, 1999	1.6084	0.8678	2.9814	0.1312
Dawson, 2000	4.4568	2.2815	8.7060	0.0000
Strandness, 2002	2.3733	1.0693	5.2678	0.0336
Hobbs, 2007 (INEXACT)	10.2294	0.4487	233.2036	0.1449
	2.5072	1.5844	3.9676	0.0001

Odds ratio and 95%CI

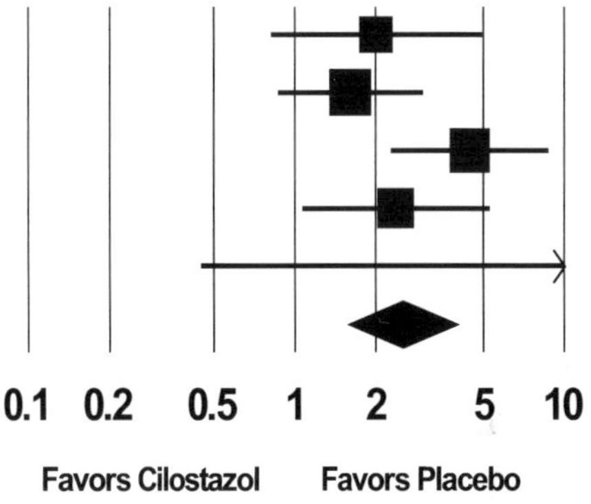

Abbreviations: CI=confidence interval.

Figure 21 shows the forest plot for the random-effects meta-analysis of the three RCTs comparing cilostazol with placebo and reporting palpitation as a side effect. The result is an estimated odds ratio of 18.11 (95% CI, 5.95 to 55.13) favoring placebo. There was no evidence of heterogeneity, with a Q-value of 0.78 for 2 degrees of freedom, p=0.68; I^2=0.00.

Figure 21. Forest plot for meta-analysis of cilostazol versus placebo on palpitation complications in the IC population

Study name	Statistics for each study			
	Odds ratio	Lower limit	Upper limit	p-Value
Beebe, 1999	30.50	1.85	502.72	0.02
Dawson, 2000	20.28	5.41	75.94	0.00
Soga, 2009	5.27	0.24	113.37	0.29
	18.11	5.95	55.13	0.00

Odds ratio and 95%CI

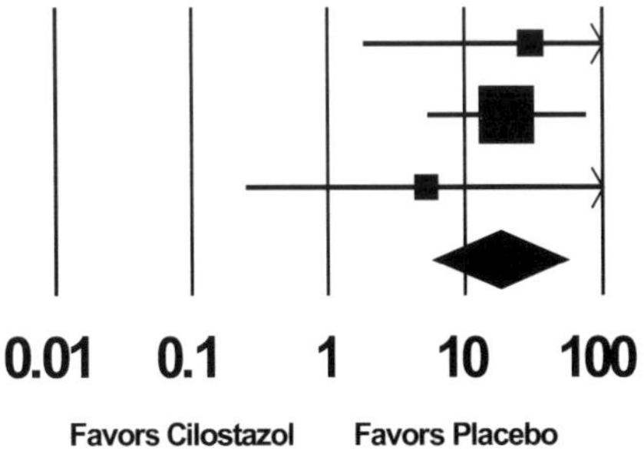

Abbreviation: CI=confidence interval.

Cilostazol increases the rate of headache (high SOE), diarrhea (moderate SOE) and palpitations (moderate SOE). No studies were identified that measured contrast nephropathy, radiation, infection, or exercise-related harms. No studies reported on whether any of the harms vary by subgroup (age, sex, race, risk factors, comorbidities, anatomic location of disease.

SOE Ratings for KQ 2

Table 21 summarizes the SOE for the outcomes outlined in KQ 2 by each treatment comparison. We found very few studies that assessed amputation, vessel patency, subgroup differences, or cardiovascular outcomes (all-cause or cardiovascular mortality, nonfatal stroke, nonfatal MI, or composite events); therefore, the evidence base is insufficient for us to draw any conclusions on these outcomes.

Table 21. Detailed SOE for IC therapies by comparator

Comparator	Number of Studies/Design (Total Patients)	Risk of Bias	Consistency	Directness	Precision	SOE and Magnitude of Effect Effect Estimate (95% CI)
All-cause mortality						
Medical therapy vs. usual care	4 RCT (2732)	3 low risk, 1 moderate risk	Inconsistent	Direct	Imprecise	OR 0.91 (0.62 to 1.35) No difference **Low SOE**
Exercise vs. usual care	2 RCT (238)	1 low risk, 1 moderate risk	Inconsistent	Direct	Imprecise	OR 0.84 (0.34 to 2.07) No difference **Low SOE**
Endovascular vs. usual care	2 RCT, 3 observational (977)	1 low risk, 4 moderate risk	Inconsistent	Direct	Imprecise	OR 0.91 (0.34 to 2.45) No difference **Low SOE**
Surgical vs. usual care	1 observational (427)	1 high risk	NA	Direct	Not reported	10.4% in surgical group, 16.7% in usual care group **Insufficient SOE**
Endovascular vs. exercise	5 RCT (710)	1 low risk, 4 moderate risk	Inconsistent	Direct	Imprecise	OR 0.77 (0.39 to 1.54) No difference **Low SOE**
Endovascular vs. surgical	2 observational (305)	2 moderate risk	Inconsistent	Direct	Not reported	Results not reported by treatment group; overall mortality rate ranged from 3 to 8% **Insufficient SOE**
Nonfatal MI						
Medical therapy vs. usual care	2 RCT (497)	2 low risk	Inconsistent	Direct	Imprecise	Low event rates in both groups Inconclusive **Insufficient SOE**
Exercise vs. usual care	1 RCT (63)	1 low risk	NA	Direct	Not reported	Only one MI total (in exercise group) **Insufficient SOE**
Endovascular vs. usual care	1 observational (479)	Moderate risk	NA	Direct	Not reported	3.0% in endovascular group, 8.8% in usual care group **Insufficient SOE**
Surgical vs. usual care	0	NA	NA	NA	NA	**Insufficient SOE**
Endovascular vs. exercise	1 RCT (106)	Moderate risk	NA	Direct	NA	No events occurred in either treatment group **Insufficient SOE**
Endovascular vs. surgical	0	NA	NA	NA	NA	**Insufficient SOE**

Table 21. Detailed SOE for IC therapies by comparator (continued)

Comparator	Number of Studies/Design (Total Patients)	Risk of Bias	Consistency	Directness	Precision	SOE and Magnitude of Effect Effect Estimate (95% CI)
Nonfatal stroke						
Medical therapy vs. usual care	3 RCT (1932)	3 low risk	Inconsistent	Direct	Imprecise	Low event rates in both groups Inconclusive **Insufficient SOE**
Exercise vs. usual care	1 RCT (63)	1 low risk	NA	Direct	Not reported	1 stroke in each group **Insufficient SOE**
Endovascular vs. usual care	2 observational (800)	2 moderate risk	NA	Direct	Not reported	One study reported 4 strokes for total study; other study reported 1 stroke in endovascular group, 2 strokes in usual care group **Insufficient SOE**
Surgical vs. usual care	0	NA	NA	NA	NA	**Insufficient SOE**
Endovascular vs. exercise	1 RCT (106)	1 moderate risk	NA	Direct	Not reported	1 stroke in each group **Insufficient SOE**
Endovascular vs. surgical	0	NA	NA	NA	NA	**Insufficient SOE**
MWD or ACD						
Medical therapy vs. usual care	6 RCT (cilostazol) (1632) 3 RCT (pentoxifylline) (797)	3 low risk, 3 moderate risk 2 moderate risk, 1 high risk	Cilostazol Consistent Pentoxifylline Inconsistent	Cilostazol Direct Pentoxifylline Direct	Cilostazol Imprecise Pentoxifylline Imprecise	ES cilostazol: 0.62 (-0.21 to 1.45) full model 0.61 (-0.20 to 1.42) sensitivity analysis No difference **Low SOE** ES pentoxifylline: 1.70 (0.36 to 3.04) Inconclusive **Insufficient SOE**
Exercise vs. usual care	9 RCT, 2 observational (624)	4 low risk, 4 moderate risk, 3 high risk	Consistent	Direct	Imprecise	ES: 0.89 (0.06 to 1.71) full model 0.98 (0.23 to 1.74) sensitivity analysis Favors exercise **Moderate SOE**
Endovascular vs. usual care	4 RCT (285)	2 low risk, 2 moderate risk	Consistent	Direct	Imprecise	ES: 0.41 (-0.54 to 1.36) full model 0.51 (-0.35 to 1.37) sensitivity analysis No difference **Low SOE**
Endovascular vs. exercise	8 RCT (695)	3 low risk, 5 moderate risk	Consistent	Direct	Imprecise	ES: -0.47 (-1.41 to 0.46) full model -0.47 (-1.31 to 0.36) sensitivity analysis No difference **Moderate SOE**

Table 21. Detailed SOE for IC therapies by comparator (continued)

Comparator	Number of Studies/Design (Total Patients)	Risk of Bias	Consistency	Directness	Precision	SOE and Magnitude of Effect Effect Estimate (95% CI)
Endovascular + exercise vs. usual care	2 RCT (248)	2 low risk	Consistent	Direct	Imprecise	ES: 1.08 (-0.37 to 2.53) full model 1.20 (-0.11 to 2.50) sensitivity analysis Favors endovascular intervention + exercise training **Low SOE**
Surgical vs. exercise + medical therapy (pentoxifylline)	1 observational (127)	1 moderate risk	NA	Direct	Imprecise	MWT improved to >15 min in surgical group and >11 min in exercise + medical therapy group **Insufficient SOE**
Endovascular vs. surgical	0	NA	NA	NA	NA	**Insufficient SOE**
Initial claudication distance or pain-free walking distance						
Medical therapy (cilostazol) vs. usual care	5 RCT (1255)	3 low risk, 2 moderate risk	Inconsistent	Direct	Imprecise	ES: 0.63 (-0.03 to 1.29) No difference **Low SOE**
Exercise vs. usual care	9 RCT, 1 observational (396)	4 low risk, 4 moderate risk, 2 high risk	Inconsistent	Direct	Imprecise	ES: 0.69 (0.22 to 1.15) Favors exercise **Low SOE**
Endovascular vs. usual care	4 RCT, 1 observational (281)	2 low risk, 2 moderate risk, 1 high risk	Inconsistent	Direct	Imprecise	ES: 0.79 (0.29 to 1.29) Favors endovascular intervention **Low SOE**
Endovascular vs. exercise	5 RCT (448)	2 low risk, 3 moderate risk	Inconsistent	Direct	Imprecise	ES: 0.10 (-0.38 to 0.58) No difference **Low SOE**
Surgical vs. exercise + medical therapy (pentoxifylline)	1 observational (127)	1 moderate risk	NA	Direct	Imprecise	COT improved to >10 min in surgical group and >7 min in exercise + medical therapy group **Insufficient SOE**
Endovascular vs. surgical	0	NA	NA	NA	NA	**Insufficient SOE**
Quality of life						
Medical theray (cilostazol) vs. usual care	2 RCT (631)	1 low risk, 1 moderate risk	Consistent	Direct	Imprecise	ES: 0.44 (0.05 to 0.83) Favors cilostazol **Low SOE**

Table 21. Detailed SOE for IC therapies by comparator (continued)

Comparator	Number of Studies/Design (Total Patients)	Risk of Bias	Consistency	Directness	Precision	SOE and Magnitude of Effect Effect Estimate (95% CI)
Exercise vs. usual care	4 RCT, 1 observational (275)	2 low risk, 1 moderate risk, 2 high risk	Consistent	Direct	Imprecise	ES: 0.56 (0.26 to 0.87) Favors exercise **Low SOE**
Endovascular vs. usual care	2 RCT, 2 observational (576)	2 low risk, 2 moderate risk	Consistent	Direct	Imprecise	ES: 0.61 (0.30 to 0.93) Favors endovascular intervention **Low SOE**
Surgical vs. usual care	2 observational (727)	2 moderate risk	Consistent	Direct	Imprecise	ES: 0.82 (0.26 to 1.39) Favors surgery **Low SOE**
Endovascular vs. exercise	4 RCT (444)	2 low risk, 2 moderate risk	Consistent	Direct	Imprecise	ES: 0.05 (-0.24 to 0.34) No difference **Low SOE**
Endovascular vs. surgical	2 observational (242)	2 moderate risk	Consistent	Direct	Imprecise	ES: 0.21 (-0.34 to 0.76) No difference **Low SOE**
Amputation						
Medical therapy vs. usual care	2 RCT (497)	2 low risk	Inconsistent	Indirect	Imprecise	Only 1 patient underwent amputation **Insufficient SOE**
Exercise vs. usual care	1 RCT (31)	1 moderate risk	NA	Indirect	Not reported	Only 1 patient underwent amputation **Insufficient SOE**
Endovascular vs. usual care	1 RCT, 1 observational (473)	2 moderate risk	Consistent	Indirect	Imprecise	Amputation was similar in endovascular and usual care groups **Insufficient SOE**
Surgical vs. usual care	0	NA	NA	NA	NA	**Insufficient SOE**
Endovascular vs. exercise	1 RCT (149)	1 moderate risk	NA	Indirect	Not reported	One amputation in endovascular group, none in exercise group **Insufficient SOE**
Endovascular vs. surgical	0	NA	NA	NA	NA	**Insufficient SOE**

Table 21. Detailed SOE for IC therapies by comparator (continued)

Comparator	Number of Studies/Design (Total Patients)	Risk of Bias	Consistency	Directness	Precision	SOE and Magnitude of Effect Effect Estimate (95% CI)
Primary patency Secondary patency						
Medical therapy vs. usual care	0	NA	NA	NA	NA	**Insufficient SOE**
Exercise vs. invasive vs. usual care (3-arm study)	1 RCT (225)	1 moderate risk	NA	Indirect	Not reported	Vessel patency was only reported in patients undergoing revascularization (endovascular group 59%, surgical group 98%) **Insufficient SOE**
Surgical vs. usual care	1 observational (427)	1 high risk	NA	Indirect	Not reported	Vessel patency was only reported in patients undergoing revascularization (aortofemoral bypass 95.5%, axillofemoral bypass 83.3%, femoropopliteal bypass 95.5%, femorofemoral bypass (AK) 67.6%, femorofemoral bypass (BK) 45.2% **Insufficient SOE**
Endovascular vs. surgical	0	NA	NA	NA	NA	**Insufficient SOE**
Modifiers of effectiveness (subgroups)						
Medical therapy vs. usual care	2 RCT (155)	2 low risk	NA (reported different outcomes)	Direct	Not reported	Inconclusive evidence due to individual studies reporting different endpoints **Insufficient SOE**
Endovascular vs. usual care	1 observational (526)	1 moderate risk	NA	Indirect	Imprecise	QOL scores were better if ABI improvement was >0.1 after successful revascularization **Insufficient SOE**
Surgical vs. usual care	1 observational (427)	1 high risk	NA	Indirect	Not reported	Patency rates lower for infrainguinal bypass and synthetic graft vs. suprainguinal and autologous vein graft **Insufficient SOE**
Endovascular vs. exercise	1 RCT (56)	1 moderate risk	NA	Indirect	Not reported	Nonsignificant MWD improvement in patients with SFA disease treated with PTA **Insufficient SOE**

Table 21. Detailed SOE for IC therapies by comparator (continued)

Comparator	Number of Studies/Design (Total Patients)	Risk of Bias	Consistency	Directness	Precision	SOE and Magnitude of Effect Effect Estimate (95% CI)
Endovascular vs. surgical	1 RCT (264)	1 moderate risk	NA	Indirect	Imprecise	Patency rates similar for suprainguinal and infrainguinal reconstruction **Insufficient SOE**
Safety concerns						
Medical therapy vs. usual care	10 RCT (3485)	5 low risk, 4 moderate risk, 1 high risk	Consistent	Direct	Precise for headache; imprecise for diarrhea and palpitations	Higher side effects on cilostazol Headache: OR 3.00 (2.29 to 3.95) **High SOE** Diarrhea: OR 2.51 (1.58 to 3.97) **Moderate SOE** Palpitations: OR 18.11 (5.95 to 55.13) **Moderate SOE**
Exercise vs. usual care	3 RCT (107)	2 low risk, 1 moderate risk	Consistent	Indirect	NA	All studies reported no adverse events in exercise or usual care groups **Insufficient SOE**
Endovascular vs. usual care	2 RCT (155)	2 low risk	Inconsistent	Direct	Imprecise	One study reported no events; other study had low rates of transfusion, dissection, and perforation in the endovascular group **Insufficient SOE**
Endovascular vs. exercise	5 RCT (282)	1 low risk, 2 moderate risk	Inconsistent	Indirect	Imprecise	Endovascular interventions were associated with higher rates of transfusion, dissection/perforation, and hematomas **Insufficient SOE**
Composite cardiovascular events **Wound healing** **Analog pain scale** **Safety concerns (subgroups)**						
All	0	NA	NA	NA	NA	**Insufficient SOE**

Abbreviations: ES=effect size; MI=myocardial infarction; MWT=mean walking time; NA=not applicable; OR=odds ratio; QOL=quality of life; RCT=randomized controlled trial; SOE=strength of evidence.

KQ 3. Comparative Effectiveness and Safety of Usual Care and Endovascular and Surgical Revascularization for CLI

KQ 3. In adults with CLI due to PAD:

a. What is the comparative effectiveness of endovascular intervention (percutaneous transluminal angioplasty, atherectomy, or stents) and surgical revascularization (endarterectomy, bypass surgery) for outcomes including cardiovascular events (e.g., all-cause mortality, myocardial infarction, stroke, cardiovascular death), amputation, quality of life, wound healing, analog pain scale score, functional capacity, repeat revascularization, and vessel patency?

b. Does the effectiveness of treatments vary by subgroup (age, sex, race, risk factors, comorbidities, or anatomic location of disease)?

c. What are the significant safety concerns associated with each treatment strategy (e.g., adverse drug reactions, bleeding, contrast nephropathy, radiation, infection, and periprocedural complications causing acute limb ischemia)? Do the safety concerns vary by subgroup (age, sex, race, risk factors, comorbidities, or anatomic location of disease)?

Key Points

Effectiveness of Interventions

- Four observational studies comparing endovascular interventions with usual care reported on mortality, amputation/limb salvage, amputation-free survival, and hospital length of stay. However, because the results were inconsistent and imprecise, SOE was insufficient.
- All-cause mortality was not different between patients treated with endovascular versus surgical revascularization (low SOE) although endovascular interventions did demonstrate a statistically nonsignificant benefit in all-cause mortality at less than 2 years in the IC-CLI population.
- Amputation-free survival was not different between patients treated with endovascular versus surgical revascularization (low SOE).
- Evidence regarding patency rates varied but secondary patency rates demonstrated a benefit of endovascular interventions compared with surgical revascularization across followup time points (low SOE).

Modifiers of Effectiveness

- Seven studies in the CLI population comparing endovascular and surgical interventions, including one RCT and six observational, reported variations in treatment effectiveness by subgroup. Subgroups reported included age (two studies), anatomic factors (two studies), type of vein graft (two studies), and one study each on diabetes and vessel patency. We found no studies reporting results by sex, race, smoking status, or presence

of renal disease. The SOE for modifiers of effectiveness was insufficient given the small number of studies and variety of subgroups that were evaluated.
- Seven studies in the mixed IC-CLI comparing endovascular and surgical interventions, including one RCT and six observational, reported variations in treatment effectiveness by subgroup. Subgroups reported include symptom class (three studies), renal failure (two studies), arterial outflow/runoff (two studies), and one study each reporting age, sex, smoking status, presence of hyperlipidemia, coronary artery disease, diabetes mellitus, hypertension, anatomic location of stenosis, and stent graft size. We found no studies reporting results by patency of intervention or type of conduit (autologous vein or prosthetic material). The SOE for modifiers of effectiveness was insufficient given the small number of studies and variety of subgroups that were evaluated.

Safety Concerns

- One observational study in the CLI population reported safety concerns. Specifically, this study reported the incidence of thrombosis at 30 days and found that the risk of thrombosis was higher in patients undergoing surgical revascularization than in those undergoing endovascular revascularization. The SOE for harms was insufficient in the studies evaluating patients with CLI given the small number of studies reporting this outcome. It may be that treatment harms are not routinely documented or collected in retrospective or prospective observational studies.
- Six studies (2 RCTs, 4 observational) in the mixed IC-CLI population reported harms of bleeding, infection, renal dysfunction, or periprocedural complications causing acute limb ischemia. There were conflicting results in the summary estimates for periprocedural complications in the IC-CLI population with the observational studies showing lower rates in those who received an endovascular intervention and RCTs showing lower rates in the surgical population; however the wide confidence intervals make the differences nonsignificant (low SOE). Infection was more common in the surgical intervention arm based on three studies (one RCT, two observational; low SOE).

Description of Included Studies

We identified 37 unique studies (3 RCTs, 34 observational) that evaluated the comparative effectiveness of usual care, endovascular intervention, and surgical revascularization in CLI or IC-CLI patients. Four observational studies compared usual care with endovascular intervention. Of the 37 studies, 23 evaluated the comparative effectiveness of endovascular and surgical revascularization in 12,779 patients with CLI.[39,99-120] Of these studies, 1 was an RCT (good quality), and 22 were observational (1 good quality, 11 fair, 10 poor). The clinical outcomes of interest included vessel patency, repeat revascularization, wound healing, analog pain scale score, cardiovascular events (e.g., all-cause mortality, MI, stroke, cardiovascular death), amputation, functional capacity, and quality of life. (Characteristics for each study are presented in Table C-3 in Appendix C.)

Of the 37 studies, 12 evaluated the comparative effectiveness of endovascular and surgical revascularization in a *mixed* population involving 565,168 PAD patients with either IC or CLI.[38,121-131] Of these studies, 2 were RCTs (both rated fair quality) and 10 were observational (4 fair, 6 poor). Similar to KQ 2, a majority of the endovascular procedures consisted of PTA with or without stent placement, and the type of stent was not specified.

The following comparisons were assessed in the included studies and are detailed in this analysis:
1. Endovascular intervention versus usual care (3 observational studies of 562 total patients with CLI and 1 observational study of 107 total patients with either IC or CLI)[99,118,132,133]
2. Endovascular intervention versus surgical revascularization (1 RCT and 22 observational studies of 12,779 total patients with CLI and 2 RCTs and 10 observational studies of 565,168 total patients with either IC or CLI)[38,39,99-131]

Detailed Synthesis

Effectiveness of Interventions

1. Endovascular Intervention Versus Usual Care

In the CLI population, three observational studies compared endovascular intervention with usual care in patients (Table 22).[99,118,133] These studies included a total of 562 patients. Of these studies, two were rated fair quality and one poor quality. Sample sizes for individual studies ranged from 70 to 304 patients. Study durations ranged from 12 to 18 months.

The mean age of study participants was 72 to 76 years of age. The proportion of female patients ranged from 30 to 43 percent. None of the studies reported the racial and ethnic demographics of the study participants.

All three studies were conducted in Europe. Funding source was reported as industry in one study,[133] and no funding source was reported in the other two studies.

In the IC-CLI population, one observational study rated fair quality compared endovascular intervention with usual care (Table 22).[132] This study included 107 patients with mean age of 71 years and 14 percent female patients. It did not report racial or ethnic demographics. This study was conducted in Japan with a government funding source.

Table 22. Endovascular intervention versus usual care

Study Population	Type of Study N Analyzed[a] Quality	Outcome Length of Followup	Results Reported by Authors
Patients with CLI			
Lawall, 2009[133] Patients with CLI	Observational N: 70 Poor	Mortality 18 mo	Endovascular intervention: 25.5% Usual care: 26.7%
		Amputation 18 mo	Endovascular intervention: 14.5% Usual care: 26.7%
		Hospital length of stay	Endovascular intervention: 20.9 ± 20.7 days Usual care: 24.4 ± 20.1 days
Varty, 1996[99] Patients with CLI	Observational N: 188 Fair	Mortality 12 mo	Endovascular intervention: 22% Usual care: 48%
		Limb salvage 12 mo	Endovascular intervention: 76% Usual care: not reported
		Hospital length of stay, median	Endovascular intervention: 4.5 days Usual care: not reported
Faglia, 2012[118] Patients with CLI	Observational N: 304 Fair	Mortality 18 mo	Endovascular intervention: 17.1% Usual care: 50%
		Amputation 18 mo	Endovascular intervention: 7.5% Usual care: 75%
		Hospital length of stay, mean	Endovascular intervention: 5.9 ± 3.5 days Usual care: 9.9 ± 2.9 days
Patients with IC or CLI			
Kamiya, 2008[132] Patients with IC or CLI	Observational N: 107 Fair	Mortality 30 mo	Endovascular intervention: 5.5% Usual care: 5.8%
		Amputation 30 mo	Endovascular intervention: 5.5% Usual care: 3.8%

[a]Number of patients in the study arms of interest.
Abbreviation: mo=month/months

Effect on All-Cause Mortality

All four observational studies reported the rate of survival/mortality during the course of followup. In the study by Lawall et al., mortality was slightly lower in the endovascular intervention group (25.5%) compared with usual care (26.7%) at 18 months of followup; however, in the study by Varty et al., mortality was much lower in the endovascular intervention group (22%) compared with usual care (48%) at 12 months of followup, and in the study by Faglia et al., mortality was also much lower in the endovascular group (17.1%) compared with the usual care group (50%) at 18 months of followup. There was no significant difference in the survival/mortality rates in the two comparison groups (5.5% in endovascular intervention and 5.8% in usual care) in Kamiya et al.[132] at 30 months of followup.

Effect on Lower Extremity Amputation/Limb Salvage

All four observational studies also reported the rate of lower extremity amputation or limb salvage (the reverse of amputation) during the course of followup. In Lawall et al. and Faglia et al., the rate of amputation was lower in the endovascular intervention group (14.5% and 7.5% respectively) compared with usual care (26.7% and 75% respectively) at 18 months. In Varty et al., the limb salvage rate was 76 percent at 12 months, but the rate was not reported in the usual care group. In Kamiya et al.,[132] there was no statistically significant difference in amputation rates between the endovascular intervention group (5.5%) compared with the usual care group (3.8%).

Effect on Amputation-Free Survival

Only Lawall et al.[133] reported the rate of amputation-free survival at 18 months of followup, showing the endovascular intervention group at 60 percent compared with the usual care group at 46.7 percent.

Effect on Vessel Patency

None of the studies reported the outcome of vessel patency.

Effect on Hospital Length of Stay

The three observational studies in the CLI population reported the hospital length of stay during the index hospitalization. In Lawall et al., the hospital length of stay was lower in the endovascular intervention group (20.9 ± 20.7 days) compared with the usual care group (24.4 ± 20.1 days) at 18 months. In Faglia et al., the hospital length of stay was also lower in the endovascular group (5.9 ± 3.5 days) compared with the usual care group (9.9 ± 2.9 days). In Varty et al.[99] the median hospital length of stay was 4.5 days at 12 months, but the duration was not reported in the usual care group.

2. Endovascular Intervention Versus Surgical Revascularization

In the CLI population, 23 studies (1 RCT, 22 observational) compared endovascular with surgical revascularization. These studies included a total of 12,779 patients. Of these studies, the RCT[134] was rated good quality, and of the observational studies, 1 was rated good quality, 11 fair quality, and 10 poor quality. Sample sizes for individual studies ranged from 73 to 4929 patients. Study durations ranged from 310 days to 84 months.

The mean age of study participants was 62 to 84 years of age. The proportion of female patients ranged from 1 to 57 percent. Only five studies (25%) reported the racial and ethnic demographics of the study participants.

Five studies (22%) were conducted within the United States or Canada, with the rest international. Funding source was reported in two studies (10%), with government agencies funding both of these studies.

In the IC-CLI population, 12 studies (2 RCTs, 10 observational) compared endovascular with surgical. These studies included a total of 565,168 patients. Of these studies, the 2 RCTs were rated fair quality, 4 of the 10 observational studies were rated fair quality and 6 were poor quality. Sample sizes for individual studies ranged from 44 to 563,143 patients. Study durations ranged from in hospital to 5 years.

The mean age of study participants was 62 to 70 years of age; median age was 66.5 years. The proportion of female patients ranged from 12 to 45 percent. Only one study reported the racial and ethnic demographics of the study participants.

Six studies (55%) were conducted within the United States or Canada, with the rest international. Funding source was reported in five studies (45%), with government, private foundation, nonprofit organization, grant and industry reported as the source of funding.

Effect on All-Cause Mortality

Twenty-four studies (18 in the CLI population and 6 in the IC-CLI population) reported the rate of survival/mortality during the course of followup (Table 23). Meta-analyses of the odds ratios were performed using Comprehensive Meta-Analysis Version 2.0 for short-term followup (≤6 months), intermediate-term followup (1 to 2 years), and long-term followup (≥3 years).

Table 23. Endovascular versus surgical revascularization: all-cause mortality

Study Population	Type of Study N Enrolled or Observed Quality	Outcome Length of Followup	Results Reported by Authors
Patients with CLI			
Adam, 2005[39] BASIL Study Patients with CLI	RCT N: 452 Good	Mortality 6 mo ≥3 yr	6 mo Endovascular: 11.6% Surgical: 13.6% ≥3 yr Endovascular: 37.5% Surgery: 36%
Ah Chong, 2009[100] Patients with CLI	Observational N: 464 Poor	Mortality In-hospital 1 yr 3 yr	In-hospital Endovascular: 3% Surgical: 8% 1yr Endovascular: 20% Surgical: 18% 3 yr Endovascular: 41% Surgical: 34%
Dorigo, 2009[101] Patients with CLI	Observational N: 73 Fair	Mortality 1 yr	Endovascular: 11% Surgical: 37%
Dosluoglu 2012[119] Patients with CLI	Observational N: 433 Fair	Mortality 1 yr 2 yr	1 yr Endovascular: 28% Surgical: 27% 2 yr Endovascular: 40% Surgical: 34%
Faglia, 2012[118] Patients with CLI	Observational N: 332 Fair	Mortality 30 days 18 mo	30 days Endovascular: 0.7% Surgical: 0% 18 mo Endovascular: 17.1% Surgical: 28%
Hynes, 2004[102] Patients with CLI	Observational N: 137 Fair	Mortality 30 days	Femoropopliteal disease (N=102) Endovascular: 0% Surgical: 4% Aortoiliac disease (N=35) Endovascular: 7% Surgical: 0%

Table 23. Endovascular versus surgical revascularization: all-cause mortality (continued)

Study Population	Type of Study N Enrolled or Observed Quality	Outcome Length of Followup	Results Reported by Authors
Johnson, 1997[120] Patients with CLI	Observational N: 150 Fair	Mortality 6 mo 1 yr	6 mo Endovascular: 23% Surgical: 18% 1 yr Endovascular: 27% Surgical: 20%
Korhonen, 2011[105] Patients with CLI	Observational N: 858 Good	Mortality 30 days 1 yr 3 yr	30 days Endovascular: 5.1% Surgical: 2.4% 1 yr Endovascular: 24.3% Surgical: 17.8% 3 yr Endovascular: 41.1% Surgical: 35.0%
Kudo, 2006[106] Patients with CLI	Observational N: 192 (237 limbs) Poor	Mortality 5 yr	Endovascular: 52% Surgical: 54%
Laurila, 2000[107] Patients with CLI	Observational N; 124 (124 limbs) Poor	Mortality 30 days 20 mo	30 days Endovascular: 0% Surgical: 5% 20 mo Endovascular: 20% Surgical: 35%
Loor, 2009[108] Patients with CLI	Observational N: 92 Fair	Mortality 1 yr	Endovascular: 13% Surgical: 24%
Soderstrom, 2010[110] Patients with CLI	Observational N: 1023 Fair	Mortality 30 days 1 yr 5 yr	30 days Endovascular: 3.5% Surgical: 5.8% 1 yr Endovascular: 26.7% Surgical: 24.2% 5 yr Endovascular: 52.5% Surgical: 56.7
Sultan, 2009[109] Patients with CLI	Observational N: 309 Fair	Mortality Perioperative 5 yr	Perioperative Endovascular: 1.6% Surgical: 3.4% 5 yr Endovascular: 78.6% Surgical: 80.1%

Table 23. Endovascular versus surgical revascularization: all-cause mortality (continued)

Study Population	Type of Study N Enrolled or Observed Quality	Outcome Length of Followup	Results Reported by Authors
Taylor, 2006[111] Patients with CLI	Observational N: 841 Poor	Mortality 5 yr	Endovascular: 40.4% Surgical: 41.9%
Varela, 2011[114] Patients with CLI	Observational N: 88 (91 limbs) Fair	Mortality 2 yr	Endovascular: 19% Surgical: 21%
Varty, 1996[99] Patients with CLI	Observational N: 188 Fair	Mortality In-hospital 1 yr	In-hospital Endovascular: 3.7% Surgical: 4% 1yr Endovascular: 22% Surgical: 9%
Wolfle, 2000[116] Patients with CLI	Observational N: 209 Poor	Mortality 30 days 84 mo	30 days Endovascular: 5.9% Surgical: 2.3% 84 mo Endovascular: 37% Surgical: 51%
Zdanowski, 1998[117] Patients with CLI	Observational N: 4929 Poor	Mortality 30 days 1 yr	30 days Endovascular: 5.0% Surgical: 5.4% 1yr Endovascular: 22.9% Surgical: 22.9%
Patients with IC or CLI			
Dosluoglu, 2010[38] Patients with IC or CLI	Observational IC: 38% in endovascular arm, 25% in surgical and hybrid arms CLI: 62% in endovascular arm, 75% in surgical and hybrid arms N: 654 Poor	Mortality 30 days	Endovascular: 1.1% Surgical: 3.1%
Janne d'Othee, 2008[122] Patients with IC or CLI	Observational IC: 97 patients CLI: Not reported N: 97 Fair	Mortality 30 days 1 yr	30 days Endovascular: 0% Surgical: 0% 1 yr Endovascular: 9.4% Surgical: 15.2%
Kashyap, 2008[131] Patients with IC or CLI	Observational IC: 54% in endovascular arm, 51% in surgical arm CLI: 46% in endovascular arm, 49% in surgical arm N: 169 Fair	Mortality 30 days	Endovascular: 4.8% Surgical: 8.1%

Table 23. Endovascular versus surgical revascularization: all-cause mortality (continued)

Study Population	Type of Study N Enrolled or Observed Quality	Outcome Length of Followup	Results Reported by Authors
Lepantalo, 2009[123] Patients with IC or CLI	RCT IC: 87% in endovascular arm, 90% in surgical arm CLI: 13% in endovascular arm, 10% in surgical arm N: 44 Fair	Mortality 30 days 18 mo	30 days Endovascular: 0% Surgical: 0% 18 mo Endovascular: 4.3% Surgical: 9.5%
McQuade, 2009[124] Patients with IC or CLI	RCT IC: 82% in endovascular arm, 62% in surgical arm CLI: 18% in endovascular arm, 38% in surgical arm N: 86 Fair	Mortality 18 mo 2 yr 4 yr	18 mo Endovascular: 8.0% Surgical: 8.0% 2 yr Endovascular: 15.4% Surgical: 12.5% 4 yr Endovascular: 28.1% Surgical: 30.8%
Rossi, 1998[125] Patients with IC or CLI	Observational IC: 24% in endovascular arm, 0% in surgical arm CLI: 76% in endovascular arm, 100% in surgical arm N: 48 Poor	Mortality 1 yr	Endovascular: 27.0% Surgical: 45.5%

Abbreviations: CLI=critical limb ischemia; IC=intermittent claudication; mo=month/months; N=number

Mortality Less Than or Equal to 6 Months After Enrollment

Figure 22 shows the forest plot for the mortality meta-analysis at the ≤6-month time point. One RCT (good quality, CLI population) and 13 observational studies (1 good quality, 6 fair, and 4 poor in the CLI population and 1 fair and 1 poor in the IC-CLI population) reporting the rate of survival/mortality less than or equal to 6 months after enrollment. One RCT[123] and one observational study[122] reported no deaths in either group at 30 days and therefore were not included in the analysis.

Summary estimates for the CLI observational studies (CLI-Obs) were OR 0.85 (95% CI, 0.57 to 1.27, p=0.43); for the CLI RCT study (CLI-RCT), OR 0.51 (CI, 0.20 to 1.35, p=0.18); and for the IC-CLI observational studies (IC-CLI-Obs), OR 0.45 (CI, 0.18 to 1.09, p=0.08). The forest plot shows the comparisons between the summary estimates by study design and population; all estimates favored endovascular intervention although did not reach statistical significance, but this was seen more in the IC-CLI observational studies and the CLI RCT. The overall SOE was rated low for all study populations and study designs, due to the large number of poor- and fair-quality observational studies, with only one good RCT, the inconsistency of the CLI-Obs studies, and imprecision of these findings.

Figure 22. Forest plot for meta-analysis of mortality at ≤6 mo in the CLI and IC-CLI populations

Group by Population	Study name	Odds ratio	Lower limit	Upper limit	p-Value	Death/Total Endovascular	Death/Total Surgical
CLI-Obs	Varty, 1996	0.92	0.19	4.44	0.92	4/108	3/68
CLI-Obs	Johnson, 1997	1.36	0.41	4.49	0.61	6/26	8/44
CLI-Obs	Zdanowski, 1998	0.92	0.69	1.24	0.59	60/1199	201/3730
CLI-Obs	Laurila, 2000	0.07	0.00	1.60	0.10	0/86	2/34
CLI-Obs	Wolfe, 2000	2.66	0.61	11.70	0.19	5/84	3/125
CLI-Obs	Hynes, 2004	0.11	0.00	2.79	0.18	0/74	1/28
CLI-Obs	Ai Chong, 2009	0.36	0.11	1.19	0.09	3/100	29/364
CLI-Obs	Sultan, 2009	0.46	0.10	2.08	0.31	3/190	4/119
CLI-Obs	Soderstrom, 2010	0.59	0.29	1.22	0.15	9/262	44/761
CLI-Obs	Korhonen, 2011	2.19	0.80	5.97	0.13	12/241	6/241
CLI-Obs	Faglia, 2012	0.71	0.03	14.96	0.83	2/292	0/40
CLI-Obs		0.85	0.57	1.27	0.43		
CLI-RCT	Adam, 2005 (BASIL)	0.51	0.20	1.35	0.18	7/237	11/197
CLI-RCT		0.51	0.20	1.35	0.18		
IC-CLI-Obs	Kashyap, 2008	0.57	0.16	2.04	0.39	4/83	7/86
IC-CLI-Obs	Dosluoglu, 2010	0.35	0.10	1.24	0.10	4/356	6/207
IC-CLI-Obs		0.45	0.18	1.09	0.08		

Favors Endovascular | Favors Surgical

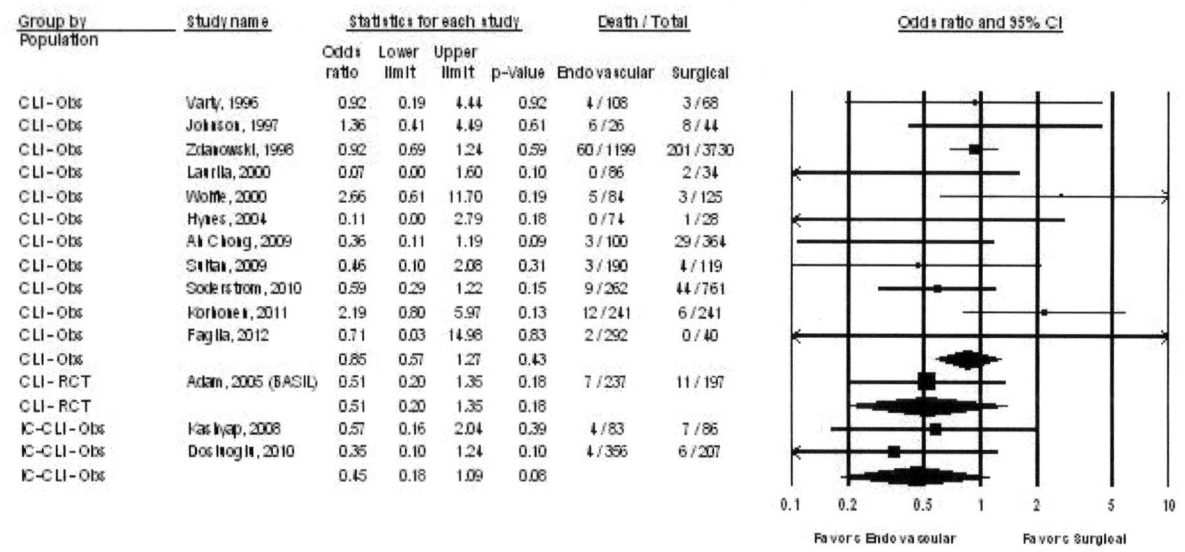

Abbreviations: CI=confidence interval; CLI=critical limb ischemia; IC=intermittent claudication; Obs=observational; RCT=randomized controlled trial.

Mortality at 1 to 2 Years After Enrollment

Figure 23 shows the forest plot for the mortality meta-analysis at the 1- to 2-year time point. Two RCTs (both fair quality in the IC-CLI population) and 14 observational studies (1 good quality, 8 fair, and 3 poor in the CLI population and 1 fair and 1 poor in the IC-CLI population) reporting the rate of survival/mortality at 1 to 2 years after enrollment.

The summary estimates for the CLI observational studies (CLI-Obs) were OR 1.01 (95% CI, 0.80 to 1.28, p=0.91); for the IC-CLI observational studies (IC-CLI-Obs), OR 0.51 (CI, 0.20 to 1.31, p=0.16); and for the IC-CLI RCT studies (IC-CLI-RCT), OR 0.81 (CI, 0.23 to 2.82, p=0.74). The forest plot shows the comparisons between the summary estimates by study design and population. The summary estimate for IC-CLI observational studies favors endovascular intervention although it did not reach statistical significance. The summary estimates of the 10 CLI observational studies and the 2 IC-CLI RCTs also failed to show a significant difference between the two procedures at 1 to 2 years. The overall SOE was rated low on the basis of two RCTs and 12 observational studies, with inconsistent results of a direct outcome and a wide confidence interval.

Figure 23. Forest plot for meta-analysis of mortality at 1-2 yr in the CLI and IC-CLI populations

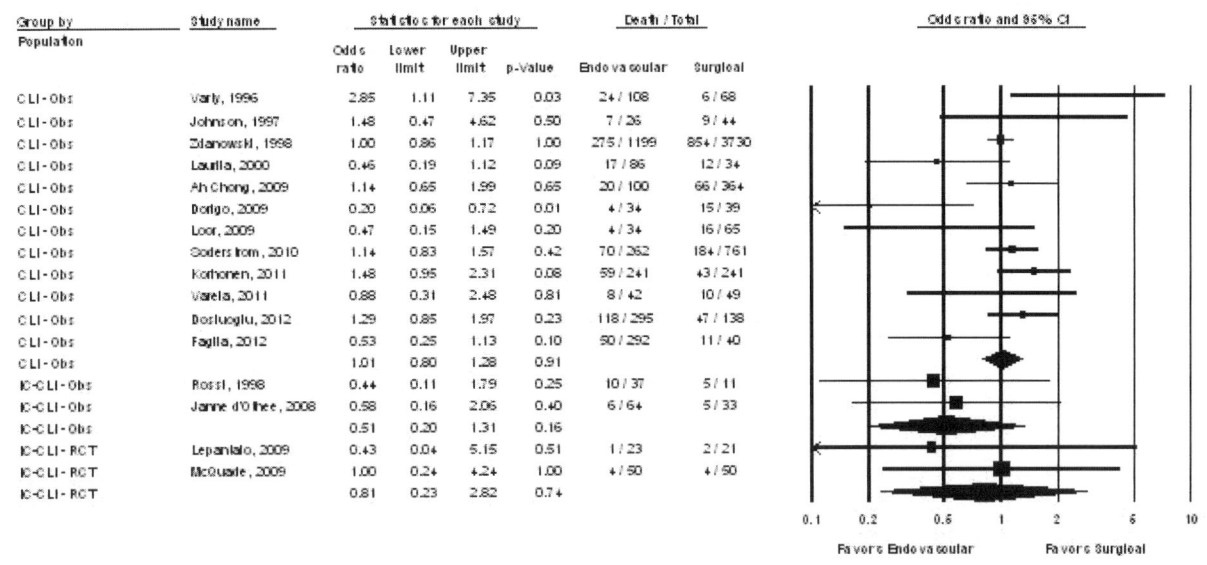

Abbreviations: CI=confidence interval; CLI=critical limb ischemia; IC=intermittent claudication; Obs=observational; RCT=randomized controlled trial.

Mortality at 3 or More Years After Enrollment

Figure 24 shows the forest plot for the mortality meta-analysis at the 3+ year time point. Two RCTs (one good-quality study in the CLI population and one fair-quality study in the IC-CLI population) and seven observational studies (one good quality, three fair, and three poor in the CLI population) reported the rate of survival/mortality at 3+ years after enrollment.

The summary estimates for the CLI observational studies (CLI-Obs) were OR 1.05 (95% CI, 0.54 to 2.06, p=0.88); for the CLI RCT (CLI-RCT), OR 1.07 (CI, 0.73 to 1.56, p=0.74); and for the IC-CLI RCT studies (IC-CLI-RCT), OR 0.88 (CI, 0.28 to 2.73, p=0.82); all demonstrating no difference between treatments. The overall SOE was rated low for the CLI population on the basis of inconsistent results of a direct outcome and a wide confidence interval. The results from the IC-CLI population are inconclusive and therefore the SOE was rated insufficient.

Figure 24. Forest plot for meta-analysis of mortality at ≥3 yr in CLI and IC-CLI populations

Abbreviations: CI=confidence interval; CLI=critical limb ischemia; IC=intermittent claudication; Obs=observational; RCT=randomized controlled trial.

Effect on Nonfatal MI

Only the BASIL study[39] reported the in-hospital rate of nonfatal MI of 3 percent in the endovascular intervention group compared with 8 percent in the surgical group.

Effect on Lower Extremity Amputation

Twenty-one studies (17 in the CLI population and 4 in the IC-CLI population) reported the rate of lower extremity amputation during the course of followup (Table 24). Meta-analyses of the odds ratios were performed using Comprehensive Meta-Analysis Version 2.0 for intermediate-term followup (1 year) and long-term followup (2 to 3 years and 5 or more years).

Table 24. Endovascular versus surgical revascularization: lower extremity amputation

Study Population	Type of Study N Analyzed[a] Quality	Outcome Length of Followup	Results Reported by Authors
Patients with CLI			
Adam, 2005[39] BASIL Study Patients with CLI	RCT N: 452 Good	Amputation 6 mo 1 yr 3 yr	6 mo Endovascular: 4.5% Surgical: 2.6% 1 yr Endovascular: 14.7% Surgical: 12.3% 3 yr Endovascular: 19.2% Surgical: 18.9%
Ah Chong, 2009[100] Patients with CLI	Observational N: 464 Poor	Limb salvage 1 yr 3 yr 5 yr	1 yr Endovascular: 93% Surgical: 82% 3 yr Endovascular: 89% Surgical: 78% 5 yr Endovascular: 77% Surgical: 76%
Dorigo, 2009[101] Patients with CLI	Observational N: 73 Fair	Limb salvage 1 yr	Endovascular: 96.8% Surgical: 88.2%
Dosluoglu 2012[119] Patients with CLI	Observational N: 433 Fair	Limb salvage 5 yr	Endovascular: 78% Surgical: 78%
Faglia, 2012[118] Patients with CLI	Observational N: 332 Fair	Major amputation 30 days 18 mo	30 days Endovascular: 2.7% Surgical: 7.5% 18 mo Endovascular: 7.5% Surgical: 20%
Hynes, 2004[102] Patients with CLI	Observational N: 137 Fair	Limb salvage 1 yr	Femoropopliteal disease (N=102) Endovascular: 97% Surgical: 82% Aortoiliac disease (N=35) Endovascular: 100% Surgical: 86%

Table 24. Endovascular versus surgical revascularization: lower extremity amputation (continued)

Study Population	Type of Study N Analyzed[a] Quality	Outcome Length of Followup	Results Reported by Authors
Korhonen, 2011[105] Patients with CLI	Observational N: 858 Good	Limb salvage 1 yr 3 yr 5 yr	1 yr Endovascular: 87% Surgical: 95% 3 yr Endovascular: 77.0% Surgical: 79.3% 5 yr Endovascular: 75.3% Surgical: 76.0%
Kudo, 2006[106] Patients with CLI	Observational N: 192 (237 limbs) Poor	Limb salvage 5 yr	Endovascular: 91% Surgical: 77%
Loor, 2009[108] Patients with CLI	Observational N: 92 Fair	Limb salvage 1 yr	Endovascular: 87% Surgical: 69%
Soderstrom, 2010[110] Patients with CLI	Observational N: 1023 Fair	Limb salvage 1 yr 3 yr 5 yr	1 yr Endovascular: 85.5% Surgical: 82.2% 3 yr Endovascular: 77.0% Surgical: 79.3% 5 yr Endovascular: 75.3% Surgical: 76.0%
Sultan, 2009[109] Patients with CLI	Observational N: 309 Fair	Major amputation 5 yr	Endovascular: 27.1% Surgical: 28.8%
Taylor, 2005[112]	Observational N: 122 Fair	Limb salvage 2-3 yr	Endovascular: 74.3% Surgical: 82.5%
Taylor, 2006[111] Patients with CLI	Observational N: 841 Poor	Limb Salvage 1 yr	Endovascular: 76.5% Surgical: 82.4%
Varela, 2011[114] Patients with CLI	Observational N: 88 (91 limbs) Fair	Limb salvage 2 yr	Endovascular: 83% Surgical: 72%
Varty, 1996[99] Patients with CLI	Observational N: 188 Fair	Limb salvage 1 yr	1 yr Endovascular: 76% Surgical: 76%
Venermo, 2011[115] Patients with CLI	Observational N: 597 Poor	Limb salvage 1 yr	Endovascular: 88.3% Surgical: 84.9%
Wolfle, 2000[116] Patients with CLI	Observational N: 209 Poor	Limb salvage 1 yr 6 yr	1 yr Endovascular: 82% Surgical: 80% 6 yr Endovascular: 63% Surgical: 69%

Table 24. Endovascular versus surgical revascularization: lower extremity amputation (continued)

Study Population	Type of Study N Analyzed[a] Quality	Outcome Length of Followup	Results Reported by Authors
Patients with IC or CLI			
Dosluoglu, 2010[38] Patients with IC or CLI	Observational IC: 38% in endovascular arm, 25% in surgical and hybrid arms CLI: 62% in endovascular arm, 75% in surgical and hybrid arms N: 654 Poor	Amputation 30 days Limb salvage 1 yr 3 yr	30 days Endovascular: 2.1% Surgical: 1.8% 1 yr Endovascular: 86% Surgical: 80% 3 yr Endovascular: 80% Surgical: 74%
Kashyap, 2008[131] Patients with IC or CLI	Observational IC: 54% in endovascular arm, 51% in surgical arm CLI: 46% in endovascular arm, 49% in surgical arm N: 169 Fair	Amputation 1 yr 2 yr 3 yr	1 yr Endovascular: 2% Surgical: 2% 2 yr Endovascular: 2% Surgical: 2% 3yr Endovascular: 2% Surgical: 2%
Lepantalo, 2009[123] Patients with IC or CLI	RCT IC: 87% in endovascular arm, 90% in surgical arm CLI: 13% in endovascular arm, 10% in surgical arm N: 44 Fair	Amputation 18 mo	Endovascular: 0% Surgical: 4.8%
McQuade, 2009[124] Patients with IC or CLI	RCT IC: 82% in endovascular arm, 62% in surgical arm CLI: 18% in endovascular arm, 38% in surgical arm N: 86 Fair	Amputation 18 mo 2 yr 4 yr	18 mo Endovascular: 3.1% Surgical: 13.5% 2 yr Endovascular: 2.6% Surgical: 12.5% 4 yr Endovascular: 3.1% Surgical: 23.1%

[a]Number of patients in the study arms of interest.
Abbreviations: CLI=critical limb ischemia; IC=intermittent claudication; mo=month/months; yr=year/years.

Amputation at Less Than 2 Years After Enrollment

Figure 25 shows the forest plot for the amputation meta-analysis at the less than 2 year time point. Three RCTs (one good quality in the CLI population and two fair quality in the IC-CLI population) and 13 observational studies (1 good quality, 6 fair, and 3 poor in the CLI population and 1 fair and 1 poor in the IC-CLI population) reported the rate of amputation at less than 2 years after enrollment.

The summary estimates did not demonstrate a difference for the CLI observational studies (CLI-Obs) OR 0.73 (95% CI, 0.48 to 1.09, p=0.12); for the CLI RCT study (CLI-RCT), OR 1.23 (CI, 0.72 to 2.11, p=0.46); or for the IC-CLI observational studies (IC-CLI-Obs), OR 1.11 (CI,

0.40 to 3.05, p=0.84). The IC-CLI RCT studies (IC-CLI-RCT) showed a trend toward a benefit of endovascular intervention but did not reach statistical significance, OR 0.22 (CI, 0.05 to 1.07, p=0.06). The forest plot shows the comparisons between the summary estimates by study design and population. There was heterogeneity within and between populations and between study designs. The observational studies are influenced by selection bias. The differences in the RCT population results are due to the PAD severity, such that the IC-CLI RCTs favor endovascular intervention (although with confidence intervals crossing 1), and the CLI RCT does not demonstrate a difference. The overall SOE was rated low for the CLI population on the basis of inconsistent results of a direct outcome and a wide confidence interval. The results from the IC-CLI population are inconclusive and therefore the SOE was rated insufficient.

Figure 25. Forest plot for meta-analysis of amputation at less than 2 years in the CLI and IC-CLI populations

Group by Population	Study name	Odds ratio	Lower limit	Upper limit	p-Value	Endovascular	Surgical
CLI-Obs	Varty, 1996	1.00	0.49	2.03	1.00	26/108	16/68
CLI-Obs	Hynes, 2004	0.14	0.03	0.73	0.02	2/74	5/28
CLI-Obs	Taylor, 2006	1.44	1.01	2.04	0.04	71/302	90/513
CLI-Obs	Ah Chong, 2009	0.34	0.15	0.77	0.01	7/100	66/364
CLI-Obs	Loor, 2009	0.33	0.11	1.03	0.06	4/34	20/65
CLI-Obs	Wolfle, 2009	0.88	0.43	1.78	0.72	15/84	25/125
CLI-Obs	Dorigo, 2009	0.25	0.03	2.11	0.20	1/34	5/39
CLI-Obs	Soderstrom, 2010	0.78	0.53	1.16	0.22	38/262	135/761
CLI-Obs	Korhonen, 2011	2.84	1.42	5.66	0.00	31/241	12/241
CLI-Obs	Venermo, 2011	0.74	0.49	1.14	0.18	44/377	54/355
CLI-Obs	Faglia, 2012	0.32	0.13	0.79	0.01	22/292	8/40
CLI-Obs		0.73	0.48	1.09	0.12		
CLI-RCT	Adam, 2005 (BASIL)	1.23	0.72	2.11	0.46	33/224	28/228
CLI-RCT		1.23	0.72	2.11	0.46		
IC-CLI-Obs	Kashyap, 2008	1.00	0.18	5.54	1.00	3/125	3/144
IC-CLI-Obs	Dosluoglu, 2010	1.17	0.33	4.10	0.81	7/356	4/207
IC-CLI-Obs		1.11	0.40	3.05	0.84		
IC-CLI-RCT	Lepantalo, 2009	0.29	0.01	7.54	0.46	0/23	1/21
IC-CLI-RCT	McQuade, 2009	0.20	0.03	1.23	0.08	2/50	7/50
IC-CLI-RCT		0.22	0.05	1.07	0.06		

Favors Endovascular   Favors Surgical

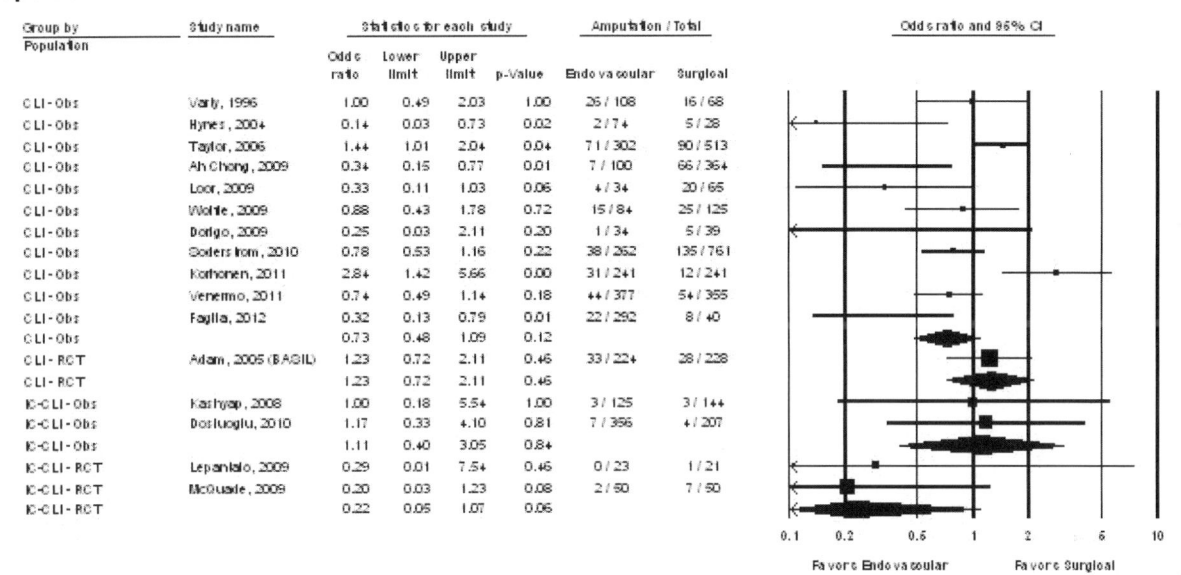

Abbreviations: CI=confidence interval; CLI=critical limb ischemia; IC=intermittent claudication; Obs=observational; RCT=randomized controlled trial.

Amputation at 2 to 3 Years After Enrollment

Figure 26 shows the forest plot for the amputation meta-analysis at the 2- to 3-year time point. Two RCTs (one good quality in the CLI population and one fair quality in the IC-CLI population) and five observational studies (one good quality, two fair, and one poor in the CLI population and one fair in the IC-CLI population) reported the rate of amputation at 2 to 3 years after enrollment.

The summary estimates for the CLI observational studies (CLI-Obs) were OR 1.08 (95% CI, 0.62 to 1.89, p=0.78); for the CLI RCT study (CLI-RCT), OR 1.02 (CI, 0.64 to 1.63, p=0.94); and for the IC-CLI observational studies (IC-CLI-Obs), OR 1.00 (CI, 0.18 to 5.54, p=1.00); all demonstrating no difference between treatments. For the IC-CLI RCT study (IC-CLI-RCT), a trend toward a benefit of endovascular interventions was seen, OR 0.18 (CI, 0.03 to 1.29, p=0.09) but it did not reach statistical significance. The forest plot shows the comparisons between the summary estimates by study design and population. Given the small number of events and total study populations in the IC-CLI observational and RCT studies, the differences in the summary estimate are likely to change with the addition of studies. The overall SOE was rated low for the CLI population. The results from the IC-CLI population are inconclusive and therefore the SOE was rated insufficient.

Figure 26. Forest plot for meta-analysis of amputation at 2 to 3 years in the CLI and IC-CLI populations

Group by Population	Study name	Statistics for each study: Odds ratio	Lower limit	Upper limit	p-Value	Amputation / Total: Endovascular	Surgical
CLI-Obs	Taylor, 2005	1.63	0.68	3.90	0.27	15 / 57	11 / 65
CLI-Obs	Ah Chong, 2009	0.44	0.22	0.86	0.02	11 / 100	80 / 364
CLI-Obs	Soderstrom, 2010	1.14	0.74	1.77	0.55	36 / 158	89 / 431
CLI-Obs	Korhonen, 2011	1.66	1.00	2.77	0.05	44 / 241	28 / 241
CLI-Obs		1.08	0.62	1.89	0.78		
CLI-RCT	Adam, 2005 (BASIL)	1.02	0.64	1.63	0.94	43 / 224	43 / 228
CLI-RCT		1.02	0.64	1.63	0.94		
IC-CLI-Obs	Kashyap, 2008	1.00	0.18	5.54	1.00	3 / 125	3 / 144
IC-CLI-Obs		1.00	0.18	5.54	1.00		
IC-CLI-RCT	McQuade, 2009	0.18	0.03	1.29	0.09	1 / 50	6 / 50
IC-CLI-RCT		0.18	0.03	1.29	0.09		

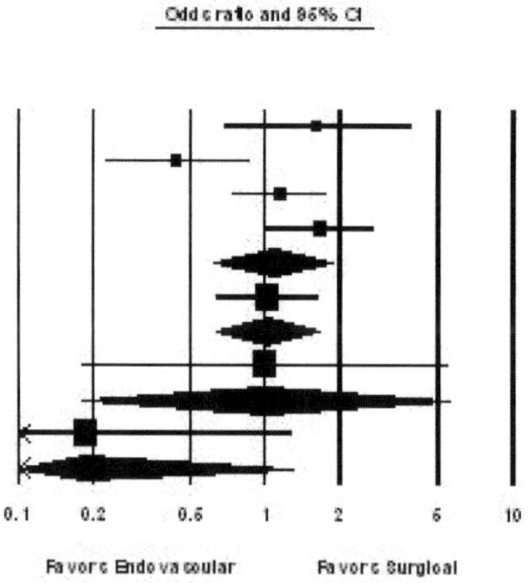

Abbreviations: CI=confidence interval; CLI=critical limb ischemia; IC=intermittent claudication; Obs=observational; RCT=randomized controlled trial.

Amputation at 5 Years After Enrollment

Figure 27 shows the forest plot for this meta-analysis in the CLI population. Seven observational studies (one good quality, three fair, and three poor) reporting the rate of lower extremity amputation after 5 years found that the odds ratio for endovascular intervention was 1.06 (95% CI, 0.70 to 1.59, p=0.79) showing no statistically significant difference in revascularization strategies in the long term. There was evidence of extreme heterogeneity, with a Q-value of 24.69 for 5 degrees of freedom, p<0.001. The cause of heterogeneity is not readily apparent since all are single-center studies comparing angioplasty with surgical bypass. In some studies, concomitant therapy with clopidogrel, aspirin, and/or LMWH was described. The overall SOE was rated low on the basis of only observational studies with inconsistent results of a direct outcome and a wide confidence interval.

Figure 27. Forest plot for meta-analysis of amputation after 5 years in the CLI population

Population	Study name	Statistics for each study: Odds ratio	Lower limit	Upper limit	p-Value	Amputation / Total: Endovascular	Surgical
CLI-Obs	Kudo, 2006	0.33	0.16	0.70	0.00	14 / 153	19 / 84
CLI-Obs	Ah Chong, 2009	0.95	0.56	1.60	0.84	23 / 100	87 / 364
CLI-Obs	Sultan, 2009	0.92	0.55	1.53	0.75	51 / 190	34 / 119
CLI-Obs	Wolfe, 2009	1.31	0.73	2.34	0.37	31 / 84	39 / 125
CLI-Obs	Soderstrom, 2010	1.04	0.68	1.59	0.86	39 / 158	103 / 431
CLI-Obs	Korhonen, 2011	3.12	1.80	5.42	0.00	53 / 241	20 / 241
CLI-Obs	Dosluoglu, 2012	1.00	0.61	1.63	1.00	65 / 295	30 / 138
		1.06	0.70	1.59	0.79		

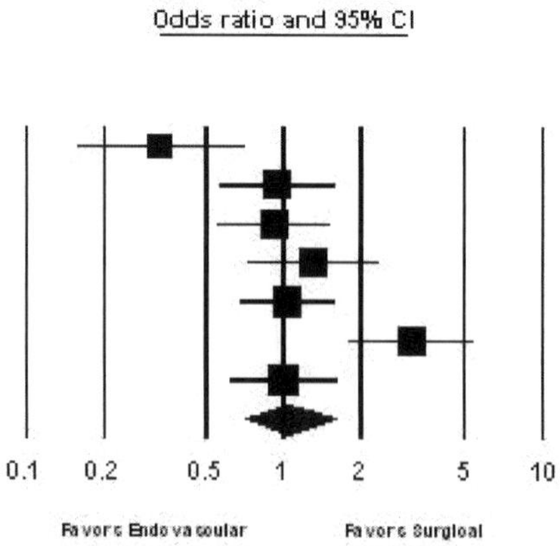

Abbreviations: CI=confidence interval; CLI=critical limb ischemia; IC=intermittent claudication; Obs=observational; RCT=randomized controlled trial.

There were no studies of the IC-CLI population with longer than 5 years of followup. The overall SOE of the amputation outcome was rated insufficient for the mixed PAD population at 5 or more years.

Effect on Amputation-Free Survival

Seven studies in the CLI population reported the rate of amputation-free survival (time to death or major amputation during followup) (Table 25). From the studies of IC-CLI population, only two reported amputation-free survival. Both studies were observational; one was a report from an administrative dataset,[126] and one was a study that reported data from a subgroup of hemodialysis-dependent patients.[121] Therefore, these studies were not included in the meta-analysis. The Zdanowski study was not included in the meta-analysis since it was the only study with a 30-day followup.[117] Meta-analyses of the odds ratios were performed using Comprehensive Meta-Analysis Version 2.0 for intermediate-term followup (1 year) and long-term followup (2 to 3 years and 5 or more years).

Table 25. Endovascular versus surgical revascularization: amputation-free survival

Study Population	Type of Study N Analyzed[a] Quality	Outcome Length of Followup	Results Reported by Authors
Patients with CLI			
Adam, 2005[39] BASIL Study Patients with CLI	RCT N: 452 Good	Amputation-free survival 1 yr 3 yr	1 yr Endovascular: 68% Surgical: 71% 3 yr Endovascular: 57% Surgical: 52%
Dosluoglu 2012[119] Patients with CLI	Observational N: 433 Fair	Amputation-free survival 5 yr	Endovascular: 30% Surgical: 39%
Korhonen, 2011[105] Patients with CLI	Observational N: 858 Good	Amputation-free survival 1 yr 2 yr 3 yr 5 yr	1 yr Endovascular: 70.0% Surgical: 79.9% 2 yr Endovascular: 60.2% Surgical: 72.6% 3 yr Endovascular: 52.1% Surgical: 61.0% 5 yr Endovascular: 42.0% Surgical: 53.7%

Table 25. Endovascular versus surgical revascularization: amputation-free survival (continued)

Study Population	Type of Study N Analyzed[a] Quality	Outcome Length of Followup	Results Reported by Authors
Soderstrom, 2010[110] Patients with CLI	Observational N: 1023 Fair	Amputation-free survival 1 yr 3 yr 5 yr	1 yr Endovascular: 64.6% Surgical: 65.9% 3 yr Endovascular: 43.6% Surgical: 49.1% 5 yr Endovascular: 37.7% Surgical: 37.3%
Sultan, 2009[109] Patients with CLI	Observational N: 309 Fair	Amputation-free survival 5 yr	Endovascular: 72.9% Surgical: 71.2%
Varela, 2011[114] Patients with CLI	Observational N: 88 (91 limbs) Fair	Amputation-free survival 2 yr	Endovascular: 73% Surgical: 66%
Zdanowski, 1998[117] Patients with CLI	Observational N: 4929 Poor	Amputation-free survival 30 days	Endovascular: 90% Surgical: 89.8%

[a]Number of patients in the study arms of interest.
Abbreviations: CLI=critical limb ischemia; IC=intermittent claudication; mo=month/months; RCT=randomized controlled trial; yr=year/years.

Amputation-Free Survival at 1 Year After Enrollment

Figure 28 shows the forest plot for this meta-analysis of two observational studies (1 good, 1 fair) and one RCT (good quality) reporting the rate of amputation-free survival. The observational studies found a summary odds ratio for endovascular versus surgical revascularization of 0.76 (95% CI, 0.48 to 1.21, p=0.24) favoring endovascular treatment at 1 year, which was not statistically significant. The odds ratio for the RCT[39] was 0.87 (CI, 0.58 to 1.30, p=0.49) and is consistent with the findings from the two observational studies. There was no evidence of heterogeneity, with a Q-value of 3.26 for 2 degrees of freedom, p=0.20. The summary estimate is provided in the figure because of the similar patient population and consistency of findings. The overall SOE was rated low.

Figure 28. Forest plot for meta-analysis of amputation-free survival at 1 year in the CLI population

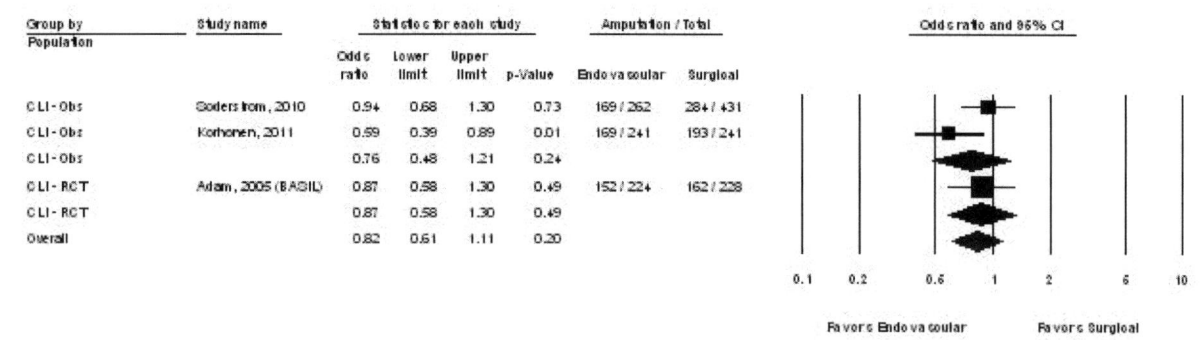

Abbreviations: CI=confidence interval; CLI=critical limb ischemia; Obs=observational; RCT=randomized controlled trial.

Amputation-Free Survival at 2 to 3 Years After Enrollment

Figure 29 shows the forest plot for this meta-analysis of one good-quality RCT and three observational studies (one good, two fair) reporting the rate of amputation-free survival at 2 to 3 years. The summary estimate for the observational studies (CLI-Obs) was OR 0.76 (95% CI, 0.53 to 1.09, p=0.13). The odds ratio for the RCT was 1.22 (CI, 0.84 to 1.77, p=0.29).

There was evidence of heterogeneity, with both the Adam (RCT)[39] and Varela[114] studies favoring surgical revascularization. In the Varela study, the event rate was based on the number of affected limbs while the other analyses were at the patient level. The Adam study is an older RCT; therefore the advances in endovascular technique may affect the summary estimate. The overall SOE was rated low on the basis of one good-quality RCT and three observational studies with inconsistent results of a direct outcome and a wide confidence interval.

Figure 29. Forest plot for meta-analysis of amputation-free survival at 2 to 3 years in the CLI population

Group by Population	Study name	Odds ratio	Lower limit	Upper limit	p-Value	Endovascular	Surgical
CLI - Obs	Soderstrom, 2010	0.80	0.59	1.09	0.16	114 / 262	212 / 431
CLI - Obs	Varela, 2011	1.34	0.58	3.11	0.50	26 / 42	27 / 49
CLI - Obs	Korhonen, 2011	0.57	0.39	0.84	0.00	145 / 241	175 / 241
CLI - Obs		0.76	0.53	1.09	0.13		
CLI - RCT	Adam, 2005 (BASIL)	1.22	0.84	1.77	0.29	128 / 224	119 / 228
CLI - RCT		1.22	0.84	1.77	0.29		

Favors Endovascular — Favors Surgical

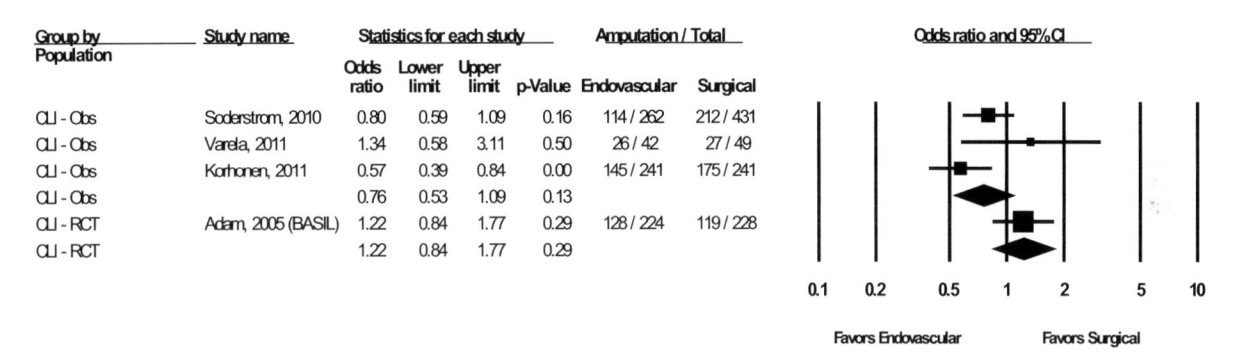

Abbreviations: CI=confidence interval; CLI=critical limb ischemia; Obs=observational; RCT=randomized controlled trial.

Amputation-Free Survival 5 Years After Enrollment

Figure 30 shows the forest plot for this meta-analysis. Four observational studies (one good quality, three fair) reporting the rate of amputation-free survival found that the odds ratio for endovascular versus surgical revascularization was 0.89 (95% CI, 0.59 to 1.34, p=0.58), showing no statistically significant difference in revascularization strategies in the long term. There was evidence of heterogeneity, with a Q-value of 12.80 for 3 degrees of freedom, p=0.005. Differences in selection bias, study location, and use of antiplatelet therapy may explain the differences among the Korhonen study,[105] the Dosluoglu study,[119] and the other studies. The overall SOE was rated low on the basis of only observational studies with inconsistent results of a direct outcome and a wide confidence interval.

Figure 30. Forest plot for meta-analysis of amputation-free survival after 5 years in the CLI population

Population	Study name	Statistics for each study: Odds ratio	Lower limit	Upper limit	p-Value	Amputation / Total: Endovascular	Surgical
CLI-Obs	Soderstrom, 2010	1.37	0.99	1.90	0.06	97 / 262	129 / 431
CLI-Obs	Korhonen, 2011	0.62	0.44	0.89	0.01	101 / 241	129 / 241
CLI-Obs	Sultan, 2011	1.09	0.65	1.81	0.75	139 / 190	85 / 119
CLI-Obs	Dosluoglu, 2012	0.67	0.44	1.02	0.06	89 / 295	54 / 138
		0.89	0.59	1.34	0.58		

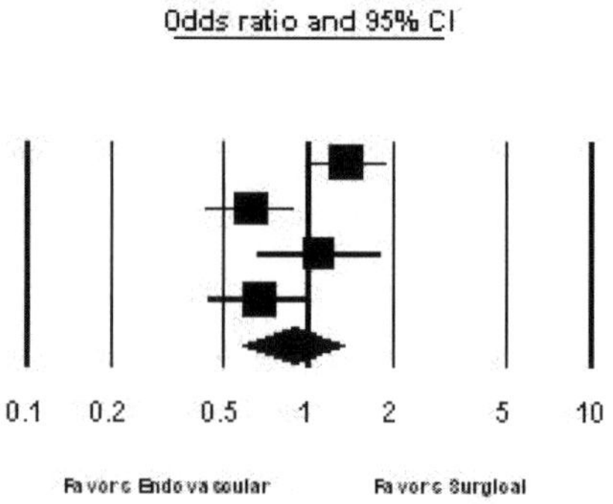

Abbreviations: CI=confidence interval; CLI=critical limb ischemia; Obs=observational; RCT=randomized controlled trial.

Effect on Wound Healing

One study in the CLI population (fair quality)[114] reported the incidence of wound healing during the study followup. The percentage of patients with wound healing and the mean time to wound healing were both improved with surgical revascularization when compared with endovascular revascularization. Due to a single study reporting this outcome, the SOE was rated insufficient.

Effect on Vessel Patency

Fourteen studies reported the rate of vessel patency during the course of followup (Table 26). Nine studies in the CLI population and five studies in the IC-CLI population reported the rate of primary patency (following initial intervention), and eight studies in the CLI population and two studies in the IC-CLI population reported the rate of secondary patency (following screening and repeat intervention, often referred to as assisted patency). Meta-analyses of the odds ratios were performed using Comprehensive Meta-Analysis Version 2.0 for intermediate-term followup (1 year) and long-term followup (2 to 3 years).

Table 26. Endovascular versus surgical revascularization: vessel patency

Study Population	Type of Study N Analyzed[a] Quality	Outcome Length of Followup	Results Reported by Authors
Patients with CLI			
Ah Chong, 2009[100] Patients with CLI	Observational N: 464 Poor	Primary patency 1 yr 3 yr Secondary patency 1 yr 3 yr	Primary patency 1 yr Endovascular: 48% Surgical: 65% 3 yr Endovascular: 27% Surgical: 65% Secondary patency 1 yr Endovascular: 61% Surgical: 74% 3 yr Endovascular: 31% Surgical: 58%
Dorigo, 2009[101] Patients with CLI	Observational N: 73 Fair	Primary patency 1 yr Secondary patency 1 yr	Endovascular: 58.9% Surgical: 67.9% Endovascular: 67.9% Surgical: 81.9%
Dosluoglu 2012[119] Patients with CLI	Observational N: 433 Fair	Primary patency 5 yr Secondary patency 5 yr	Endovascular: 50% Surgical: 48% Endovascular: 73% Surgical: 64%
Hynes, 2004[102] Patients with CLI	Observational N: 137 Fair	Primary patency 2 yr Secondary patency 2 yr	Femoropopliteal disease (N=102) Endovascular: 84% Surgical: 68% Aortoiliac disease (N=35) Endovascular: 93% Surgical:81% Femoropopliteal disease (N=102) Endovascular: 98% Surgical: 100% Aortoiliac disease (N=35) Endovascular: 100% Surgical: 95%
Jerabek, 2003[103] Patients with CLI	Observational N: 131 Poor	Primary patency 18 mo	Endovascular: 83.3% Surgical: 87.4%
Kudo, 2006[106] Patients with CLI	Observational N: 192 (237 limbs) Poor	Primary patency 5 yr Secondary patency 5 yr	Endovascular: 44% Surgical: 28% Endovascular: 88% Surgical: 57%

Table 26. Endovascular versus surgical revascularization: vessel patency (continued)

Study Population	Type of Study N Analyzed[a] Quality	Outcome Length of Followup	Results Reported by Authors
Loor, 2009[108] Patients with CLI	Observational N: 92 Fair	Primary patency 1 yr Secondary patency 1 yr	Endovascular: 63% Surgical: 64% Endovascular: 76% Surgical: 75%
Taylor, 2005[112] Patients with CLI	Observational N: 122 Fair	Primary patency 1 yr 2 yr 3 yr Secondary patency 1 yr 2 yr 3 yr	Primary patency 1 yr Endovascular: 62.0% Surgical: 67.7% 2 yr Endovascular: 55.3% Surgical: 63.3% 3 yr Endovascular: 48.4% Surgical: 60.5% Secondary patency 1 yr Endovascular: 74.1% Surgical: 87.4% 2 yr Endovascular: 70.7% Surgical: 80.1% 3 yr Endovascular: 63.7% Surgical: 80.1%
Varela, 2011[114] Patients with CLI	Observational N: 88 (91 limbs) Fair	Primary patency 2 yr Secondary patency 2 yr	Endovascular: 76% Surgical: 72% Endovascular: 82% Surgical: 82%
Patients with IC or CLI			
Janne d'Othee, 2008[122] Patients with IC or CLI	Observational IC: 97 patients CLI: Not reported N: 97 Fair	Primary patency Secondary patency 30 days 1 yr	Primary patency 30 day Endovascular: 98% Surgical: 100% 1 yr Endovascular: 94% Surgical: 95% Secondary patency 30 day Endovascular: 100% Surgical: 100%

108

Table 26. Endovascular versus surgical revascularization: vessel patency (continued)

Study Population	Type of Study N Analyzed[a] Quality	Outcome Length of Followup	Results Reported by Authors
Kashyap, 2008[131] Patients with IC or CLI	Observational IC: 54% in endovascular arm, 51% in surgical arm CLI: 46% in endovascular arm, 49% in surgical arm N: 169 Fair	Primary patency 1 yr 2 yr 3 yr	1 yr Endovascular: 90% Surgical: 93% 2 yr Endovascular: 92% Surgical: 93% 3 yr Endovascular: 74% Surgical: 93%
Lepantalo, 2009[123] Patients with IC or CLI	RCT IC: 87% in endovascular arm, 90% in surgical arm CLI: 13% in endovascular arm, 10% in surgical arm N: 44 Fair	Primary patency 1 yr	Primary patency Endovascular: 46% Surgical: 84% Secondary patency Endovascular: 63% Surgical: 100%
McQuade, 2009[124] Patients with IC or CLI	RCT IC: 82% in endovascular arm, 62% in surgical arm CLI: 18% in endovascular arm, 38% in surgical arm N: 86 Fair	Primary patency 1 yr 2 yr 3 yr 4 yr	1 yr Endovascular: 72% Surgical: 76% 2 yr Endovascular: 63% Surgical: 63% 3 yr Endovascular: 63% Surgical: 63% 4 yr Endovascular: 59% Surgical: 58%
Timaran, 2003[129] Patients with IC or CLI	Observational IC: 59% of total population CLI: 41% of total population N: 62 patients (68 procedures) Poor	Primary patency 1 yr 3 yr	1 yr Endovascular: 85% Surgical: 89% 3 yr Endovascular: 72% Surgical: 86%

[a]Number of patients in the study arms of interest.
Abbreviations: CLI=critical limb ischemia; IC=intermittent claudication; mo=month/months; yr=year/years.

Primary Patency at 1 Year After Enrollment

Figure 31 shows the forest plot for the primary patency meta-analysis at the 1-year time point. Two RCTs (both fair quality in the IC-CLI population) and eight observational studies (three fair and two poor in the CLI population and three fair in the IC-CLI population) reported the rate of primary patency at 1 year after enrollment.

The summary estimates for the CLI observational studies (CLI-Obs) were OR 0.63 (95% CI, 0.46 to 0.86, p=0.00); for the IC-CLI observational studies (IC-CLI-Obs), OR 0.71 (CI, 0.40 to 1.28, p=0.26); and for the IC-CLI RCT studies (IC-CLI-RCT), OR 0.40 (CI, 0.08 to 1.93, p=0.26). The forest plot shows the comparisons between the summary estimates by study design and population. The CLI observational studies (three fair quality and two poor) are consistent, direct, and precise (moderate SOE). The overall SOE was rated low for the IC-CLI observational studies and RCTs due to the inconsistency and imprecision.

Figure 31. Forest plot for meta-analysis of primary patency at 1 year in the CLI and IC-CLI populations

Group by Population	Study name	Odds ratio	Lower limit	Upper limit	p-Value	Endovascular	Surgical
CLI-Obs	Jerabek, 2003	0.72	0.25	2.10	0.55	30/36	83/95
CLI-Obs	Taylor, 2005	0.78	0.37	1.64	0.51	40/65	39/57
CLI-Obs	Ah Chong, 2009	0.50	0.32	0.78	0.00	48/100	237/364
CLI-Obs	Dorigo, 2009	0.68	0.26	1.77	0.43	20/34	26/39
CLI-Obs	Loor, 2009	0.96	0.40	2.27	0.92	21/34	42/65
CLI-Obs		0.63	0.46	0.86	0.00		
IC-CLI-Obs	Timaran, 2003	0.70	0.26	1.88	0.48	116/136	46/52
IC-CLI-Obs	d'O hee, 2008	0.82	0.22	3.16	0.78	104/111	65/68
IC-CLI-Obs	Kashyap, 2008	0.68	0.28	1.61	0.38	113/125	134/144
IC-CLI-Obs		0.71	0.40	1.28	0.26		
IC-CLI-RCT	Lepantalo, 2009	0.16	0.04	0.69	0.01	10/21	18/21
IC-CLI-RCT	McQuade, 2009	0.81	0.33	1.99	0.65	36/50	38/50
IC-CLI-RCT		0.40	0.08	1.93	0.25		

Favors Endovascular   Favors Surgical

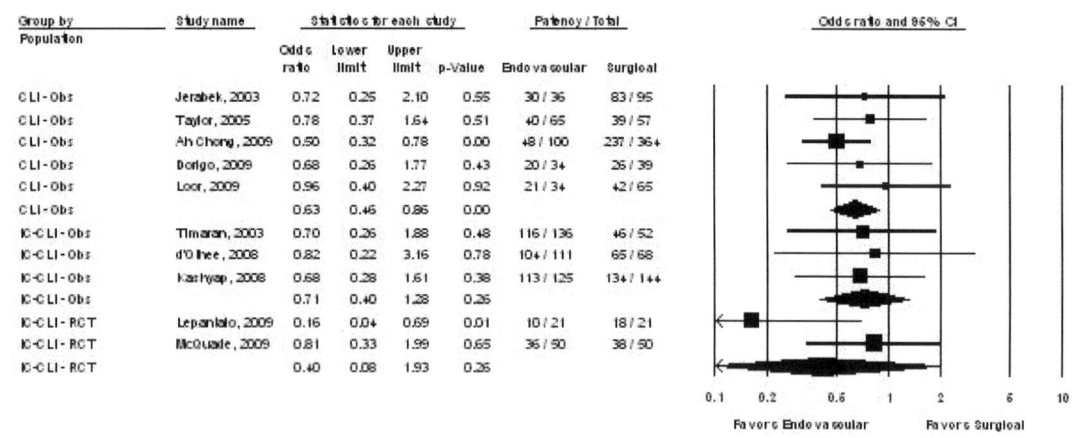

Abbreviations: CI=confidence interval; CLI=critical limb ischemia; IC=intermittent claudication; Obs=observational; RCT=randomized controlled trial.

Primary Patency at 2 to 3 Years After Enrollment

Figure 32 shows the forest plot for the primary patency meta-analysis at the 2- to 3-year time point. One RCT (fair quality in the IC-CLI population) and six observational studies (three fair and one poor in the CLI population and two fair in the IC-CLI population) reporting the rate of primary patency at 2-3 years after enrollment.

The summary estimate for the CLI observational studies (CLI-Obs) was inconclusive, OR 0.77 (95% CI, 0.24 to 2.42, p=0.65). The summary estimate showed a trend toward a benefit of endovascular intervention for the IC-CLI observational studies (IC-CLI-Obs), OR 0.29 (CI, 0.15 to 0.55, p=0.00). The summary estimate did not demonstrate a difference for the IC-CLI RCT study (IC-CLI-RCT), OR 0.96 (CI, 0.42 to 2.16, p=0.92). The forest plot shows the comparisons between the summary estimates by study design and population. The overall SOE was rated insufficient for the CLI and IC-CLI populations on the basis of inconsistent results with wide confidence intervals.

Figure 32. Forest plot for meta-analysis of primary patency at 2 to 3 years in the CLI and IC-CLI populations

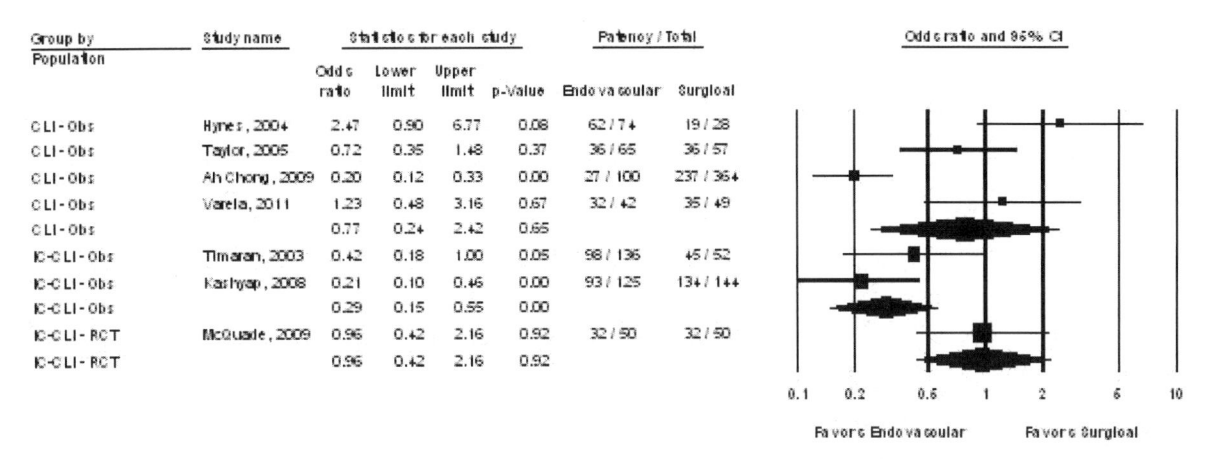

Group by Population	Study name	Odds ratio	Lower limit	Upper limit	p-Value	Endovascular	Surgical
CLI-Obs	Hynes, 2004	2.47	0.90	6.77	0.08	62/74	19/28
CLI-Obs	Taylor, 2005	0.72	0.35	1.48	0.37	36/65	36/57
CLI-Obs	Ah Chong, 2009	0.20	0.12	0.33	0.00	27/100	237/364
CLI-Obs	Varela, 2011	1.23	0.48	3.16	0.67	32/42	35/49
CLI-Obs		0.77	0.24	2.42	0.65		
IC-CLI-Obs	Timaran, 2003	0.42	0.18	1.00	0.05	98/136	45/52
IC-CLI-Obs	Kashyap, 2008	0.21	0.10	0.46	0.00	93/125	134/144
IC-CLI-Obs		0.29	0.15	0.55	0.00		
IC-CLI-RCT	McQuade, 2009	0.96	0.42	2.16	0.92	32/50	32/50
IC-CLI-RCT		0.96	0.42	2.16	0.92		

Abbreviations: CI=confidence interval; CLI=critical limb ischemia; IC=intermittent claudication; Obs=observational; RCT=randomized controlled trial.

Secondary Patency at 1 Year After Enrollment

Figure 33 shows the forest plot for the secondary patency meta-analysis at the 1 year time point. One additional RCT was excluded from this analysis because both the endovascular and surgical groups had 100 percent secondary patency.[122] One RCT (fair quality in the IC-CLI population) and four observational studies (three fair and one poor in the CLI population) reporting the rate of secondary patency at 1 year after enrollment.

The summary estimates for the CLI observational studies (CLI-Obs) were OR 0.57 (95% CI, 0.40 to 0.82, p=0.002) and for the IC-CLI RCT study (IC-CLI-RCT), OR 0.04 (CI, 0.00 to 0.73, p=0.03). The forest plot shows the comparisons between the summary estimates by study design and population. The overall SOE was rated low for the CLI population and insufficient for the IC-CLI population.

Figure 33. Forest plot for meta-analysis of secondary patency at 1 year in the CLI and IC-CLI populations

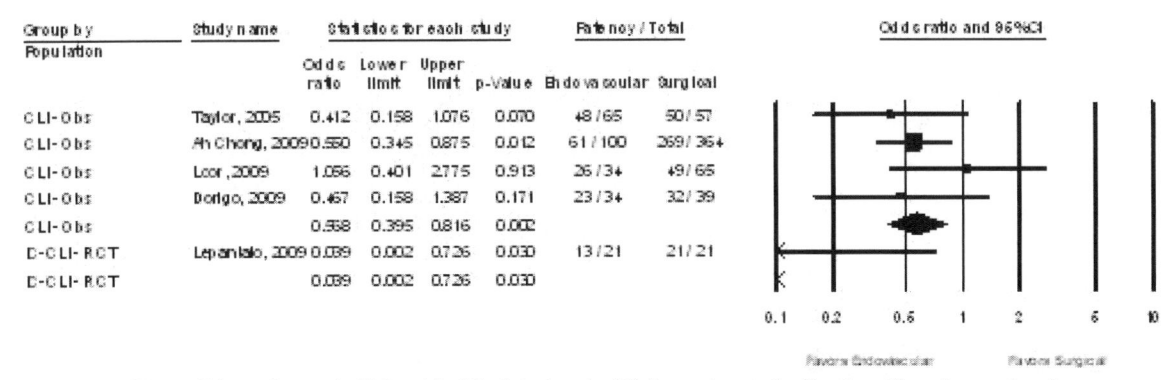

Group by Population	Study name	Odds ratio	Lower limit	Upper limit	p-Value	Endovascular	Surgical
CLI-Obs	Taylor, 2005	0.412	0.158	1.076	0.070	48/65	50/57
CLI-Obs	Ah Chong, 2009	0.550	0.345	0.875	0.012	61/100	269/364
CLI-Obs	Loor, 2009	1.056	0.401	2.775	0.913	26/34	49/65
CLI-Obs	Dorigo, 2009	0.467	0.158	1.387	0.171	23/34	32/39
CLI-Obs		0.568	0.395	0.816	0.002		
IC-CLI-RCT	Lepantalo, 2009	0.039	0.002	0.726	0.030	13/21	21/21
IC-CLI-RCT		0.039	0.002	0.726	0.030		

Abbreviations: CI=confidence interval; CLI=critical limb ischemia; IC=intermittent claudication; Obs=observational; RCT=randomized controlled trial.

Secondary Patency at 2 to 3 Years After Enrollment

Figure 34 shows the forest plot for this meta-analysis. Four observational studies (three fair and one poor) in the CLI population reporting the rate of secondary patency found that the odds ratio for surgical versus endovascular revascularization was 0.49 (95% CI, 0.28 to 0.85, p=0.01) favoring endovascular revascularization at 2 to 3 years after enrollment. There was evidence of moderate heterogeneity, with a Q-value of 6.13 for 3 degrees of freedom, p=0.10, I^2=51.10. The overall SOE was rated low on the basis of observational studies with inconsistent results of an indirect outcome and a wide confidence interval.

Figure 34. Forest plot for meta-analysis of secondary patency at 2 to 3 years in the CLI population

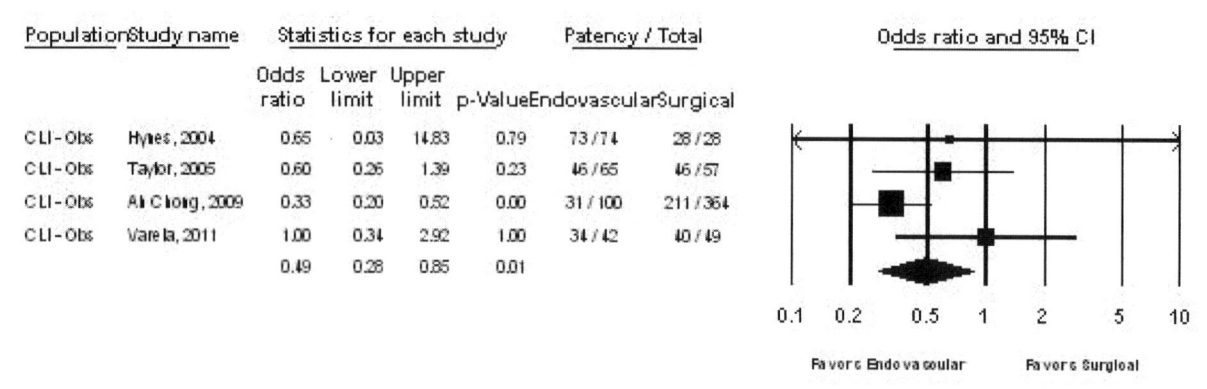

Population	Study name	Odds ratio	Lower limit	Upper limit	p-Value	Endovascular	Surgical
CLI-Obs	Hynes, 2004	0.65	0.03	14.83	0.79	73/74	28/28
CLI-Obs	Taylor, 2005	0.60	0.26	1.39	0.23	46/65	46/57
CLI-Obs	Ah Chong, 2009	0.33	0.20	0.52	0.00	31/100	211/364
CLI-Obs	Varela, 2011	1.00	0.34	2.92	1.00	34/42	40/49
		0.49	0.28	0.85	0.01		

Abbreviations: CI=confidence interval; CLI=critical limb ischemia; Obs=observational.

Effect on Hospital Length of Stay

Fourteen studies (nine in the CLI population and five in the IC-CLI population) reported hospital length of stay during the index hospitalization (Table 27). Some studies reported mean days without standard deviations (SD), and in those studies that did report the SD, the value varied such that we did not consider the data robust enough to calculate a summary estimate of the effect. The range of hospital stay was 1 to 15 days in the endovascular group and 2 to 37 days in the surgical group. Therefore, the SOE was rated insufficient.

Table 27. Endovascular versus surgical revascularization: hospital length of stay

Study Population	Type of Study N Analyzed[a] Quality	Length of Stay	Results Reported by Authors
Patients with CLI			
Adam, 2005[39] BASIL Study Patients with CLI	RCT N: 452 Good	Days, mean (SD)	Endovascular: 2.06 (1.5) Surgical: 2.14 (1.3)
Ah Chong, 2009[100] Patients with CLI	Observational N: 464 Poor	Days, mean	Endovascular: 4 Surgical: 24
Faglia, 2012[118] Patients with CLE	Observational N: 332 Fair	Days, mean (SD)	Endovascular: 5.9 (3.5) Surgical: 10.0 (3.5)
Hynes, 2004[102] Patients with CLI	Observational N: 137 Fair	Days, mean	Endovascular: 15 Surgical: 37

Table 27. Endovascular versus surgical revascularization: hospital length of stay (continued)

Study Population	Type of Study N Analyzed[a] Quality	Length of Stay	Results Reported by Authors
Jerabek, 2003[103] Patients with CLI	Observational N: 131 Poor	Days, mean	Endovascular: 9.47 Surgical: 20.69
Kudo, 2006[106] Patients with CLI	Observational N: 192 (237 limbs) Poor	Days, mean (SD)	Endovascular: 2.6 (4.9) Surgical: 7.7 (8.3)
Loor, 2009[108] Patients with CLI	Observational N: 92 Fair	Days, mean (SD)	Endovascular: 3.7 (1.3) Surgical: 6.8 (1.3)
Sultan, 2009[109] Patients with CLI	Observational N: 309 Fair	Days, mean (SD)	Endovascular: 14 (16) Surgical: 24 (23)
Varela, 2011[114] Patients with CLI	Observational N: 88 (91 limbs) Fair	Days, mean (SD)	Endovascular: 13 (12) Surgical: 19 (14)
Patients with IC or CLI			
Dosluoglu, 2010[38] Patients with IC or CLI	Observational IC: 38% in endovascular arm, 25% in surgical and hybrid arms CLI: 62% in endovascular arm, 75% in surgical and hybrid arms N: 654 Poor	Days, mean (SD)	Endovascular: 3.6 (7.0) Surgical: 9.2 (10.1)
Lepantalo, 2009[123] Patients with IC or CLI	RCT IC: 87% in endovascular arm, 90% in surgical arm CLI: 13% in endovascular arm, 10% in surgical arm N: 44 Fair	Days, mean (range)	Endovascular: 1.7 (0-7) Surgical: 4.5 (2-10)
McQuade, 2009[124] Patients with IC or CLI	RCT IC: 82% in endovascular arm, 62% in surgical arm CLI: 18% in endovascular arm, 38% in surgical arm N: 86 Fair	Days, mean (SD)	Endovascular: 0.9 (0.8) Surgical: 3.1 (1.8)
Sachs, 2011[126] Patients with IC or CLI	Observational IC: NR CLI: NR N: 563,143 Poor	Days, mean (SD)	Endovascular: 1.0 (0.2) Surgical (aortofem): 5.88 (0.31) Surgical (peripheral): 4.52 (0.31)

Table 27. Endovascular versus surgical revascularization: hospital length of stay (continued)

Study Population	Type of Study N Analyzed[a] Quality	Length of Stay	Results Reported by Authors
Whatling, 2000[130] Patients with IC or CLI	Observational IC: 121 patients of total population CLI: 17 patients of total population N: 138 Poor	Days, mean (SE)	Endovascular: 2.5 (0.6) Surgical: 5.8 (0.6)

[a]Number of patients in the study arms of interest.
Abbreviations: CLI=critical limb ischemia; IC=intermittent claudication; mo=month/months; RCT=randomized controlled trial; SD=standard deviation; SE=standard error.

Modifiers of Effectiveness

Seven studies in the CLI population, including one RCT[39] and six observational,[104,108,110,112,117,119] reported variations in treatment effectiveness by subgroup (Table 28). All subgroup analyses were performed in studies comparing the effect of endovascular intervention with surgical revascularization. Two studies reported the effect of age.[112,117] Two studies reported the effect of treatment based on anatomic factors.[104,119] One study reported on the effect of treatment based on the patency of intervention.[104] One study reported the effect of treatment based on the presence of tissue loss and the presence of diabetes.[108] One study reported the effect of use of autologous vein versus prosthetic bypass material and use of subintimal versus standard angioplasty on amputation-free survival and overall survival.[39] One study reported effect of use of autologous versus nonautologous vein grafts.[119] We found no studies reporting results by the following subgroups: sex, race, smoking status, or the presence of renal disease. The SOE for modifiers of effectiveness was insufficient given the few number of studies and variety of subgroups that were evaluated.

In the mixed IC-CLI population, seven studies, including one RCT[124] and six observational studies[38,121,126-128,131] reported variations in treatment effectiveness by subgroup (Table 28). All subgroup analyses were performed in studies comparing the effect of endovascular intervention with surgical revascularization. Three studies reported the effect of symptom class.[126,127,131] Two studies reported the effect of renal failure.[121,131] Two studies reported the effect of arterial outflow or runoff.[128,131] One study reported the effect of age, sex, smoking status, presence of hyperlipidemia, coronary artery disease, diabetes mellitus, hypertension,[131] anatomic location of stenosis,[131] and stent graft size.[124]

We found no studies reporting results by the following subgroups: patency of intervention or type of conduit (autologous vein or prosthetic material). The SOE for modifiers of effectiveness was insufficient for the other modifiers given the small number of studies and variety of subgroups that were evaluated.

In the single RCT of CLI patients, the use of autologous vein was associated with improved outcomes when compared with prosthetic conduit. Additionally, the performance of subintimal angioplasty was associated with statistically nonsignificant worse outcomes when compared with standard angioplasty. Data derived from the observational studies had a high likelihood of bias but did show that with advanced age, renal failure, and higher Rutherford classification, patients generally fared worse in terms of mortality and amputation.

Table 28. Modifiers of effectiveness for KQ 3

Study Population	Type of Study N Analyzed[a] Comparison Quality	Subgroup	Results Reported by Authors
Patients with CLI			
Adam, 2005[39] BASIL Study Patients with CLI	RCT N: 452 Endovascular vs. surgical revascularization Good	Patients treated with autologous vein or prosthetic material	Amputation free-survival at 1 yr: Autologous vein: 73% Prosthetic graft: 63% Overall survival at 1 yr: Autologous vein: 79% Prosthetic graft: 78% Amputation free-survival at 2 yr: Autologous vein: 67% Prosthetic graft: 51% Overall survival at 2 yr: Autologous vein: 71% Prosthetic graft: 63% Amputation free-survival at 5 yr: Autologous vein: 47% Prosthetic graft: 19% Overall survival at 5 yr: Autologous vein: 53% Prosthetic graft: 45%
		Patients treated with subintimal angioplasty vs. standard angioplasty	Amputation free-survival at 1 yr: Subintimal angioplasty: 77% Standard angioplasty: 78% Overall survival at 1 yr: Subintimal angioplasty: 77% Standard angioplasty: 78% Amputation free-survival at 2 yr: Subintimal angioplasty: 64% Standard angioplasty: 66%
			Overall survival at 2 yr: Subintimal angioplasty: 64% Standard angioplasty: 66% Amputation free-survival at 5 yr: Subintimal angioplasty: 33% Standard angioplasty: 40% Overall survival at 5 yr: Subintimal angioplasty: 33% Standard angioplasty: 40%

Table 28. Modifiers of effectiveness for KQ 3 (continued)

Study Population	Type of Study N Analyzed[a] Comparison Quality	Subgroup	Results Reported by Authors
Dosluoglu 2012[119] Patients with CLI	Observational N: 433 Endovascular vs. surgical revascularization Fair	Patients treated with autologous vein vs. nonautologous vein	Survival at 5 yr: Autologous: 59% Nonautologous: 35% Endovascular: 36% Limb salvage at 5 yr: Autologous: 91% Nonautologous: 67% Endovascular: 78% Amputation-free survival at 5 yr: Autologous: 55% Nonautologous: 25% Endovascular: 30%
		Only patients with TASC-D lesions	Primary patency at 5 yr: Endovascular: 39% Surgical: 47% Autologous vein: 66% Assisted primary patency at 5 yr: Endovascular: 55% Surgical: 58% Autologous vein: 80% Secondary patency at 5 yr: Endovascular: 60% Surgical: 63% Autologous vein: 83% Limb salvage at 5 yr: Endovascular: 77% Surgical: 78% Autologous vein: 91% Amputation-free survival at 5 yr: Endovascular: 29% Autologous vein: 54%
Khan, 2009[104] Patients with CLI	Observational N: 358 patients, 412 limbs Endovascular vs. surgical revascularization Poor	Anatomy-specific factors Patency of treated segment	Survival at 1 yr: Patients with patent endovascular-treated segment: 67% Patients with patent surgical revascularization bypass(es): 86% Major amputation at 3 mo: Patients with patent endovascular-treated segment: 58% Patients with patent surgical revascularization bypass(es): 36% Major amputation at 12 mo: Patients with patent endovascular-treated segment: 88% Patients with patent surgical revascularization bypass(es): 86%

Table 28. Modifiers of effectiveness for KQ 3 (continued)

Study Population	Type of Study N Analyzed[a] Comparison Quality	Subgroup	Results Reported by Authors
Loor, 2009[108] Patients with CLI	Observational N: 92 Endovascular vs. surgical revascularization Fair	Patients with tissue loss	Limb Salvage at 1 yr: Endovascular: 82% Surgical: 71%
		Presence of diabetes mellitus	Amputation-free survival at 1 yr: Endovascular: 60% Surgical: 79%
Soderstrom, 2010[110] Patients with CLI	Observational N: 1023 Endovascular vs. surgical revascularization Fair	Presence of diabetes mellitus	Survival at 5 yr: Endovascular: 44.3% Surgical: 39.2% Limb Salvage at 5 yr: Endovascular: 75.3% Surgical: 72.3% Amputation-free Survival at 5 yr: Endovascular: 34.4% Surgical: 32.7% Freedom from any revascularization at 5 yr: Endovascular: 77.8% Surgical: 77.7% Freedom from surgical revascularization at 5 yr: Endovascular: 85.6% Surgical: 93.5%

Table 28. Modifiers of effectiveness for KQ 3 (continued)

Study Population	Type of Study N Analyzed[a] Comparison Quality	Subgroup	Results Reported by Authors
Taylor, 2005[112] Patients with CLI	Observational N: 122 Endovascular vs. surgical revascularization Fair	Age: Patients > 80 yr	Mortality at 6 mo: Endovascular: 15.4% Surgical: 3.5% Mortality at 1 yr: Endovascular: 24.9% Surgical: 7.4% Mortality at 2 yr: Endovascular: 32.3% Surgical: 18.9% Mortality at 3 yr: Endovascular: 50.3% Surgical: 26.9% Limb Salvage at 6 mo: Endovascular: 81.4% Surgical: 87.6% Limb Salvage at 1 yr: Endovascular: 77.4% Surgical: 87.6% Limb Salvage at 2 yr: Endovascular: 74.3% Surgical: 82.5% Limb Salvage at 3 yr: Endovascular: 74.3% Surgical: 82.5%
			Amputation-free survival at 6 mo: Endovascular: 64.9% Surgical: 84.9% Amputation-free survival at 1 yr: Endovascular: 54.8% Surgical: 79.8% Amputation-free survival at 2 yr: Endovascular: 50.4% Surgical: 71.0% Amputation-free survival at 3 yr: Endovascular: 33.6% Surgical: 63.4% Primary Patency at 6 mo: Endovascular: 68.7% Surgical: 79.9%

Table 28. Modifiers of effectiveness for KQ 3 (continued)

Study Population	Type of Study N Analyzed[a] Comparison Quality	Subgroup	Results Reported by Authors
Taylor, 2005[112] (continued)			Primary Patency at 1 yr: Endovascular: 62.0% Surgical: 67.7% Primary Patency at 2 yr: Endovascular: 55.3% Surgical: 63.3% Primary Patency at 3 yr: Endovascular: 60.5% Surgical: 48.4% Secondary Patency at 6 mo: Endovascular: 80.1% Surgical: 90.4% Secondary Patency at 1 yr: Endovascular: 74.1% Surgical: 87.4% Amputation-free survival at 2 yr: Endovascular: 50.4% Surgical: 71.0% Amputation-free survival at 3 yr: Endovascular: 33.6% Surgical: 63.4%
Zdanowski, 1998[117] Patients with CLI	Observational N: 4929 Endovascular vs. surgical revascularization Poor	Age: Patients <76 yr and >76 yr	Mortality at 30 days: <76 yr, endovascular: 3.1% <76 yr, surgical: 4.0% >76 yr, endovascular: 6.0% >76 yr, surgical: 6.5% Mortality at 1 yr: <76 yr, endovascular: 17.6% <76 yr, surgical: 17.6% >76 yr, endovascular: 25.8% >76 yr, surgical: 26.6% Amputation-free survival at 30 days: <76 yr, endovascular: 91.5% <76 yr, surgical: 89.3% >76 yr, endovascular: 89.2% >76 yr, surgical: 89.0% Amputation-free survival at 1 yr: <76 yr, endovascular: 73.2% <76 yr, surgical: 72.4% >76 yr, endovascular: 64.1% >76 yr, surgical: 63.2%

Table 28. Modifiers of effectiveness for KQ 3 (continued)

Study Population	Type of Study N Analyzed[a] Comparison Quality	Subgroup	Results Reported by Authors
Patients with IC or CLI			
Dosluoglu, 2010[38] Patients with IC or CLI	Observational N: 654 Endovascular revascularization vs. surgical revascularization vs. hybrid revascularization Poor	Presence of aortoiliac stenosis	Primary patency at 12 mo Endovascular: 41/45 Surgical: 29/35 Secondary patency at 12 mo Endovascular: 41/48 Surgical: 31/35
Hoshino, 2010[121] Patients with IC or CLI	Observational N: 180 Endovascular revascularization vs. surgical revascularization Fair	Hemodialysis vs. nonhemodialysis	Amputation free survival Hemodialysis: HR 1.69 (0.63-4.99) Nonhemodialysis: HR 1.13 (0.48-2.60) Survival Hemodialysis: HR 2.48 (0.89-8.00) Nonhemodialysis: HR 1.13 (0.48-2.60)
Kashyap, 2008[131] Patients with IC or CLI	Observational N: 169 Endovascular revascularization vs. surgical revascularization Fair (Unless specified by treatment group, some subgroup findings include the entire study cohort.)	Age	Survival at 3 yr >60 (N=103): 76%, HR 1.0 <60 (N=56): 87%, HR 0.6 (0.3-1.2) Vessel patency >60 Endovascular revascularization (N=91 limbs): 75%, HR 1.0 Surgical revascularization (N=76 limbs): 92% (85-99) HR 1.0 <60 Endovascular revascularization (N=34 limbs): 71%, HR 1.8 (0.8-3.7) Surgical revascularization (N=68 limbs): 94%, HR 0.9 (0.2-3.3)
		Sex	<u>Survival at 3 yr</u> Male (N=103): 75%, HR 1.0 Female (N=62): 87%, HR 0.7 (0.4-1.3) <u>Vessel patency</u> Male Endovascular revascularization (N=73 limbs): 71%, HR 1.0 Surgical revascularization (N=94 limbs): 93%, HR 1.0 Female Endovascular revascularization (N=52 limbs): 81%, HR 1.8 (0.8-3.7) Surgical revascularization (N=50 limbs): 91%, HR 0.7 (0.2-3.5)
		Hyperlipidemia	<u>Survival at 3 yr</u> Hyperlipidemia (N=89): 90%, HR 0.4 (0.2-0.8) No hyperlipidemia (N=69): 68%, HR 1.0

Table 28. Modifiers of effectiveness for KQ 3 (continued)

Study Population	Type of Study N Analyzed[a] Comparison Quality	Subgroup	Results Reported by Authors
Kashyap, 2008[131] (continued)		CAD status	Survival at 3 yr CAD low (N=57): 80%, HR 1.0 CAD intermediate (N=75): 85%, HR 0.9 CAD high (N=27): 66%, HR 1.5 (0.7-3.4)
		Diabetes	Survival at 3 yr No diabetes (N=124): 83%, HR 1.0 NIDDM (N=29): 72%, HR 2.1 (1.1-4.1) IDDM (N=5): 60%, HR 1.8 (0.4 - 7.7) Vessel patency No diabetes Endovascular revascularization (N=102 limbs): 74%, HR=1.0 Surgical revascularization (N=105 limbs): 95%, HR 1.0 NIDDM Endovascular revascularization (N=21 limbs): 72%, HR 1.5 (0.7-3.5) Surgical revascularization (N=29 limbs): 97%, HR 0.8 (0.1-6.9) IDDM Endovascular revascularization (N=2 limbs): HR 5.3(2.8-10.0) Surgical revascularization (N=8 limbs): 0%, HR 11.6 (3.6-37.6)
		Hypertension	Survival at 3 yr Hypertension (N=91): 81%, HR 1.1 (0.6-2.1) No hypertension (N=53): 79%, HR 1.0
		Smoking	Survival at 3 yr Smoking (N=91): 81%, HR 0.9 (0.5-1.7) No smoking (N=53): 83%, HR=1.0 Vessel patency Smoking Endovascular revascularization (N=58 limbs): 75%, HR 0.8 (0.4-1.7) Surgical revascularization (N=102 limbs): 92%, HR 1.2 (0.1-13.9) No smoking Endovascular revascularization (N=65 limbs): 74%, HR 1.0 Surgical revascularization (N=14 limbs): 92%, HR 1.0
		Renal failure	Survival at 3 yr Renal failure (N=18): 595, HR 2.5 (1.1-5.7) No renal failure (N=141): 83%, HR=1.0

Table 28. Modifiers of effectiveness for KQ 3 (continued)

Study Population	Type of Study N Analyzed[a] Comparison Quality	Subgroup	Results Reported by Authors
Kashyap, 2008[131] (continued)		Poor outflow	<u>Survival at 3 yr</u> Poor outflow (N=56): 71%, HR 2.0 (1.1-3.7) Good outflow (N=98): 84%, HR 1.0 <u>Vessel patency</u> Poor outflow Endovascular revascularization (N=38 limbs): 66%, HR 1.3 (0.5-3.1) Surgical revascularization (N=56 limbs): 90%, HR 1.3(0.4-4.5) Good outflow Endovascular revascularization (N=85 limbs): 77%, HR 1.0 Surgical revascularization (N=80 limbs): 95%, HR=1.0
		Claudication vs. rest pain vs. tissue loss vs. ALI	<u>Survival at 3 yr</u> Claudication (N=84): 91%, HR 1.0 Rest pain (N=45): 77%, HR 2.5 (1.1-5.7) Tissue loss (N=19): 63%, HR 8.1 (3.5-18.7) Acute limb ischemia (N=11): 34%, HR 10.5 (4.0-27.7)
		TASC classification	<u>Vessel patency</u> TASC B Endovascular revascularization (N=20 limbs): 53%, HR 1.0 Surgical revascularization (N=32 limbs): 96%, HR 1.0 TASC C Endovascular revascularization (N=37 limbs): 61%, HR 0.8 (0.3-1.8) Surgical revascularization (N=32 limbs): 91%, HR 0.8 (0.2-3.6) TASC D Endovascular revascularization (N=68 limbs): 90%, HR 0.2 (0.1-0.7) Surgical revascularization (N=32 limbs): 90%, HR 0.4 (0.1-2.7)

Table 28. Modifiers of effectiveness for KQ 3 (continued)

Study Population	Type of Study N Analyzed[a] Comparison Quality	Subgroup	Results Reported by Authors
Kashyap, 2008[131] (continued)		Femoral management	Vessel patency Native Endovascular revascularization (N=100 limbs): 74%, HR 1.0 Surgical revascularization (N=57 limbs): 95%, HR 1.0 Unilateral common femoral endarterectomy and / or profundaplasty Endovascular revascularization (N=15 limbs): 67%, HR 0.3 (0.1-1.6) Surgical revascularization (N==28 limbs): 100%, HR not estimable Bilateral common femoral endarterectomy and/or profundaplasty Endovascular revascularization (N=4 limbs): Patency not estimable Surgical revascularization (N=46 limbs): 95%, HR 1.2 (0.3 to 5.1) Bypass Endovascular revascularization (N=6 limbs): Patency not estimable, HR 2.4 (0.3 to 20.0) Surgical revascularization (N=11 limbs): 61%, HR 7.4 (1.4 to 38.1)
McQuade, 2009[124] Kedora, 2007[135] McQuade, 2010[136] Patients with IC or CLI	RCT N: 86 Endovascular revascularization vs. surgical revascularization Fair	Stent graft size	Vessel patency Primary patency at 24 mo: Smaller diameter stent graft (5 mm): 54% Larger diameter stent graft (6-7 mm): 69% Surgical bypass: 64% Primary patency at 48 mo: Smaller diameter stent graft (5 mm): 54% Larger diameter stent graft (6-7 mm): 62% Surgical bypass: 58% Secondary patency at 24 mo: Smaller diameter stent graft (5 mm): 70% Larger diameter stent graft (6-7 mm): 77% Surgical bypass: 76% Secondary patency at 48 mo: Smaller diameter stent graft (5 mm): 70% Larger diameter stent graft (6-7 mm): 77% Surgical bypass: 71%

Table 28. Modifiers of effectiveness for KQ 3 (continued)

Study Population	Type of Study N Analyzed[a] Comparison Quality	Subgroup	Results Reported by Authors
Sachs, 2011[126] Patients with IC or CLI	Observational N: 563,143 Endovascular revascularization vs. surgical revascularization Poor	CLI	In-hospital mortality Endovascular revascularization: 2.1% Aortofemoral bypass: 4.1% Peripheral bypass: 2.6% Major amputation Endovascular revascularization: 7.0% Aortofemoral bypass: 3.0% Peripheral bypass: 3.9%
Stoner, 2008[127] Patients with IC or CLI	Observational N: 359 Endovascular revascularization vs. surgical revascularization Poor	IC vs. CLI	Vessel patency Primary assisted patency at 12 mo IC Endovascular revascularization: 80% +/- 0.04% Surgical revascularization 93% +/- 0.03% CLI Endovascular revascularization: 54% +/- 0.05% Surgical revascularization: 66% +/- 0.05%
Timaran, 2003[128] Patients with IC or CLI	Observational N: 188 Endovascular revascularization vs. surgical revascularization Fair	Patients with poor run-off	Vessel patency Primary patency at 1 yr Endovascular revascularization: 74% Surgical revascularization: 80% Primary patency at 3 yr Endovascular revascularization: 36% Surgical revascularization: 75% Primary patency at 5 yr Endovascular revascularization: 36% Surgical revascularization: 68%

[a] Number of patients in the study arms of interest.
Abbreviations: CLI=critical limb ischemia; IC=intermittent claudication; mo=month/months; PAD=peripheral artery disease; yr=year/years.

Safety Concerns

In the CLI population, one observational study (fair quality)[101] reported safety concerns. Specifically, this study reported the incidence of thrombosis at 30 days and found that the risk of thrombosis was higher in patients undergoing surgical revascularization than in patients undergoing endovascular revascularization.

We found no studies in this population reporting harms of adverse drug reactions, bleeding, contrast nephropathy, radiation, infection, or periprocedural complications causing acute limb ischemia. The SOE for harms was insufficient given the small number of studies reporting this outcome. It may be that treatment harms are not routinely documented or collected in retrospective or prospective observational studies.

In the IC-CLI population, six studies including two RCTs[123,124] and four observational studies[38,122,125,131] reported safety concerns. Six studies[38,122-125,131] reported the incidence of periprocedural complications in patients undergoing endovascular and surgical revascularization. Three studies[38,123,131] reported the incidence of infection, one study[38] reported the incidence of bleeding, and one study[131] reported the incidence of renal dysfunction following endovascular and surgical revascularization (Table 29).

Table 29. Safety concerns in the IC-CLI population

Study	Type of Study N Analyzed[a] Comparison Quality	Harm	Results Reported by Authors
Patients with IC or CLI			
Dosluoglu, 2010[38]	Observational N: 654 Endovascular revascularization vs. surgical revascularization vs. hybrid revascularization Poor	1. Bleeding 2. Infection 3. Periprocedural complications (graft/stent occlusion)	1. Endovascular: 0.2% Surgical: 1.3% 2. Endovascular: 0.2% Surgical: 15.4% 3. Endovascular: 0.5% Surgical: 1.8%
Janne d'Othee, 2008[122]	Observational N: 97 Endovascular vs. surgical revascularization Fair	1. Periprocedural complications (complications requiring medical care within 30 days)	Endovascular: 0.5% Surgical: 1.8%
Kashyap, 2008[131]	Observational N: 169 Endovascular revascularization vs. surgical revascularization Fair	1. Renal dysfunction 2. Infection 3. Periprocedural complications (no definition given)	1. Endovascular: 4.8% Surgical: 1.1% 2. Endovascular: 2.4% Surgical: 5.8% 3. Endovascular: 0% Surgical: 3.5%
Lepantalo, 2009[123]	RCT N: 44 Endovascular vs. surgical revascularization Fair	1. Infection 2. Periprocedural complications (graft/stent occlusion)	1. Endovascular: 0% Surgical: 19.0% 2. Endovascular: 8.7% Surgical: 0%
McQuade, 2009[124] Kedora, 2007[135] McQuade, 2010[136]	RCT N: 86 Endovascular revascularization vs. surgical revascularization Fair	Periprocedural complications (vascular dissection, leg edema, thigh pain)	Endovascular: 8.0% Surgical: 6.0%
Rossi, 1998[125]	Observational N: 48 Endovascular vs. surgical revascularization Poor	Periprocedural complications (cardiac event)	Endovascular: 16.2% Surgical: 45.5%

[a]Number of patients in the study arms of interest.
Abbreviation: RCT=randomized controlled trial.

Periprocedural Complications by 30 Days

Figure 35 shows the forest plot for the meta-analysis of the two RCTs[123,124] and four observational studies[38,122,125,131] comparing the effect of surgical revascularization versus endovascular revascularization on periprocedural complications by 30 days in IC-CLI patients. Periprocedural complications may have included graft or stent occlusion, limb ischemia, wound dehiscence, arterial dissection or any repeat revascularization procedure.

In the observational studies, the between-group estimate was OR 1.87 (95% CI, 0.63 to 5.49) favoring the endovascular strategy; however, in the RCTs the estimated odds ratio was 0.57 (CI,

0.14 to 2.26) favoring a surgical strategy, both being considered inconclusive in their findings. The differences in results between the observational studies and RCTs may be due to the types of periprocedural complications reported and the definition of those complications across studies. Patient selection bias in the observational studies is likely a factor where healthier patients (higher proportion of IC patients) are chosen for an endovascular procedure, whereas in the RCTs the distribution of PAD severity would have been equally distributed. The SOE is insufficient given the high number of observational studies and two fair-quality RCTs, inconsistent results, differing definitions of a periprocedural complication, and imprecise results.

Figure 35. Forest plot for meta-analysis of surgical versus endovascular revascularization on periprocedural complications by 30 days in IC-CLI population

Group by Population	Study name	Odds ratio	Lower limit	Upper limit	p-Value	Surgical	Endovascular
IC-CLI-Obs	Rossi, 1998	4.30	0.99	18.79	0.05	5/11	6/37
IC-CLI-Obs	Kashyap, 2008	0.31	0.06	1.56	0.15	2/86	6/83
IC-CLI-Obs	Janne d'Othee, 2008	2.27	0.80	6.45	0.12	9/33	9/64
IC-CLI-Obs	Dosluoglu, 2010	3.65	0.61	21.94	0.16	4/207	2/356
IC-CLI-Obs		1.87	0.63	5.49	0.26		
IC-CLI-RCT	Lepantalo, 2009	0.20	0.01	4.41	0.31	0/21	2/23
IC-CLI-RCT	McQuade, 2009	0.73	0.16	3.46	0.70	3/50	4/50
IC-CLI-RCT		0.57	0.14	2.26	0.42		
Overall		1.19	0.51	2.79	0.69		

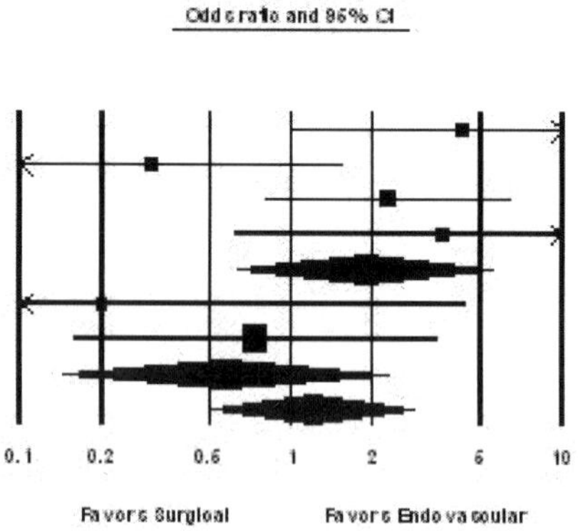

Abbreviations: CI=confidence interval; CLI=critical limb ischemia; IC=intermittent claudication; Obs=observational; RCT=randomized controlled trial.

Infection by 30 Days

Figure 36 shows the forest plot for the meta-analysis of the three studies[38,123,131] (one fair-quality RCT; two observational studies, one fair, one poor) comparing surgical versus endovascular revascularization on periprocedural complications by 30 days in IC-CLI patients.

In the observational studies, the between-group estimate was OR 14.10 (95% CI, 0.43 to 460.70), and in the RCT the estimated OR was 12.09 (CI, 0.61 to 239.54) with both favoring an endovascular strategy although not reaching statistical significance. The overall estimated OR was 12.90 (CI, 1.34 to 124.65). There was some evidence of heterogeneity, with a Q-value of 5.52 for 2 degrees of freedom, p=0.06; I^2=63.78. The heterogeneity is likely due to the patient selection bias in the observational studies, although it is plausible that surgical revascularization will cause more wound infections when compared to endovascular intervention. Given the small number of studies, moderate heterogeneity, and imprecision, the SOE is low.

Figure 36. Forest plot for meta-analysis of surgical versus endovascular revascularization on infections by 30 days in IC-CLI population

Group by Population	Study name	Odds ratio	Lower limit	Upper limit	p-Value	Surgical	Endovascular
IC-CLI - Obs	Kashyap, 2008	2.58	0.42	15.87	0.31	4/86	2/83
IC-CLI - Obs	Dosluoglu, 2010	90.83	8.61	957.74	0.00	32/207	1/356
IC-CLI - Obs		14.10	0.43	460.70	0.14		
IC-CLI - RCT	Lepantalo, 2009	12.09	0.61	239.54	0.10	4/21	0/23
IC-CLI - RCT		12.09	0.61	239.54	0.10		
Overall		12.90	1.34	124.65	0.03		

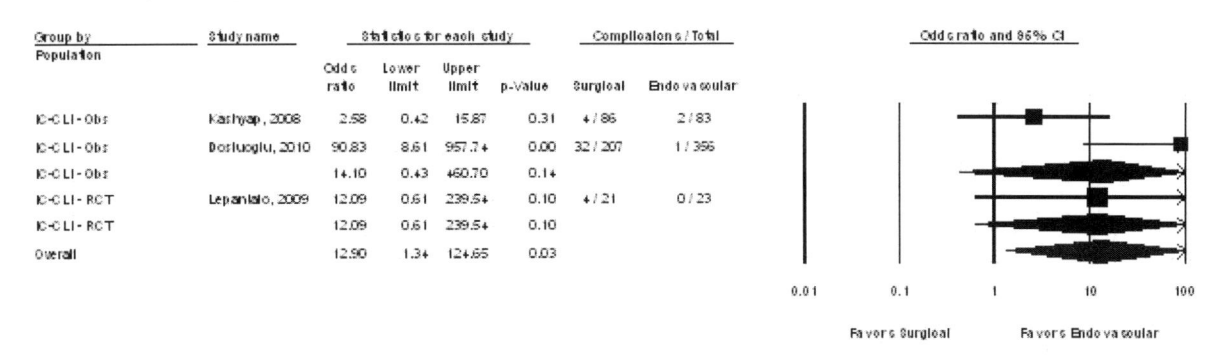

Abbreviations: CI=confidence interval; CLI=critical limb ischemia; IC=intermittent claudication; Obs=observational; RCT=randomized controlled trial.

Also, in the IC-CLI population, we found no studies reporting harms of adverse drug reactions and radiation. The SOE for the remaining safety concerns was insufficient given the small number of studies reporting these outcomes. It may be that treatment harms are not routinely documented or collected in retrospective or prospective observational studies.

SOE Ratings for KQ 3

Tables 30–31 summarize the SOE for the outcomes across the four domains outlined in the KQ by each treatment comparison. Any outcomes not reported in either the CLI or IC-CLI population are grouped together and labeled as insufficient evidence. The tables list outcomes for the type of PAD population and study design if they are reported in the literature; therefore assume that any PAD population or study design not listed under that outcome constitutes no (or insufficient) evidence.

Table 30. Detailed SOE for endovascular intervention versus usual care in CLI and IC-CLI populations

Population Study Design Number of Studies (Total Patients)	Risk of Bias	Consistency	Directness	Precision	SOE and Magnitude of Effect Effect Estimate (95% CI)
All-cause mortality					
CLI Observational 3 (562)	2 moderate risk, 1 high risk	Consistent	Direct	Imprecise	Mortality higher in usual care group when compared with endovascular group **Insufficient SOE**
IC-CLI Observational 1 (107)	1 moderate risk	NA	Direct	Imprecise	Endovascular intervention: 5.5% Usual care: 5.8% **Insufficient SOE**
Amputation					
CLI Observational 3 (562)	2 moderate risk, 1 high risk	Inconsistent	Direct	Imprecise	Amputation rate was higher in usual care group in two studies, and it was only reported in the revascularization group in the other study **Insufficient SOE**

Table 30. Detailed SOE for endovascular intervention versus usual care in CLI and IC-CLI populations (continued)

Population Study Design Number of Studies (Total Patients)	Risk of Bias	Consistency	Directness	Precision	SOE and Magnitude of Effect Effect Estimate (95% CI)
IC-CLI Observational 1 (107)	1 moderate risk	NA	Direct	Imprecise	Endovascular intervention: 5.5% Usual care: 3.8% **Insufficient SOE**
Amputation-free survival					
CLI Observational 1 (70)	1 high risk	NA	Direct	Imprecise	Amputation-free survival was better in endovascular group (60% vs. 47%) **Insufficient SOE**
Length of stay					
CLI Observational 3 (562)	2 moderate risk, 1 high risk	Inconsistent	Indirect	Imprecise	LOS was lower in the endovascular group in two studies, and it was only reported in the revascularization group in the other study **Insufficient SOE**
Nonfatal stroke Nonfatal MI Composite cardiovascular events MWD or ACD Initial claudication distance or pain-free walking distance Quality of life Primary patency Secondary patency Wound healing Analog pain scale Modifiers of effectiveness (subgroups) Safety concerns Safety concerns (subgroups)					
All 0	NA	NA	NA	NA	**Insufficient SOE**

Abbreviations: ACD=absolute claudication distance; CI=confidence interval; CLI=critical limb ischemia; IC=intermittent claudication; LOS=hospital length of stay; MI=myocardial infarction; MWD=masimal walking distance; NA=not applicable; RCT=randomized controlled trial; SOE=strength of evidence.

Table 31. Detailed SOE of evidence for endovascular versus surgical revascularization in CLI and IC-CLI populations

Population	Study Design Number of Studies (Total Patients)	Risk of Bias	Consistency	Directness	Precision	SOE and Magnitude of Effect Effect Estimate (95% CI)
All-cause mortality ≤6 mo						
CLI	Observational: 11 (8249) RCT: 1 (452)	Observational: 1 low risk, 6 moderate risk, 4 high risk RCT: 1 low risk	Inconsistent	Direct	Imprecise	Observational OR 0.85 (0.57 to 1.27) RCT OR 0.51 (0.20 to 1.35) Favors endovascular **Low SOE**
IC-CLI	Observational: 2 (823)	1 moderate risk, 1 high risk	Consistent	Direct	Imprecise	OR 0.45 (0.18 to 1.09) Favors endovascular **Low SOE**
All-cause mortality at 1–2 yr						
CLI	Observational: 12 (7850)	1 low risk, 8 moderate risk, 3 high risk	Consistent	Direct	Imprecise	OR 1.01 (0.80 to 1.28) No difference **Low SOE**
IC-CLI	Observational: 2 (145) RCT: 2 (130)	Observational: 1 moderate risk, 1 high risk RCT: 2 moderate risk	Inconsistent	Direct	Imprecise	Observational OR 0.51 (0.20 to 1.31) RCT OR 0.81 (0.23 to 2.82) Favors endovascular **Low SOE**
All-cause mortality at ≥3 yr						
CLI	Observational: 7 (7176) RCT: 1 (452)	Observational: 1 low risk, 3 moderate risk, 3 high risk RCT: 1 low risk	Inconsistent	Direct	Imprecise	Observational: OR 1.05 (0.54 to 2.06) RCT: OR 1.07 (0.73 to 1.56) No difference **Low SOE**
IC-CLI	RCT: 1 (58)	1 moderate risk	NA	Direct	Imprecise	OR 0.88 (0.28 to 2.73) Inconclusive **Insufficient SOE**
Nonfatal MI						
CLI	RCT: 1 (452)	1 low risk	NA	Direct	Imprecise	Endovascular group had fewer MIs than surgical group (3% vs. 8%) **Insufficient SOE**

Table 31. Detailed SOE of evidence for endovascular versus surgical revascularization in CLI and IC-CLI populations (continued)

Population	Study Design Number of Studies (Total Patients)	Risk of Bias	Consistency	Directness	Precision	SOE and Magnitude of Effect Effect Estimate (95% CI)
Amputation at <2 yr						
CLI	Observational: 11 (4490) RCT: 1 (452)	Observational: 1 low risk, 6 moderate risk, 4 high risk RCT: 1 low risk	Inconsistent	Direct	Imprecise	Observational: OR 0.73 (0.48 to 1.09) RCT OR 1.23 (0.72 to 2.11) No difference **Low SOE**
IC-CLI	Observational: 2 (823) RCT: 2 (130)	Observational: 1 moderate risk, 1 high risk RCT: 2 moderate risk	Inconsistent	Direct	Imprecise	Observational OR 1.11 (0.40 to 3.05) RCT OR 0.22 (0.05 to 1.07) Inconclusive **Insufficient SOE**
Amputation at 2–3 yr						
CLI	Observational: 4 (3187) RCT: 1 (452)	Observational: 1 low risk, 2 moderate risk, 1 high risk RCT: 1 low risk	Inconsistent	Direct	Imprecise	Observational OR 1.08 (0.62 to 1.89) RCT OR 1.02 (0.64 to 1.63) No difference **Low SOE**
IC-CLI	Observational: 1 (169) RCT: 1 (86)	Observational: 1 moderate risk RCT: 1 moderate risk	Inconsistent	Direct	Imprecise	Observational OR 1.00 (0.18 to 5.54) RCT OR 0.18 (0.03 to 1.29) Inconclusive **Insufficient SOE**
Amputation after 5 yr						
CLI	Observational: 7 (3101)	1 low risk, 3 moderate risk, 3 high risk	Inconsistent	Direct	Imprecise	OR 1.06 (0.70 to 1.59) No difference **Low SOE**
Amputation-free survival at 1 yr						
CLI	Observational: 2 (1881) RCT: 1 (452)	Observational: 1 low risk, 1 moderate risk RCT: 1 low risk	Consistent	Direct	Precise	Observational OR 0.76 (0.48 to 1.21) RCT OR 0.87 (0.58 to 1.30) No difference **Low SOE**

Table 31. Detailed SOE of evidence for endovascular versus surgical revascularization in CLI and IC-CLI populations (continued)

Population	Study Design Number of Studies (Total Patients)	Risk of Bias	Consistency	Directness	Precision	SOE and Magnitude of Effect Effect Estimate (95% CI)
Amputation-free survival at 2–3 yr						
CLI	Observational: 3 (1972) RCT: 1 (452)	Observational: 1 low risk, 2 moderate risk RCT: 1 low risk	Inconsistent	Direct	Imprecise	Observational OR 0.76 (0.53 to 1.09) RCT OR 1.22 (0.84 to 1.77) No difference **Low SOE**
Amputation-free survival after 5 yr						
CLI	Observational: 4 (2190)	1 low risk, 3 moderate risk	Inconsistent	Direct	Imprecise	OR 0.89 (0.59 to 1.34) No difference **Low SOE**
Wound healing						
CLI	Observational: 1 (91)	1 moderate risk	NA	Indirect	Imprecise	Surgical revascularization (83%) endovascular revascularization (80%) **Insufficient SOE**
Primary patency at 1 yr						
CLI	Observational: 5 (890)	3 moderate risk, 2 high risk	Consistent	Indirect	Precise	OR 0.63 (0.46 to 0.86) No difference **Moderate SOE**
IC-CLI	Observational: 3 (328) RCT: 2 (130)	Observational: 3 moderate risk RCT: 2 moderate risk	Consistent	Indirect	Imprecise	Observational OR 0.71 (0.40 to 1.28) RCT OR 0.40 (0.08 to 1.93) Favors endovascular **Low SOE**
Primary patency at 2–3 yr						
CLI	Observational: 4 (768)	3 moderate risk, 1 high risk	Inconsistent	Indirect	Imprecise	OR 0.77 (0.24 to 2.42) Inconclusive **Insufficient SOE**

Table 31. Detailed SOE of evidence for endovascular versus surgical revascularization in CLI and IC-CLI populations (continued)

Population	Study Design Number of Studies (Total Patients)	Risk of Bias	Consistency	Directness	Precision	SOE and Magnitude of Effect Effect Estimate (95% CI)
IC-CLI	Observational: 2 (231) RCT: 1 (86)	Observational: 2 moderate risk RCT: 1 moderate risk	Inconsistent	Indirect	Imprecise	Observational OR 0.29 (0.15 to 0.55) RCT OR 0.96 (0.42 to 2.16) Inconclusive **Insufficient SOE**
Secondary patency at 1 yr						
CLI	Observational: 4 (759)	3 moderate risk, 1 high risk	Inconsistent	Indirect	Imprecise	OR 0.57 (0.40 to 0.82) Favors endovascular **Low SOE**
IC-CLI	RCT: 1 (44)	1 moderate risk	NA	Indirect	Imprecise	OR 0.04 (0.00 to 0.73) Inconclusive **Insufficient SOE**
Secondary patency at 2–3 yr						
CLI	Observational: 4 (815)	3 moderate risk, 1 high risk	Inconsistent	Indirect	Imprecise	OR 0.49 (0.28 to 0.85) Favors endovascular **Low SOE**
Length of stay						
CLI	Observational: 8 (1745) RCT: 1 (452)	Observational: 5 moderate risk, 3 high risk RCT: 1 low risk	Inconsistent	Indirect	Imprecise	LOS longer in surgical group with large SD in 3 observational studies and no variability reported in 4 observational studies and one RCT **Insufficient SOE**
IC-CLI	Observational: 3 (563,935) RCT: 2 (130)	Observational: 3 high risk RCT: 2 moderate risk	Consistent	Indirect	Imprecise	LOS longer in surgical group with large SD in the observational studies and RCTs **Insufficient SOE**

Table 31. Detailed SOE of evidence for endovascular versus surgical revascularization in CLI and IC-CLI populations (continued)

Population	Study Design Number of Studies (Total Patients)	Risk of Bias	Consistency	Directness	Precision	SOE and Magnitude of Effect Effect Estimate (95% CI)
Modifiers of effectiveness (subgroups)						
All	2 RCTs, 12 observational (572,188)	1 low risk, 8 moderate risk, 5 high risk	NA	NA	NA	One RCT showed higher survival in autologous vein graft compared to prosthetic graft. An observational study showed worse survival in advanced age, renal failure and with higher PAD severity. **Insufficient SOE**
Safety concerns: periprocedural complications						
IC-CLI	Observational: 4 (968) RCT: 2 (130)	Observational: 2 moderate risk, 2 high risk RCT: 2 moderate risk	Inconsistent	Direct	Imprecise	Observational OR 1.87 (0.63 to 5.49) RCT OR 0.57 (0.14 to 2.26) Observational studies favored endovascular while the RCTs favored surgical revascularization **Insufficient SOE**
Safety concerns: infection						
IC-CLI	Observational: 2 (823) RCT: 1 (44)	Observational: 1 moderate risk, 1 high risk RCT: 1 moderate risk	Consistent	Direct	Imprecise	Observational OR 14.10 (0.43 to 460.70) RCT OR 12.09 (0.61 to 239.54) Favors endovascular **Low SOE**

Table 31. Detailed SOE of evidence for endovascular versus surgical revascularization in CLI and IC-CLI populations (continued)

Population	Study Design Number of Studies (Total Patients)	Risk of Bias	Consistency	Directness	Precision	SOE and Magnitude of Effect Effect Estimate (95% CI)
Nonfatal stroke Composite cardiovascular events MWD or ACD ICD or PFWD Quality of life Analog pain scale Safety concerns (subgroups)						
All	0	NA	NA	NA	NA	Insufficient SOE

Abbreviations: ACD=absolute claudication distance; CI=confidence interval; CLI=critical limb ischemia; IC=intermittent claudication; ICD=initial claudication distance; LOS=hospital length of stay; MI=myocardial infarction; MWD=maximal walking distance; NA=not applicable; Obs=observational; PFWD=pain-free walking distance; RCT=randomized controlled trial; SOE=strength of evidence.

Discussion

Key Findings and SOE

In this comparative effectiveness review, we identified the following studies:

- Eleven studies (10 RCTs, 1 observational), involving 15,150 patients, that assessed the effectiveness of aspirin, clopidogrel, or other antiplatelet agents on cardiovascular outcomes in the PAD population (KQ 1)
- Thirty-five studies (27 RCTs, 8 observational), involving 7475 patients with IC, that assessed the effectiveness of exercise training, medication, endovascular intervention, and/or surgical revascularization on functional outcomes, quality of life, and cardiovascular events (KQ 2)
- Thirty-seven studies (3 RCTs, 34 observational) that assessed the effectiveness of usual care, endovascular intervention, or surgical revascularization on vessel patency, amputation, mortality, and amputation-free survival (KQ 3). Of these, 23 studies (1 RCT, 22 observational) involved 12,779 patients with CLI and 12 studies (2 RCTs, 10 observational) involved 565,168 patients with IC or CLI.

KQ 1. Comparative Effectiveness and Safety of Antiplatelet Therapy in Adults With PAD

Our review of antiplatelet agents shows that the comparative effectiveness for prevention of cardiovascular disease appears to vary by PAD severity and medication. In asymptomatic PAD patients with no previous cardiovascular disease, including asymptomatic PAD patients with diabetes, aspirin 100 mg daily did not reduce vascular events or mortality compared with placebo from two good quality RCTs. In PAD patients with IC, aspirin reduced the rates of fatal and nonfatal MI as well as other vascular events when compared to placebo in one fair quality RCT.

The comparative effectiveness of clopidogrel versus aspirin has been studied in one good-quality RCT (CAPRIE), which found clopidogrel more effective at reducing cardiovascular mortality, nonfatal MI, and composite vascular events. Clopidogrel and aspirin appeared to be equivalent for prevention of nonfatal stroke, but the confidence interval was wide, making this conclusion less certain.

DAPT with clopidogrel plus aspirin has been compared with aspirin monotherapy. In a predominately IC population, the CHARISMA RCT showed no difference between aspirin and dual therapy (clopidogrel plus aspirin) for outcomes of all-cause mortality, nonfatal stroke, cardiovascular mortality, or composite vascular events; however, it showed a statistically significant benefit favoring dual therapy compared with aspirin for reducing nonfatal MI. In a mixed IC and CLI population randomized to dual antiplatelet versus aspirin therapy after unilateral bypass graft, DAPT resulted in no difference in nonfatal stroke and composite vascular events. In patients with IC or CLI after endovascular procedure, the MIRROR study showed no difference between dual therapy and aspirin in cardiovascular events or mortality at 6 months but was insufficiently powered for those outcomes.

Four additional studies assessed other antiplatelet comparisons. One poor-quality retrospective study of 113 CLI patients after infrainguinal bypass comparing aspirin with no-aspirin therapy showed no differences in the rate of graft failure or vascular death between the groups. One good-quality RCT in 103 IC patients after PTA comparing DAPT with aspirin showed no differences in adverse events (bleeding, rash, hematoma, or bruising); the main finding was greater platelet function inhibition with dual therapy. Two fair-quality RCTs assessed other antiplatelet comparisons (aspirin or iloprost versus no antiplatelet agent, n=38; and aspirin 1000 mg versus aspirin 10 mg, n=216) in IC and CLI patients after PTA. Both RCTs reported no differences in vessel patency or restenosis between the treatment groups and were underpowered.

Four RCTs reported subgroup analyses of demographic or clinical factors that modify the effect of antiplatelet agents in PAD and involved a total of 5053 patients. Two of these RCTs included asymptomatic or symptomatic patients, and two included patients with either IC or CLI. Subgroups analyzed included diabetes (one RCT), age (one RCT), sex (two RCT), and PAD characteristics (two studies assessing ABI or type of bypass graft). The small number of and variation in subgroup analyses precluded the calculation of any overall estimate. One study of patients with IC or CLI showed a benefit of clopidogrel plus aspirin for reducing composite vascular events in patients with a prosthetic bypass graft compared to those with a venous bypass graft. Another study showed similar clinical outcomes in men and women treated with antiplatelet agents.

Seven RCTs reported safety concerns from antiplatelet treatment in the PAD population and involved a total of 8297 patients. All seven studies reported bleeding—GI bleeding, transfusion, any bleeding—as a harm. In general, use of antiplatelet agents was associated with higher rates of minor and moderate bleeding compared with placebo, ranging from 2 to 4 percent with aspirin, 2 percent with dual antiplatelet (no procedure), and 16.7 percent with dual antiplatelet (postbypass grafting).

Table 32 summarizes the SOE for the outcomes of all-cause mortality, nonfatal MI, nonfatal stroke, and composite vascular events. No studies reported results on functional outcomes or quality of life. Very few studies reported modifiers of effectiveness or safety outcomes.

Table 32. Summary SOE for KQ 1: Comparative effectiveness and safety of antiplatelet therapy for adults with PAD[a]

Comparison	Population	Outcome SOE	Results or Effect Estimate (95% Confidence Interval)
Aspirin vs. placebo in adults with asymptomatic or symptomatic PAD at 2+ years	Asymptomatic population	All-cause mortality SOE=High	2 RCTs, 3,986 patients HR 0.93 (0.71 to 1.24) HR 0.95 (0.77 to 1.16) No difference
		Nonfatal MI SOE=High	2 RCTs, 3,986 patients HR 0.98 (0.68 to 1.42) HR 0.91 (0.65 to 1.29) No difference
		Nonfatal stroke SOE=High	2 RCTs, 3,986 patients HR 0.71 (0.44 to 1.14) HR 0.97 (0.62 to 1.53) No difference
		Cardiovascular mortality SOE=Moderate	2 RCTs, 3,986 patients HR 1.23 (0.79 to 1.92) HR 0.95 (0.77 to 1.17) No difference
		Composite vascular events SOE=High	2 RCTs, 3,986 patients HR 0.98 (0.76 to 1.26) HR 1.00 (0.85 to 1.17) No difference

Table 32. Summary SOE for KQ 1: Comparative effectiveness and safety of antiplatelet therapy for adults with PAD[a] (continued)

Comparison	Population	Outcome SOE	Results or Effect Estimate (95% Confidence Interval)
Aspirin vs. placebo in adults with asymptomatic or symptomatic PAD at 2+ years (continued)		Functional outcomes Quality of life Safety concerns (subgroups) **SOE=Insufficient**	0 studies
		Modifiers of effectiveness (subgroups) **SOE=Insufficient**	2 RCTs, 3,986 patients Inconclusive evidence due to imprecision, with 1 study reporting similar rates of cardiovascular outcomes by age, sex, or baseline ABI and 1 study reporting similar rates of cardiovascular mortality and stroke by diabetic status.
		Safety concerns **SOE=Insufficient**	2 RCTs, 3,986 patients Inconclusive evidence due to heterogeneous results between aspirin and placebo in regard to major hemorrhage and GI bleeding rates.
	IC population	Nonfatal MI **SOE=Low**	1 RCT, 181 patients HR 0.18 (0.04 to 0.82) Favors aspirin.
		Nonfatal stroke **SOE=Insufficient**	1 RCT, 181 patients HR 0.54 (0.16 to 1.84) Inconclusive evidence due to imprecision.
		Cardiovascular mortality **SOE=Insufficient**	1 RCT, 181 patients HR 1.21 (0.32 to 4.55) Inconclusive evidence due to imprecision.
		Composite vascular events **SOE=Low**	1 RCT, 181 patients HR 0.35 (0.15 to 0.82) Favors aspirin
		Functional outcomes Quality of life Safety concerns (subgroups **SOE=Insufficient**	0 studies
		Modifiers of effectiveness (subgroups) **SOE=Insufficient**	1 RCT, 216 patients Inconclusive evidence due to imprecision, with 1 study reporting similar rates in vessel patency by sex.
		Safety concerns **SOE=Insufficient**	1 RCT, 181 patients Inconclusive evidence due to imprecision, with 1 study reporting a bleeding rate of 3% in aspirin group and 0% in placebo group.
	CLI population	Nonfatal MI **SOE=Insufficient**	1 observational study, 113 patients Inconclusive evidence due to imprecision, with 1 study reporting MI rate of 1.2% in aspirin group and 5.9% in no-aspirin group.
		Nonfatal stroke **SOE=Insufficient**	1 observational study, 113 patients Inconclusive evidence due to imprecision, with 1 study reporting stroke rate of 2.5% in aspirin group and 8.8% in no-aspirin group.

Table 32. Summary SOE for KQ 1: Comparative effectiveness and safety of antiplatelet therapy for adults with PAD[a] (continued)

Comparison	Population	Outcome SOE	Results or Effect Estimate (95% Confidence Interval)
Aspirin vs. placebo in adults with asymptomatic or symptomatic PAD at 2+ years (continued)		Cardiovascular mortality SOE=Insufficient	1 observational study, 113 patients Inconclusive evidence due to imprecision, with 1 study reporting cardiovascular mortality rate of 33% in aspirin group and 26% in no-aspirin group..
		Functional outcomes Quality of life Modifiers of effectiveness (subgroups) Safety concerns Safety concerns (subgroups) SOE=Insufficient	0 studies
Clopidogrel vs. aspirin in adults with IC at 2 years (CAPRIE)		Nonfatal MI SOE=Moderate	1 RCT, 6,452 patients HR 0.62 (0.43 to 0.88) Favors clopidogrel
		Nonfatal stroke SOE=Low	1 RCT, 6,452 patients HR 0.95 (0.68 to 1.31) No difference
		Cardiovascular mortality SOE=Moderate	1 RCT, 6,452 patients HR 0.76 (0.64 to 0.91) Favors clopidogrel.
		Composite cardiovascular events SOE=Moderate	1 RCT, 6,452 patients HR 0.78 (0.65 to 0.93) Favors clopidogrel.
		All-cause mortality Functional outcomes Quality of life Modifiers of effectiveness (subgroups) Safety concerns Safety concerns (subgroups) SOE=Insufficient	0 studies
Clopidogrel/aspirin vs. aspirin in adults with PAD at 2 years	Symptomatic–asymptomatic population (CHARISMA)	All-cause mortality SOE=Moderate	1 RCT, 3,096 patients HR 0.89 (0.68 to 1.16) No difference.
		Nonfatal MI SOE=Low	1 RCT, 3,096 patients HR 0.63 (0.42 to 0.95) Favors dual antiplatelet.
		Nonfatal stroke SOE=Low	1 RCT, 3,096 patients HR 0.79 (0.51 to 1.22) No difference.
		Cardiovascular mortality SOE=Low	1 RCT, 3,096 patients HR 0.92 (0.66 to 1.29) No difference.
		Composite cardiovascular events SOE=Moderate	1 RCT, 3,096 patients HR 0.85 (0.66 to 1.09) No difference.

Table 32. Summary SOE for KQ 1: Comparative effectiveness and safety of antiplatelet therapy for adults with PAD[a] (continued)

Comparison	Population	Outcome SOE	Results or Effect Estimate (95% Confidence Interval)
Clopidogrel/aspirin vs. aspirin in adults with PAD at 2 years (continued)		Functional outcomes Quality of life Safety concerns (subgroups) Modifiers of effectiveness (subgroups) **SOE=Insufficient**	0 studies
		Safety concerns **SOE=Insufficient**	1 RCT, 3,096 patients Inconclusive evidence due to low rates of severe and moderate bleeding, although minor bleeding was significantly higher with DAPT (34.4%) vs. ASA (20.8%).
	IC–CLI population (CASPAR, MIRROR, Cassar)	All-cause mortality **SOE=Insufficient**	2 RCTs, 931 patients CASPAR, HR 1.44 (0.77 to 2.69) MIRROR, OR 0.33 (0.01 to 8.22) Inconclusive evidence due to imprecision.
		Nonfatal MI **SOE=Insufficient**	1 RCT, 851 patients CASPAR, HR 0.81 (0.32 to 2.06) Inconclusive evidence due to imprecision.
		Nonfatal stroke **SOE=Low**	1 RCT, 851 patients CASPAR, HR 1.02 (0.41 to 2.55) No difference.
		Cardiovascular mortality **SOE=Insufficient**	1 RCT, 851 patients CASPAR, HR 1.44 (0.77 to 2.69) Inconclusive evidence due to imprecision.
		Composite cardiovascular events **SOE=Low (CASPAR)** **SOE=Insufficient (MIRROR)**	2 RCTs, 931 patients CASPAR, HR 1.09 (0.65 to 1.82), No difference MIRROR, OR 0.71 (0.28 to 1.81), Inconclusive evidence due to imprecision.
		Functional outcomes Quality of life Safety concerns (subgroups) **SOE=Insufficient**	0 studies
		Modifiers of effectiveness (subgroups) **SOE=Insufficient**	1 RCT, 851 patients Inconclusive evidence due to imprecision, with 1 study reporting that patients with prosthetic graft had lower cardiovascular events on DAPT.

Table 32. Summary SOE for KQ 1: Comparative effectiveness and safety of antiplatelet therapy for adults with PAD[a] (continued)

Comparison	Population	Outcome SOE	Results or Effect Estimate (95% Confidence Interval)
Clopidogrel/aspirin vs. aspirin in adults with PAD at 2 years (continued)		Safety concerns SOE=Insufficient	3 RCTs, 1,034 patients Inconclusive evidence due to inconsistent results from individual studies: CASPAR study showed statistically significant higher rates of moderate and minor bleeding with DAPT; Cassar study showed more bruising with DAPT but no significant difference in gastrointestinal bleeding or hematoma; MIRROR study showed no significant difference in bleeding.

[a] Gray highlights insufficient strength of evidence.
Abbreviations: ABI=ankle-brachial index; CLI=critical limb ischemia; DAPT=dual antiplatelet therapy; HR=hazard ratio; IC=intermittent claudication; MI=myocardial infarction; OR=odds ratio; RCT=randomized controlled trial; SOE=strength of evidence

KQ 2. Comparative Effectiveness and Safety of Exercise, Medications, and Endovascular and Surgical Revascularization for IC

Thirty-five (27 RCT, 8 observational; 7475 patients) evaluated the effectiveness of exercise, medical therapy, endovascular or surgical revascularization for IC. The following comparisons were assessed in the included studies: (1) medical therapy (cilostazol) versus placebo (10 RCTs; 4103 total patients); (2) exercise training versus usual care (10 RCTs, two observational; 754 total patients); (3) endovascular intervention versus usual care (5 RCTs, 4 observational; 1593 total patients); (4) surgical revascularization versus usual care (1 observational; 427 total patients); (5) endovascular intervention versus exercise training (9 RCTs; 1005 total patients); (6) surgical revascularization versus exercise training plus medical therapy (1 observational; 127 total patients); and (7) endovascular versus surgical revascularization (3 observational studies; 421 total patients). A majority of the endovascular procedures consisted of PTA with or without stent placement, and the type of stent was not specified. Differences in the treatment comparisons, measures, and followup time points reduced the number of studies that could be pooled for analysis of direct comparisons.

In a random-effects meta-analysis of 12 RCTs that compared the effect of multiple treatments on all-cause mortality, no specific treatment was found to have a statistically significant effect.

In a random-effects meta-analysis of 16 RCTs that compared the effect of multiple treatments on MWD or ACD, exercise training was associated with a statistically significant improvement when compared with usual care; endovascular intervention was associated with a statistically significant improvement in ACD when compared with usual care. None of the other treatments were found to have a statistically significant effect when compared with usual care or against each other. A sensitivity analysis removing the pentoxifylline studies (due to inconsistency and imprecision) resulted in effect size estimates that are slightly increased for the remaining treatment modalities. Studies that measured peak walking time rather than distance showed similar results across treatment comparisons.

In a random-effects meta-analysis of 12 RCTs that compared the effect of multiple treatments on initial claudication distance or pain-free walking distance, cilostazol was associated with a statistically nonsignificant improvement when compared with usual care;

however, exercise training and endovascular revascularization was associated with a statistically significant improvement when compared with usual care. When directly compared in head-to-head studies, there was no difference between the three treatments. Again, studies not included in the meta-analysis due to measurement of claudication onset time rather than distance found similar results across treatment comparisons.

A meta-analysis of 13 RCTs examining the difference in the SF-36 measure of physical functioning among exercise training, endovascular intervention, and usual care measured between 3 months and 6 months showed a significant improvement in quality of life from cilostazol, exercise training, endovascular intervention, and surgical revascularization compared with usual care. However, the comparisons of all active treatments with each other showed that none of the treatments are significantly different from each other.

Vessel patency, repeat revascularization, wound healing, analog pain scale score, cardiovascular events (e.g., all-cause mortality, MI, stroke, cardiovascular death), and amputation were infrequently reported.

Six studies (4 RCTs, 2 observational) reported variations in the treatment effectiveness by subgroup including severity of symptoms, functional limitations, anatomic location of disease, and success of revascularization. There were no studies reporting results by the following subgroups: age, sex, race, presence of diabetes mellitus or renal disease, smoking status, or prior revascularization. Despite limited data to draw definitive conclusions, one study reported improvements in quality-of-life measures and ABI in patients with successful endovascular revascularization when compared with patients without successful endovascular revascularization. Another study reported improvement in ABI in patients with successful surgical revascularization when compared with patients treated with exercise and medical therapy. One other study reported a statistically nonsignificant improvement in MWD favoring exercise training over endovascular revascularization in patients with SFA stenosis when compared with patients with iliac stenosis. Last, a single study reported variability in the patency of surgical revascularization based on anatomic location and graft type.

Seventeen RCTs reported safety concerns. A single study of exercise therapy versus usual care did not identify side effects from exercise. Studies of cilostazol had higher rates of headache, dizziness, and diarrhea. Studies of endovascular interventions reported more transfusions, arterial dissection/perforation, and hematomas compared to the usual care groups but the complication rates were low (1 to 2%). No studies were identified that measured contrast nephropathy, radiation, infection, or exercise-related harms. No studies reported on whether any of the harms vary by subgroup (age, sex, race, risk factors, comorbidities, anatomic location of disease).

Table 33 summarizes the SOE for the outcomes outlined in the KQ by each treatment strategy. We found very few studies that assessed cardiovascular outcomes (all-cause or cardiovascular mortality, nonfatal MI, nonfatal stroke, or composite events); therefore, the evidence base is insufficient for us to draw any conclusions on these outcomes. Similar to KQ 1, very few studies reported modifiers of effectiveness or safety outcomes.

Table 33. Summary SOE for KQ 2: Comparative effectiveness and safety of treatments for IC[a]

Comparison	Outcome SOE	Results or Effect Estimate (95% Confidence Interval)
Medical therapy vs. usual care	All-cause mortality SOE=Low	4 RCTs, 2,732 patients OR 0.91 (0.62 to 1.35) No difference.
	Nonfatal MI SOE=Insufficient	2 RCTs, 497 patients Inconclusive evidence due to low event rates in both groups.
	Nonfatal stroke SOE=Insufficient	3 RCTs, 1,932 patients Inconclusive evidence due to low event rates in both groups.
	Amputation SOE=Insufficient	2 RCTs, 497 patients Inconclusive evidence due to sparse data, with only 1 patient who underwent amputation in the 2 RCTs.
	Quality of life SOE=Low	2 RCTs, 631 patients ES: 0.44 (0.05 to 0.83) Favors cilostazol.
	MWD or ACD SOE=Low (cilostazol) SOE=Insufficient (pentoxifylline)	Cilostazol (6 RCTs, 1,632 patients) ES: 0.62 (-0.21 to 1.45) full model; 0.61 (-0.20 to 1.42) sensitivity analysis No difference. Pentoxifylline (3 RCTs, 797 patients) ES: 1.70 (0.36 to 3.04) full model Inconclusive evidence due to imprecision.
	Initial claudication distance or pain-free walking distance SOE=Low (cilostazol)	5 RCTs, 1,255 patients ES: 0.63 (-0.03 to 1.29) No difference.
	Modifiers of effectiveness (subgroups) SOE=Insufficient	2 RCTs, 155 patients Inconclusive evidence due to individual studies reporting different endpoints.
	Safety concerns SOE=High (headache) SOE=Moderate (diarrhea) SOE=Moderate (palpitations)	Higher side effects on cilostazol Headache 10 RCTs, 3,485 patients OR 3.00 (2.29 to 3.95) Diarrhea 10 RCTs, 3,485 patients OR 2.51 (1.58 to 3.97) Palpitations 10 RCTs, 3,485 patients OR 18.11 (5.95 to 55.13)
	Primary patency Secondary patency Composite cardiovascular events Wound healing Analog pain scale Safety concerns (subgroups) SOE=Insufficient	0 studies

Table 33. Summary SOE for KQ 2: Comparative effectiveness and safety of treatments for IC[a] **(continued)**

Comparison	Outcome SOE	Results or Effect Estimate (95% Confidence Interval)
Exercise training vs. usual care	All-cause mortality SOE=Low	2 RCTs, 238 patients OR 0.84 (0.34 to 2.07) No difference.
	Nonfatal MI SOE=Insufficient	1 RCT, 63 patients Inconclusive evidence due to sparse data, with only 1 MI in exercise group.
	Nonfatal stroke SOE=Insufficient	1 RCT, 63 patients Inconclusive evidence due to sparse data, with only 1 stroke in each group.
	Amputation SOE=Insufficient	1 RCT; 31 patients Inconclusive evidence due to sparse data, with only 1 patient who underwent amputation.
	Quality of life SOE=Low	4 RCTs, 1 observational study, 275 patients ES: 0.56 (0.26 to 0.87) Favors exercise.
	MWD or ACD SOE=Moderate	9 RCTs, 2 observational studies, 624 patients ES: 0.89 (0.06 to 1.71) full model; 0.98 (0.23 to 1.74) sensitivity analysis Favors exercise.
	Initial claudication distance or pain-free walking distance SOE=Low	9 RCTs, 1 observational studies, 396 patients ES: 0.69 (0.22 to 1.15) Favors exercise.
	Safety concerns SOE=Insufficient	3 RCTs, 107 patients Inconclusive evidence due to sparse data, with studies reporting no adverse events in exercise or usual care groups.
	Composite cardiovascular events Wound healing Analog pain scale Safety concerns (subgroups) SOE=Insufficient	0 studies
Endovascular intervention vs. usual care	All-cause mortality SOE=Low	2 RCTs, 3 observational studies, 977 patients OR 0.91 (0.34 to 2.45) No difference.
	Nonfatal MI SOE=Insufficient	1 observational study; 479 patients Inconclusive evidence due to imprecision, with 1 study reporting 3.0% in endovascular group and 8.8% in usual care group.
	Nonfatal stroke SOE=Insufficient	2 observational studies; 800 patients Inconclusive evidence due to sparse data, with 1 study reporting 4 strokes for total study, and 1 study reporting 1 stroke in endovascular group, 2 strokes in usual care group.
	Amputation SOE=Insufficient	1 RCT, 1 observational study, 73 patients Inconclusive evidence due to imprecision, with 1 study reporting similar amputation rates in the endovascular and usual care groups.
	Quality of life SOE=Low	2 RCTs, 2 observational studies, 576 patients ES: 0.61 (0.30 to 0.93) Favors endovascular intervention.

Table 33. Summary SOE for KQ 2: Comparative effectiveness and safety of treatments for IC[a] (continued)

Comparison	Outcome SOE	Results or Effect Estimate (95% Confidence Interval)
Endovascular intervention vs. usual care (continued)	MWD or ACD SOE=Low	4 RCTs, 285 patients ES: 0.41 (-0.54 to 1.36) full model; 0.51 (-0.35 to 1.37) sensitivity analysis No difference.
	Initial claudication distance or pain-free walking distance SOE=Low	5 RCTs, 281 patients ES: 0.79 (0.29 to 1.29) Favors endovascular intervention.
	Modifiers of effectiveness (subgroups) SOE=Insufficient	1 observational study, 526 patients Inconclusive evidence due to imprecision, with 1 study reporting better quality-of-life scores if ABI improvement was >0.1 after successful revascularization.
	Safety concerns SOE=Insufficient	2 RCTs, 155 patients Inconclusive evidence due to sparse data, with 1 study reporting no events, and 1 study reporting low rates of transfusion, dissection, and perforation in the endovascular group.
	Composite cardiovascular events Wound healing Analog pain scale Safety concerns (subgroups) SOE=Insufficient	0 studies
Surgical revascularization vs. usual care	All-cause mortality SOE=Insufficient	1 observational study, 427 patients Inconclusive evidence due to imprecision, with mortality rates of 10.4% in surgical group and 16.7% in usual care group.
	Quality of life SOE=Low	2 observational studies, 727 patients ES: 0.82 (0.26 to 1.39) Favors surgery.
	Primary patency Secondary patency SOE=Insufficient	1 observational study, 427 patients Inconclusive evidence due to imprecision, with 1 study reporting vessel patency only in patients undergoing revascularization (aortofemoral bypass 95.5%, axillofemoral bypass 83.3%, femorofemoral bypass 95.5%, femoropopliteal bypass [AK] 67.6%, femorofemoral bypass [BK] 45.2%).
	Modifiers of effectiveness (subgroups) SOE=Insufficient	1 observational study, 427 patients Inconclusive evidence due to results from 1 study where patency rates were significantly lower for infrainguinal bypass and synthetic graft vs. suprainguinal and autologous vein graft.
	Nonfatal MI Nonfatal stroke Amputation Composite cardiovascular events Wound healing Analog pain scale Safety concerns (subgroups) SOE=Insufficient	0 studies

Table 33. Summary SOE for KQ 2: Comparative effectiveness and safety of treatments for IC[a] (continued)

Comparison	Outcome SOE	Results or Effect Estimate (95% Confidence Interval)
Endovascular intervention vs. exercise training	All-cause mortality SOE=Low	5 RCTs, 710 patients OR 0.77 (0.39 to 1.54) No difference.
	Nonfatal MI SOE=Insufficient	1 RCT, 106 patients Inconclusive evidence due to sparse data, with no events occurring in either treatment group.
	Nonfatal stroke SOE=Insufficient	1 RCT, 106 patients Inconclusive evidence due to sparse data, with only 1 stroke in each group.
	Amputation SOE=Insufficient	1 RCT, 149 patients Inconclusive evidence due to sparse data, with 1 amputation in endovascular group and none in exercise group.
	Quality of life SOE=Low	4 RCTs, 444 patients ES: 0.05 (-0.24 to 0.34) No difference.
	MWD or ACD SOE=Moderate	4 RCTs, 695 patients ES: -0.47 (-1.41 to 0.46) full model; -0.47 (-1.31 to 0.36) sensitivity analysis No difference.
	ICD or PFWD SOE=Low	5 RCTs, 448 patients ES: 0.10 (-0.38 to 0.58) No difference.
	Modifiers of effectiveness (subgroups) SOE=Insufficient	1 RCT, 56 patients Inconclusive evidence due to indirect results from 1 study reporting a statistically nonsignificant improvement in MWD in patients with superficial femoral artery (SFA) disease treated with percutaneous transluminal angioplasty (PTA).
	Safety concerns SOE=Insufficient	5 RCTs, 282 patients Inconclusive evidence due to heterogeneity of reporting, with individual studies reporting that endovascular interventions were associated with higher rates of transfusion, dissection/perforation, and hematomas.
	Composite cardiovascular events Wound healing Analog pain scale Safety concerns (subgroups) SOE=Insufficient	0 studies
Surgical intervention vs. exercise + medical therapy (pentoxifylline)	MWD or ACD SOE=Insufficient	1 observational study, 127 patients Inconclusive evidence due to imprecision, with 1 study reporting that MWT improved to >15 min in surgical group and >11 min in exercise plus medical therapy group.
	Initial claudication distance or pain-free walking distance SOE=Insufficient	1 observational study, 127 patients Inconclusive evidence due to imprecision, with 1 study reporting that COT improved to >10 min in surgical group and >7 min in exercise plus medical therapy group.

Table 33. Summary SOE for KQ 2: Comparative effectiveness and safety of treatments for IC[a] (continued)

Comparison	Outcome SOE	Results or Effect Estimate (95% Confidence Interval)
Surgical intervention vs. exercise + medical therapy (pentoxifylline) (continued)	Composite cardiovascular events Wound healing Analog pain scale Safety concerns (subgroups) SOE=Insufficient	0 studies
Endovascular intervention vs. surgical revascularization	All-cause mortality SOE=Insufficient	2 observational studies, 305 patients Inconclusive evidence due to inadequate reporting, with neither study reporting results by treatment group; overall mortality rate ranged from 3 to 8%.
	Quality of life SOE=Low	2 observational studies, 242 patients ES: 0.21 (-0.34 to 0.76) No difference.
	MWD or absolute claudication distance SOE=Insufficient	0 studies
	ICD or PFWD SOE=Insufficient	0 studies
	Modifiers of effectiveness (subgroups) SOE=Insufficient	1 RCT, 264 patients Inconclusive evidence due to indirect results from 1 study, with similar patency rates for suprainguinal and infrainguinal reconstruction.
	Nonfatal MI Nonfatal stroke Amputation Primary patency Secondary patency Composite cardiovascular events Wound healing Analog pain scale Safety concerns (subgroups) SOE=Insufficient	0 studies
Endovascular intervention + exercise training vs. usual care	MWD or ACD SOE=Low	2 RCTs, 248 patients ES: 1.08 (-0.37 to 2.53) full model; 1.20 (-0.11 to 2.50) sensitivity analysis Favors endovascular intervention plus exercise training.
	Composite cardiovascular events Wound healing Analog pain scale Safety concerns (subgroups) SOE=Insufficient	0 studies

Table 33. Summary SOE for KQ 2: Comparative effectiveness and safety of treatments for IC[a] (continued)

Comparison	Outcome SOE	Results or Effect Estimate (95% Confidence Interval)
Exercise training vs. invasive therapy vs. usual care	Primary patency Secondary patency SOE=Insufficient	1 RCT, 225 patients Inconclusive evidence due to biased reporting where vessel patency was only reported in patients undergoing revascularization (endovascular group 59%, surgical group 98%).
	Composite cardiovascular events Wound healing Analog pain scale Safety concerns (subgroups) SOE=Insufficient	0 studies

[a] Grey background indicates insufficient SOE.
Abbreviations: ACD=absolute claudication distance; ES=effect size; ICD=initial claudication distance; MI=myocardial infarction; MWD=maximal walking distance; OR=odds ratio; PFWD=pain-free walking distance; PTA=percutaneous transluminal angioplasty; RCT=randomized controlled trial; SFA=superficial femoral artery; SOE=strength of evidence.

KQ 3. Comparative Effectiveness and Safety of Usual Care and Endovascular and Surgical Revascularization for CLI

We identified 37 unique studies (3 RCT, 34 observational) that evaluated the comparative effectiveness of usual care, endovascular intervention, and surgical revascularization in CLI or IC-CLI patients. Of these, four observational studies compared usual care with endovascular intervention. Of the 37 studies, 23 (1 RCT, 22 observational) evaluated the comparative effectiveness of endovascular and surgical revascularization in 12,779 patients with CLI, and 12 (2 RCT, 10 observational) evaluated the comparative effectiveness of endovascular and surgical revascularization in a *mixed* population of 565,168 PAD patients with either IC or CLI. The clinical outcomes of interest included vessel patency, repeat revascularization, wound healing, analog pain scale score, cardiovascular events (e.g., all-cause mortality, MI, stroke, cardiovascular death), amputation, functional capacity, and quality of life.

In the four observational studies that compared endovascular interventions with usual care, the reported outcomes included mortality (four studies), amputation/limb salvage (four studies), amputation-free survival (one study), and hospital length of stay (two studies). Most clinical outcomes were improved with endovascular therapy however the results were nonsignificant and inconsistent. None of these studies reported the rates of stroke, MI, functional outcomes, quality of life, vessel patency, wound healing, pain scores, subgroup differences, or harms. Similar to KQ 2, a majority of the endovascular procedures consisted of PTA with or without stent placement, and the type of stent was not specified.

Meta-analysis of endovascular versus surgical revascularization studies showed all-cause mortality was not different between patients treated with endovascular versus surgical revascularization although endovascular interventions did demonstrate a statistically nonsignificant benefit in all-cause mortality at less than 6 months in the CLI and IC-CLI populations and at 1 to 2 years in the IC-CLI population. Evidence regarding patency rates varied, but secondary patency rates demonstrated a benefit of endovascular interventions compared with surgical revascularization across all followup time points in the CLI population. There were few studies that assessed functional outcomes, quality of life, or cardiovascular outcomes (cardiovascular mortality, nonfatal stroke, nonfatal MI, or composite events). Fourteen studies reported hospital length of stay during the index hospitalization. The range of hospital stay was 1 to 15 days in the endovascular group and 2 to 37 days in the surgical group.

Variations in treatment effectiveness by subgroup were reported in 14 studies (2 RCT, 12 observational; 7 CLI and 7 IC-CLI populations). Subgroups reported included age (three studies), symptom class (three studies), renal failure (two studies), anatomic factors (four studies), type of vein graft (two studies), and one study each on diabetes, smoking status, hyperlipidemia, and hypertension. In the single RCT of CLI patients, the use of autologous vein was associated with improved outcomes when compared with prosthetic conduit. Additionally, the performance of subintimal angioplasty was associated with statistically nonsignificant worse outcomes when compared with standard angioplasty. Data derived from the observational studies had a high likelihood of bias but did show that with advanced age, renal failure, and higher Rutherford classification, patients generally fared worse in terms of mortality and amputation.

Only one observational study in the CLI population reported safety concerns. Specifically, this study reported the incidence of thrombosis at 30 days and found that the risk of thrombosis was higher in patients undergoing surgical revascularization than in patients undergoing endovascular revascularization. Six studies (2 RCT, 4 observational) in the mixed IC-CLI population reported harms of bleeding, infection, renal dysfunction, or periprocedural complications causing acute limb ischemia. There were conflicting results in the summary estimates for periprocedural complications in the IC-CLI population with the observational studies showing lower rates in those who received an endovascular intervention and RCTs showing lower rates in the surgical population; however the wide confidence intervals make the differences nonsignificant. Infection was more common in the surgical intervention arm based on three studies.

Table 34 summarizes the SOE for the outcomes from the endovascular versus surgical revascularization studies. We found very few studies that assessed functional outcomes, quality of life, or cardiovascular outcomes (cardiovascular mortality, nonfatal MI, nonfatal stroke, or composite events), therefore the evidence base is insufficient for us to draw any conclusions on these outcomes. Like the other KQs, very few studies reported modifiers of effectiveness or safety outcomes.

Table 34. Summary SOE for KQ 3: Comparative effectiveness and safety of treatments for CLI[a]

Comparison	Outcome SOE	Results or Effect Estimate (95% Confidence Interval)
Endovascular intervention vs. usual care in CLI and IC-CLI populations	All-cause mortality SOE=Insufficient	CLI-Obs (3 studies, 562 patients) Inconclusive evidence due to imprecision. IC-CLI-Obs (1 study, 107 patients) Inconclusive evidence due to imprecision, with 1 study reporting similar mortality rates.
	Amputation SOE=Insufficient	CLI-Obs (3 studies, 562 patients) Inconclusive evidence due to heterogeneity in reporting amputation rates across studies. IC-CLI-Obs (1 study, 107 patients) Inconclusive evidence due to imprecision, with 1 study reporting a nonsignificant difference.
	Amputation-free survival SOE=Insufficient	CLI-Obs (1 study, 70 patients) Inconclusive evidence due to imprecision, with 1 study reporting AFS rates (endovascular group 60%, usual care 47%).

Table 34. Summary SOE for KQ 3: Comparative effectiveness and safety of treatments for CLI[a] (continued)

Comparison	Outcome SOE	Results or Effect Estimate (95% Confidence Interval)
Endovascular intervention vs. usual care in CLI and IC-CLI populations (continued)	Length of stay SOE=Insufficient	CLI-Obs (3 studies, 562 patients) Inconclusive evidence due to inconsistent and imprecise results across studies.
	Nonfatal stroke Nonfatal MI Composite cardiovascular events MWD or absolute claudication distance Initial claudication distance or pain-free walking distance Quality of life Primary patency Secondary patency Wound healing Analog pain scale Modifiers of effectiveness (subgroups) Safety concerns Safety concerns (subgroups) SOE=Insufficient	All PAD populations and study design (0 studies)
Endovascular vs. surgical revascularization in CLI and IC-CLI populations	All-cause mortality less than or equal to 6 months SOE=Low	CLI-Obs (11 studies, 8,249 patients), OR 0.85 (0.57 to 1.27) CLI-RCT (1 study, 452 patients), OR 0.51 (0.20 to 1.35) Favors endovascular. IC-CLI-Obs (2 studies, 823 patients), OR 0.45 (0.18 to 1.09) Favors endovascular.
	All-cause mortality at 1 to 2 years SOE=Low	CLI-Obs (12 studies, 7,850 patients), OR 1.01 (0.80 to 1.28) No difference. IC-CLI-Obs (2 studies, 145 patients), OR 0.51 (0.20 to 1.31) IC-CLI-RCT (2 studies, 130 patients), OR 0.81 (0.23 to 2.82) Favors endovascular.
	All-cause mortality at 3 or more years SOE=Low (CLI) SOE=Insufficient (IC-CLI)	CLI-Obs (7 studies, 7,176 patients), OR 1.05 (0.54 to 2.06) CLI-RCT (1 study, 452 patients), OR 1.07 (0.73 to 1.56) No difference. IC-CLI-RCT (1 study, 58 patients) OR 0.88 (0.28 to 2.73) Inconclusive evidence due to imprecision.
	Nonfatal MI SOE=Insufficient	CLI-RCT (1 study, 452 patients) Inconclusive evidence due to imprecision, with 1 study reporting MI rates (endovascular group 3% and surgical group 8%).

Table 34. Summary SOE for KQ 3: Comparative effectiveness and safety of treatments for CLI[a] (continued)

Comparison	Outcome SOE	Results or Effect Estimate (95% Confidence Interval)
Endovascular vs. surgical revascularization in CLI and IC-CLI populations (continued)	Amputation at <2 years SOE=Low (CLI) SOE=Insufficient (IC-CLI)	CLI-Obs (11 studies, 4490 patients), OR 0.73 (0.48 to 1.09) CLI-RCT (1 study, 452 patients), OR 1.23 (0.72 to 2.11) No difference. IC-CLI-Obs (2 studies, 823 patients), OR 1.11 (0.40 to 3.05) IC-CLI-RCT (2 studies, 130 patients), OR 0.22 (0.05 to 1.07) Inconclusive evidence due to imprecision.
	Amputation at 2 to 3 years SOE=Low (CLI) SOE=Insufficient (IC-CLI)	CLI-Obs (4 studies, 3187 patients), OR 1.08 (0.62 to 1.89) CLI-RCT (1 study, 452 patients), OR 1.02 (0.64 to 1.63) No difference. IC-CLI-Obs (1 study, 169 patients), OR 1.00 (0.18 to 5.54) IC-CLI-RCT (1 study, 86 patients), OR 0.18 (0.02 to 1.29) Inconclusive evidence due to imprecision.
	Amputation after 5 years SOE=Low	CLI-Obs (7 studies, 3101 patients), OR 1.06 (0.70 to 1.59) No difference.
	Amputation-free survival at 1 year SOE=Low	CLI-Obs (2 studies, 1881 patients), OR 0.76 (0.48 to 1.21) CLI-RCT (1 study, 452 patients), OR 0.87 (0.58 to 1.30) No difference.
	Amputation-free survival at 2 to 3 years SOE=Low	CLI-Obs (3 studies, 1972 patients), OR 0.75 (0.53 to 1.09) CLI-RCT (1 study, 452 patients), OR 1.22 (0.84 to 1.77) No difference.
	Amputation-free survival after 5 years SOE=Low	CLI-Obs (4 studies, 2190 patients), OR 0.89 (0.59 to 1.34) No difference.
	Wound healing SOE=Insufficient	CLI-Obs (1 study, 91 patients) Inconclusive evidence due to imprecision, with 1 study reporting similar rates of wound healing in the surgical revascularization group (83%) and endovascular revascularization group (80%).
	Primary patency at 1 year SOE=Moderate (CLI) SOE=Low (IC-CLI)	CLI-Obs (5 studies, 890 patients), OR 0.63 (0.46 to 0.86) No difference. IC-CLI-Obs (3 studies, 328 patients), OR 0.71 (0.40 to 1.28) IC-CLI-RCT (2 studies, 130 patients), OR 0.40 (0.08 to 1.93) Favors endovascular intervention.

Table 34. Summary SOE for KQ 3: Comparative effectiveness and safety of treatments for CLI[a] (continued)

Comparison	Outcome SOE	Results or Effect Estimate (95% Confidence Interval)
Endovascular vs. surgical revascularization in CLI and IC-CLI populations (continued)	Primary patency at 2 to 3 years SOE=Insufficient	CLI-Obs (4 studies, 768 patients), OR 0.77 (0.24 to 2.42) Inconclusive evidence due to imprecision. IC-CLI-Obs (2 studies, 231 patients), OR 0.29 (0.15 to 0.55) IC-CLI-RCT (1 study, 86 patients), OR 0.96 (0.42 to 2.16) Inconclusive evidence due to imprecision.
	Secondary patency at 1 year SOE=Low (CLI) SOE=Insufficient (IC-CLI)	CLI-Obs (4 studies, 759 patients), OR 0.57 to (0.40 to 0.82) Favors endovascular intervention. IC-CLI-RCT (1 study, 44 patients), OR 0.04 (0.00 to 0.73) Inconclusive evidence due to imprecision.
	Secondary patency at 2 to 3 years SOE=Low	CLI-Obs (4 studies, 815 patients), OR 0.49 (0.28 to 0.85) Favors endovascular intervention.
	Length of stay SOE=Insufficient	CLI-Obs (8 studies, 1745 patients) CLI-RCT (1 study, 452 patients) Inconclusive evidence due to inconsistency and imprecision, with individual studies reporting LOS longer in surgical group with large SD in 3 observational studies and no variability reported in 4 observational studies and one RCT. IC-CLI-Obs (3 studies, 563,935 patients) IC-CLI-RCT (2 studies, 130 patients) Inconclusive evidence due to imprecision, with individual studies reporting LOS longer in surgical group with large SD in the observational studies and RCTs.
	Modifiers of effectiveness (subgroups) SOE=Insufficient	All PAD populations and study design (14 studies, 572,188 patients) Inconclusive evidence due to heterogeneity in subgroups assessed across individual studies and inability to quantitatively synthesize results. One RCT showed higher survival in autologous vein graft compared with prosthetic graft. An observational study showed worse survival in advanced age, renal failure, and with higher PAD severity.
	Safety concerns: periprocedural complications SOE=Insufficient	IC-CLI-Obs (4 studies, 968 patients), OR 1.87 (0.63 to 5.49) IC-CLI-RCT (2 studies, 130 patients), OR 0.57 (0.14 to 2.26) Inconclusive evidence due to inconsistency and imprecision with observational studies favoring endovascular while the RCTs favor surgical revascularization.
	Safety concerns: infection SOE=Low	IC-CLI-Obs (2 studies, 823 patients), OR 14.10 (0.43 to 460.70) IC-CLI-RCT (1 study, 44 patients), OR 12.09 (0.61 to 239.54) Favors endovascular intervention.

Table 34. Summary SOE for KQ 3: Comparative effectiveness and safety of treatments for CLI[a] (continued)

Comparison	Outcome SOE	Results or Effect Estimate (95% Confidence Interval)
Endovascular vs. surgical revascularization in CLI and IC-CLI populations (continued)	Nonfatal stroke Composite cardiovascular events MWD or absolute claudication distance Initial claudication distance or pain-free walking distance Quality of life Analog pain scale Safety concerns (subgroups) SOE=Insufficient	All PAD populations and study design (0 studies)

[a] Grey background indicates insufficient SOE.
Abbreviations: ACD=absolute claudication distance; CLI=critical limb ischemia; IC=intermittent claudication; ICD=initial claudication distance; MI=myocardial infarction; MWD=maximal walking distance; Obs=observational; PFWD=pain-free walking distance; RCT=randomized controlled trial; SOE=strength of evidence; yr=year(s).

Findings in Relation to What Is Already Known

For KQ 1, which addresses antiplatelet therapy in PAD patients, our findings on the effectiveness of aspirin are similar to a meta-analysis of 18 studies published in 2009 by Berger et al.[44] In the subset treated with aspirin alone compared with placebo, they found a nonsignificant reduction in cardiovascular events (defined as nonfatal MI, nonfatal stroke, and cardiovascular mortality; RR 0.75; 95% CI, 0.48 to 1.18); a significant reduction in nonfatal stroke (RR 0.64; CI, 0.42 to 0.99); and no statistically significant reductions in nonfatal MI, cardiovascular mortality, or major bleeding.

In this review, we excluded studies published prior to 1995 (n=15) and did not include studies with the combination of aspirin and dipyridamole (n=9). Also, 12 of the 18 studies in the previous meta-analysis[44] were in patients who were treated prior to or after a revascularization procedure. We felt this represented a population with evidence of clinical disease and possible interaction with revascularization therapies. The study by Fowkes et al.[56] was published after that meta-analysis and is the largest study of asymptomatic patients with PAD who have no established cardiovascular disease. Therefore, our review of three aspirin versus placebo studies[54-56] contains the most recent evidence for the effectiveness of aspirin in an era where secondary prevention of cardiovascular events includes treatment of hypertension, diabetes, hyperlipidemia, and tobacco use with current guideline recommendations to reach specific blood pressure, hemoglobin A1c, and lipid-lowering goals as well as access to nicotine replacement therapy for smoking cessation. Additionally, the current meta-analysis includes more asymptomatic patients treated with aspirin for PAD and may represent a treatment effect by symptom status. The lack of clinical effectiveness of 100 mg daily of aspirin in addition to better (aggressive) management of cardiovascular risk factors is of clinical note and consistent with the meta-analysis by Berger et al. when viewed with regard to background therapy. The findings for clopidogrel monotherapy or DAPT were evaluated within subgroups of large RCTs.

Our finding that clopidogrel monotherapy is superior or equivalent to aspirin monotherapy in reducing adverse cardiovascular outcomes from one good-quality RCT in a PAD subgroup population represents current clinical practice and helps reinforce the current guideline recommendations for patients with PAD. The role for DAPT compared with aspirin monotherapy is less certain. From the PAD subgroup analysis of one large RCT[60] and a smaller study on a postrevascularization population,[63] the combination of clopidogrel with aspirin as DAPT did not show a significant benefit in reducing stroke events or cardiovascular mortality in IC patients. In patients with symptomatic or asymptomatic PAD (92% IC, 8% asymptomatic), the PAD subgroup analysis of the CHARISMA study did however show a statistically significant benefit favoring dual therapy (clopidogrel plus aspirin) compared with aspirin for reducing nonfatal MI but showed no difference between aspirin and dual therapy for other outcomes. In the only other systematic review of antiplatelet agents for IC by the Cochrane group,[137] the report included the results of the CAPRIE study, but did not contain the results of the CHARISMA or CASPAR studies. That review also included other antiplatelet agents such as indobufen, picotamide, ticlopidine, and triflusal, which are not prescribed in the United States. Recently, several new antiplatelet agents have been studied in patients with coronary artery disease, and the effects of these agents in patients with PAD is not known.

For KQ 2, our review found that exercise training improved functional measures for walking distance when indirectly compared with usual care or medical therapy. Endovascular therapy in our review was found to lead to a statistically nonsignificant functional improvement, although these studies again were limited by the multiple comparisons and possibility of bias. Patients treated with a combination of endovascular intervention and exercise training had better outcomes than patients treated with either exercise training or endovascular intervention alone in a study by Frans et al.[138] These findings again highlight the need for more studies when viewed in context of the recent CLEVER RCT of exercise versus endovascular therapy for aortoiliac disease, which found greater functional improvement with exercise and greater quality-of-life improvement with endovascular therapy.[77]

Our findings for KQ 2 are consistent with existing systematic reviews of exercise therapy in patients with IC[139,140] and with the systematic review for the NICE guidelines[141] of medical therapy, supervised exercise, angioplasty, and surgical bypass for patients with IC. Current practice for patients with symptomatic PAD is to maximize medical and behavioral treatments prior to more invasive treatment with endovascular or surgical treatment. To examine the effectiveness of more invasive treatments, this review included any studies that assessed endovascular or surgical treatments versus usual care since 1995, which is when more effective medical treatments such as statins, ACE inhibitors, and adequate control of hypertension and diabetes were used as standard practice. Unfortunately, few surgical studies have been published since 1995. The endovascular studies in this review found mixed results on functional improvement except when combined with exercise training. The few studies that compared surgical treatment with usual care since 1995 provided little information on functional outcomes.

Our analysis also found evidence for improved walking function with medical therapy such as cilostazol, which is similar to a Cochrane review in 2008.[142] In contrast to the few RCTs showing little functional effect over placebo with pentoxifylline leading to the Class IIB recommendation in the PAD guidelines, the current analysis incorporates RCTs and multiple comparison studies and shows a functional benefit of pentoxifylline, which is similar to the benefit seen in a meta-analysis by Girolami et al.[143]

The NICE guidelines focused on direct comparisons of specific therapies, and therefore the number of studies identified for each comparison was low and limited the authors' conclusions. In our systematic review, we used an effect size meta-analysis to assess the comparative effectiveness across all treatment strategies—medications, exercise training, endovascular interventions, and surgical revascularization—on the clinical outcomes outlined in KQ 2.

For KQ 3 in the CLI population, the current findings should serve as a call to action for further studies. This review found 1 RCT and 22 observational studies in the CLI population and 2 RCTs and 10 observational studies in a mixed IC-CLI population evaluating endovascular therapy versus surgical revascularization. The RCTs were performed in the balloon angioplasty-only era, and the observational studies suffer from risk of bias based on treatment decisions and patient inclusion. A Cochrane review of bypass surgery for CLI also concluded that there was limited evidence for the effectiveness of bypass surgery compared with angioplasty.[144] The NICE evidence statements for the comparison of angioplasty and bypass surgery are primarily based on the only RCT conducted in the CLI population (i.e., the BASIL study). We understand that the subgroup analysis from the BASIL study found survival benefit of open bypass surgery for patients who survived longer than 2 years, but this subgroup analysis does not provide the level of evidence to make a key point and should instead be considered hypothesis-generating, rather than conclusive.[145] Therefore, our findings the current variability and lack of a consistently agreed upon treatment approach for patients with CLI, as evidenced by the recommendations from current guidelines to perform revascularization based on best clinical judgment.

For assessing same-treatment strategy comparisons, the draft guidelines from NICE in March 2012[141] and a previous AHRQ report on invasive interventions for lower extremity PAD in 2008[146] contain meta-analyses regarding stent versus angioplasty, bare metal stent versus drug-eluting stent, angioplasty with selective stent placement versus angioplasty with primary stent placement, and autologous vein versus prosthetic bypass comparisons. The NICE report reviewed 10 RCTs comparing stent placement with angioplasty and found very low to low evidence of a difference in those modalities for any clinical outcomes, thus leading to the guideline recommendation to not offer primary stent placement for treating people with IC caused by aortoiliac disease (except complete occlusion) or femoropopliteal disease. The NICE report found one study (120 patients) that compared bare metal stents with drug-eluting stents, and the evidence was rated very low that vessel patency at 1 and 2 years was better with drug-eluting stents. Also there was no difference in clinical outcomes; therefore their recommendation was to use bare metal stents for IC. The AHRQ PAD report identified 10 RCTs and 11 observational studies evaluating stent versus PTA, primarily for femoropopliteal disease. Most RCTs used balloon-expandable stents, and two RCTs compared different stents. Overall, the RCTs and comparative observational studies failed to find a difference in the type of endovascular intervention for any clinical outcome. In addition, the studies were too heterogeneous to pool into a meta-analysis to estimate the relative differences in event rates. This review did not assess the comparative effectiveness of same-treatment strategies.

Challenges in Evaluating the Existing Literature in PAD Patients

Comparing endovascular with surgical revascularization techniques in published studies has the following challenges:
1. *Population differences*: Inclusion and exclusion criteria have varied among studies, and stratification based on symptom status and procedural risk is important.
2. *Endpoint differences*: These differences include variable functional endpoints for evaluation of claudication therapies and the surgical literature that defines success by

primary and secondary patency while the endovascular literature measures success by the lack of need for target lesion or target vessel revascularization.
3. *Length of followup*: Studies have been biased toward shorter duration of followup, thus heavily influencing differential ascertainment including the important clinical endpoint of amputation-free survival.
4. *Evolution of revascularization techniques*: Improvements in surgical and endovascular techniques have made direct comparisons between "state-of-the-art" strategies more challenging; we were unable to account for this in our analyses.
5. *Crossover between surgical and endovascular therapies*: Patients often undergo both surgical and endovascular revascularization in studies as well as in clinical practice, either as part of a hybrid approach to revascularization or because of treatment failure.

Applicability

We used 1995 as the start date for the literature search to improve the applicability of the findings to current clinical practice where secondary prevention of cardiovascular events includes treatment of hypertension, diabetes, hyperlipidemia, and tobacco use. Current guideline recommendations include reaching specific blood pressure, hemoglobin A1c, and lipid-lowering goals as well as providing access to nicotine replacement therapy for smoking cessation. By removing studies prior to 1995, we acknowledge that earlier comparative studies of aspirin, dipyridamole, pentoxifylline, and surgical bypass were not included in this review. Including older studies with outdated background medical therapy for cardiovascular risk factors would have biased the results to favor active treatment over suboptimal usual care treatment.

The data available for antiplatelet agents in PAD treatment fell into two categories: (1) subgroup analysis of PAD patients in large antiplatelet RCTs and (2) smaller antiplatelet RCTs in patients who recently had an endovascular intervention or bypass surgery. There are no studies that specifically evaluate the role of antiplatelet agents in a population of patients representing the full spectrum of PAD (asymptomatic, IC, and CLI).

In the analysis of treatments for the IC population, there were a number of single-center and multicenter studies conducted outside the United States (primarily Europe). There were several RCTs comparing exercise training, medical therapies, and endovascular interventions. More of the studies comparing endovascular interventions with usual care or surgical revascularization were based on observational studies.

In the analysis of treatments for the CLI population, only one RCT of endovascular versus surgical revascularization has been conducted, with the majority of the literature based on observational, single-center studies. Subsequently, the introduction of stents, drug-eluting stents, and drug-coated balloons has likely changed the definition and results of the endovascular therapy group. Therefore, the available evidence for CLI revascularization is significantly limited with regard to applicability to current practice.

Implications for Clinical and Policy Decisionmaking

PAD was identified by the Institute of Medicine as one of the top 100 priorities for comparative effectiveness research because of the large population of patients affected with significant morbidity and mortality, the multiple potential treatment options, and the high costs of care to the health care system. The current analysis provides an important evidence review that must be put in context with current clinical practice so that it may inform both future research and clinical and policy decisionmaking.

The findings for antiplatelet therapy demonstrate that monotherapy with clopidogrel 75 mg daily may be more effective than aspirin 100 mg daily for the prevention of cardiovascular events in the PAD population. The available evidence of aspirin monotherapy does not show a significant reduction in cardiovascular events compared with placebo. Additionally, from a large PAD subgroup of an RCT, clopidogrel and aspirin did not significantly reduce cardiovascular events compared with aspirin alone but did increase minor bleeding. These findings favor clopidogrel as the antiplatelet therapy for patients with PAD and, with introduction of the generic drug into clinical practice, may have important implications for health plans and medical systems. Finally, for studies aimed at improving the outcomes of patients with PAD, clopidogrel monotherapy seems justified as the current standard of care. It should be noted that the current AHA/ACC guidelines[12] recommend an antiplatelet therapy with either aspirin or clopidogrel for patients with PAD based on both randomized data and some of the older observational studies.

Regarding the treatment of patients with IC, this review found that several therapies—exercise training, medical therapy, and endovascular therapy—were effective at improving functional status and walking time. However, these data are limited by many single-treatment comparisons, multiple functional endpoints, and the lack of rigorous strategy treatment studies where exercise and/or medical therapy are provided as background therapy. Since both the Centers for Medicare and Medicaid Services and most insurers do not currently cover supervised exercise for PAD, these types of studies and data are needed to build the evidence base regarding supervised exercise. Additionally, with increasing innovation of endovascular therapy, current well-performed multicenter RCTs and registry analysis of actual utilization are needed to determine efficacy.

Perhaps the largest and most important gap with implications for health policy and national funding may be seen in the evaluation of endovascular versus surgical therapy for CLI. Our analysis found one older RCT comparing balloon angioplasty to surgical bypass for patients with CLI, a condition that carries a significant morbidity and mortality. The remaining observational studies are at high risk for bias, have heterogeneous results, and highlight the need for further comparative effectiveness studies to determine the best current care for these patients. Such studies would need to enroll a broad population of patients with all available endovascular and surgical therapies.

Limitations of the Review Process

The current review was limited to English-language–only studies and focused on those that compared two treatment modalities. This limited and excluded the single-arm studies examining endovascular or surgical therapy—most of which populate the current literature on PAD. Although some of these studies used objective performance criteria for comparison to existing or historical controls of practice, they were excluded for not having a direct comparison. However, it is unlikely these studies would have provided substantial additional information given the quality and SOE of the studies reviewed.

Limitations of the Evidence Base

As we have noted, there are several limitations to the available evidence for the treatment of PAD. First and foremost, the majority of the available literature is single-arm observational studies without true direct comparisons with other treatment modalities or even with placebo. Additionally, when comparisons are made, many comparisons are within similar treatment modalities (i.e., endovascular therapy with stent A versus stent B, surgery with graft A versus graft B, or supervised versus structured home exercise). These comparisons may be meaningful; however, the current care pattern for patients with PAD demonstrates large variability. Several important treatment strategy studies are needed. Furthermore, the literature was insufficient to allow evaluation of the anatomic locations and severity of arterial disease that are often important in treatment decisionmaking. We found and reported subgroup findings from the small number of studies that did publish outcomes for these important patient factors. In addition, we were not able to assess the effectiveness of treatment strategies that were delivered if another modality had failed.

Regarding endpoints, there are numerous and heterogeneous measures reported, often with no clear agreed upon definition for patients with IC and CLI. The time points for followup are variable and often the ascertainment is not standardized. Finally, there are little data on important subgroups of harms.

Research Gaps

The current literature search for PAD revealed many single-center, single-modality observational studies that could not be included for this comparative effectiveness review on the basis of our inclusion/exclusion criteria. In addition, there were many within-treatment comparisons; for example, studies comparing two types of surgical bypass, two types of endovascular interventions, or two types of exercise modalities. Studies that evaluated direct comparisons between treatments, unfortunately, were limited. From the ones we were able to identify, there was a notable variation in (1) outcome measures used to assess functional capacity and quality life, (2) followup assessment time points, and (3) type of outcomes reported (i.e., surrogate and hard clinical endpoints). Therefore, there are numerous areas of evidence gaps and areas for potential future research in PAD. We used the framework recommended by Robinson[147] to identify gaps in the evidence and classify why these gaps exist using the PICOTS approach (Table 35). Gaps were classified as secondary to (1) insufficient or imprecise information, (2) biased information, (3) inconsistency or unknown consistency, and (4) not the right information.

KQ 1 Research Gaps

For KQ 1, the primary limitation of the available evidence was the low number of studies that compare the effectiveness of aspirin, clopidogrel, and new antiplatelet agents. A single RCT has compared clopidogrel with aspirin, and three RCTs have compared clopidogrel plus aspirin to aspirin alone. More RCTs on asymptomatic or symptomatic patients with PAD are needed to firmly conclude whether antiplatelet monotherapy or DAPT is warranted in this high-risk cardiovascular population. Most of the studies were also subgroup analyses of larger antiplatelet RCTs. Additionally, newer antiplatelet agents are available that have not been studied in the PAD population. RCTs that solely focus on enrollment of the PAD population are encouraged since much of the existing literature is based on PAD subgroups (often with an inclusion criteria for the main RCT of known coronary artery, cerebrovascular, or PAD).

KQ 2 Research Gaps

For KQ 2, the primary limitation of the available evidence was the heterogeneity of outcome measures used to assess functional capacity in the IC population such that an effect size analysis had to be performed across the treatment strategies for this report. Some studies failed to report the variability of the mean, median, or percentage change result and so had to be excluded from the random-effects model. Also, the quality-of-life measures used varied among five instruments (SF-36, EQ-5D, WIQ, PAQ and VascuQOL). We focused on the results of the SF-36 physical functioning score since it was most commonly reported. Generic health-related quality-of-life measures, such as the SF-36 physical functioning score, are often thought to be less responsive to change than a disease-specific measure is. From the limited studies we analyzed, it appears that there was a large effect of various therapies on improving quality of life. Validation in future research using both general and disease-specific quality-of-life measures is encouraged, and treatment studies that evaluate exercise, medical therapy, and invasive approaches are needed.

KQ 3 Research Gaps

For KQ 3, the primary limitation of the available evidence was the plethora of observational studies (only one RCT) comparing endovascular with surgical revascularization. A majority of these studies were rated poor quality due to insufficient reporting of study methodology and variability in the reporting of results. Since most of the studies were retrospective studies, there was a lack of assessment of functional capacity or quality-of-life measures. All-cause mortality and amputation (or limb salvage) rates were commonly reported. Newer studies have started to report amputation-free survival, but very few reported other vascular events such as MI or stroke, or minor amputations. The relationship between vessel patency and functional outcomes or quality of life is not well established, so this is viewed more as a surrogate clinical outcome and not a direct clinical outcome. More RCTs or prospective cohort studies with assessment of functional capacity, quality of life, and additional vascular outcomes are needed.

Underreporting of Subgroup Results Across All KQs

Across all KQs, the underreporting of results for subgroups that may modify the comparative effectiveness was common. Given the limited space in publications, it would be helpful to have online, supplementary appendices that report the outcomes by age, race, sex, PAD classification, and comorbidities. The representation of women and the reporting of race/ethnicity were also low in these studies. Future studies that oversample for women and minority populations are needed to address subpopulation questions.

In addition, the reporting of safety concerns such as bleeding, exercise-related harms, infection, and adverse drug reactions was sparse in these studies. Underreporting may be expected in retrospective observational studies since medical documentation of safety issues are often lacking. However, we would expect that RCTs or prospective cohort studies would make this a priority to measure during the course of the study and to report in a published manuscript. Harms related to antiplatelet therapy (monotherapy or DAPT), endovascular procedures, and surgical interventions should be reported along with the treatment effectiveness results to determine the net benefit of therapies. Finally, although not a focus of this review, there was a lack of studies about health care utilization and costs associated with the various therapies. Observational studies using administrative datasets, or RCTs and prospective studies collecting and reporting resource use data are needed to address this evidence gap.

Table 35. Research gaps

Criteria	Evidence Gap	Reason	Type of Studies To Consider
Patients	Comparative effectiveness of therapies for PAD subpopulations of interest, including subgroups based on: age, sex, race, risk factors, comorbidities and PAD classification (all KQs)	Insufficient information	RCTs and potentially patient-level meta-analyses of existing/future RCTs
	Low representation of women and minorities (all KQs)	Insufficient information	RCTs and prospective registries with oversampling of female and minority populations
Interventions/ comparators	Comparative effectiveness of new antiplatelet medications to aspirin or clopidogrel (KQ 1)	Insufficient information	RCTs
	Comparative effectiveness of DAPT to antiplatelet monotherapy (KQ 1)	Imprecise and inconsistent information	RCTs
	Comparative effectiveness of endovascular and surgical revascularization in CLI (KQ 3)	Imprecise and inconsistent information	RCTs
Outcomes	Comparative effectiveness of available therapies on functional capacity, quality of life in IC patients (KQ 2)	Imprecise and inconsistent information	RCTs or prospective cohort studies using standardized measures of patient-centered outcomes
	Comparative effectiveness of available therapies on functional capacity, quality of life in CLI patients (KQ 3)	Insufficient information	RCTs or prospective cohort studies using standardized measures of patient-centered outcomes
	Comparative effectiveness of available therapies on mortality (all-cause or cardiovascular), nonfatal MI, nonfatal stroke, and composite vascular events in the IC and CLI populations (KQ 2 and KQ 3)	Insufficient information	RCTs adequately powered to assess short- and long-term cardiovascular outcomes
	Comparative effectiveness of available therapies in impacting healthcare utilitization (KQ 2 and KQ 3)	Insufficient information	Observational studies
	Comparative safety of available therapies, focusing on harms such as such as bleeding, infection, and adverse drug reactions (KQ 2 and KQ 3, especially the exercise, endovascular, and surgical therapies)	Insufficient information	Reporting from RCTs and observational studies
Settings	Limited settings need larger real world populations represented (all KQs)	Insufficient information	Large, real-world registries

Abbreviations: CLI=critical limb ischemia; IC=intermittent claudication; RCTs=randomized controlled trials.

Conclusions

The available evidence for treatment of patients with PAD is limited by few RCTs that provide comparisons of meaningful treatment options. Several advances in care in both medical therapy and invasive therapy have not been rigorously tested. With respect to antiplatelet therapy for the prevention of cardiovascular events in patients with PAD, we found from a limited number of studies that it appears that aspirin has no benefit over placebo in asymptomatic patients with PAD; clopidogrel monotherapy is more beneficial or equivalent to aspirin; and

DAPT is not significantly better than aspirin on reducing cardiovascular events in patients with PAD. For IC patients, exercise, medical therapy, and endovascular or surgical revascularization all had an effect on improving functional status and quality of life; the impact of these therapies on cardiovascular events is uncertain. Additionally, the potential additive effects of these therapies are unknown. There does not appear to be significant differences in mortality or limb outcomes between endovascular and surgical revascularization in CLI patients. However, these data are derived from one RCT and many observational studies, and the presence of clinical heterogeneity of these results makes conclusions for clinical outcomes uncertain and provides an impetus for further research.

References

1. Hiatt WR, Goldstone J, Smith SC, Jr., et al. Atherosclerotic Peripheral Vascular Disease Symposium II: nomenclature for vascular diseases. Circulation. 2008;118(25):2826-9. PMID: 19106403.

2. Hirsch AT, Haskal ZJ, Hertzer NR, et al. ACC/AHA 2005 Practice Guidelines for the management of patients with peripheral arterial disease (lower extremity, renal, mesenteric, and abdominal aortic): a collaborative report from the American Association for Vascular Surgery/Society for Vascular Surgery, Society for Cardiovascular Angiography and Interventions, Society for Vascular Medicine and Biology, Society of Interventional Radiology, and the ACC/AHA Task Force on Practice Guidelines (Writing Committee to Develop Guidelines for the Management of Patients With Peripheral Arterial Disease): endorsed by the American Association of Cardiovascular and Pulmonary Rehabilitation; National Heart, Lung, and Blood Institute; Society for Vascular Nursing; TransAtlantic Inter-Society Consensus; and Vascular Disease Foundation. Circulation. 2006;113(11):e463-654. PMID: 16549646.

3. Hirsch AT, Criqui MH, Treat-Jacobson D, et al. Peripheral arterial disease detection, awareness, and treatment in primary care. JAMA. 2001;286(11):1317-24. PMID: 11560536.

4. Meijer WT, Hoes AW, Rutgers D, et al. Peripheral arterial disease in the elderly: The Rotterdam Study. Arterioscler Thromb Vasc Biol. 1998;18(2):185-92. PMID: 9484982.

5. Hiatt WR. Medical treatment of peripheral arterial disease and claudication. N Engl J Med. 2001;344(21):1608-21. PMID: 11372014.

6. Norgren L, Hiatt WR, Dormandy JA, et al. Inter-Society Consensus for the Management of Peripheral Arterial Disease (TASC II). European Journal of Vascular and Endovascular Surgery. 2007;33 Suppl 1:S1-75. PMID: 17140820.

7. Criqui MH, Ninomiya JK, Wingard DL, et al. Progression of peripheral arterial disease predicts cardiovascular disease morbidity and mortality. Journal of the American College of Cardiology. 2008;52(21):1736-42. PMID: 19007695.

8. Criqui MH, Langer RD, Fronek A, et al. Mortality over a period of 10 years in patients with peripheral arterial disease. New England Journal of Medicine. 1992;326(6):381-6. PMID: 1729621.

9. Remes L, Isoaho R, Vahlberg T, et al. Quality of life among lower extremity peripheral arterial disease patients who have undergone endovascular or surgical revascularization: a case-control study. European Journal of Vascular and Endovascular Surgery. 2010;40(5):618-25. PMID: 20418121.

10. Nehler MR, McDermott MM, Treat-Jacobson D, et al. Functional outcomes and quality of life in peripheral arterial disease: current status. Vascular Medicine. 2003;8(2):115-26. PMID: 14518614.

11. Kannel WB. Risk factors for atherosclerotic cardiovascular outcomes in different arterial territories. Journal of Cardiovascular Risk. 1994;1(4):333-9. PMID: 7621317.

12. Rooke TW, Hirsch AT, Misra S, et al. 2011 ACCF/AHA focused update of the guideline for the management of patients with peripheral artery disease (updating the 2005 guideline): a report of the American College of Cardiology Foundation/American Heart Association Task Force on Practice Guidelines: developed in collaboration with the Society for Cardiovascular Angiography and Interventions, Society of Interventional Radiology, Society for Vascular Medicine, and Society for Vascular Surgery. J Vasc Surg. 2011;54(5):e32-58. PMID: 21958560.

13. Resnick HE, Lindsay RS, McDermott MM, et al. Relationship of high and low ankle brachial index to all-cause and cardiovascular disease mortality: the Strong Heart Study. Circulation. 2004;109(6):733-9. PMID: 14970108.

14. Mehler PS, Coll JR, Estacio R, et al. Intensive blood pressure control reduces the risk of cardiovascular events in patients with peripheral arterial disease and type 2 diabetes. Circulation. 2003;107(5):753-6. PMID: 12578880.

15. Ware JE, Jr., Sherbourne CD. The MOS 36-item short-form health survey (SF-36). I. Conceptual framework and item selection. Med Care. 1992;30(6):473-83. PMID: 1593914.

16. Spronk S, Bosch JL, den Hoed PT, et al. Intermittent claudication: clinical effectiveness of endovascular revascularization versus supervised hospital-based exercise training--randomized controlled trial. Radiology. 2009;250(2):586-95. PMID: 19188327.

17. Dolan P. Modeling valuations for EuroQol health states. Med Care. 1997;35(11):1095-108. PMID: 9366889.

18. Morgan MB, Crayford T, Murrin B, et al. Developing the Vascular Quality of Life Questionnaire: a new disease-specific quality of life measure for use in lower limb ischemia. J Vasc Surg. 2001;33(4):679-87. PMID: 11296317.

19. McDermott MM, Liu K, Guralnik JM, et al. Measurement of walking endurance and walking velocity with questionnaire: validation of the walking impairment questionnaire in men and women with peripheral arterial disease. J Vasc Surg. 1998;28(6):1072-81. PMID: 9845659.

20. Spertus J, Jones P, Poler S, et al. The peripheral artery questionnaire: a new disease-specific health status measure for patients with peripheral arterial disease. Am Heart J. 2004;147(2):301-8. PMID: 14760329.

21. Bernardi D, Bartoli P, Ferreri A, et al. Assessment of captopril and nicardipine effects on chronic occlusive arterial disease of the lower extremity using Doppler ultrasound. Angiology. 1988;39(11):942-52. PMID: 3052183.

22. Roberts DH, Tsao Y, McLoughlin GA, et al. Placebo-controlled comparison of captopril, atenolol, labetalol, and pindolol in hypertension complicated by intermittent claudication. Lancet. 1987;2(8560):650-3. PMID: 2887941.

23. Van de Ven LL, Van Leeuwen JT, Smit AJ. The influence of chronic treatment with betablockade and angiotensin converting enzyme inhibition on the peripheral blood flow in hypertensive patients with and without concomitant intermittent claudication. A comparative cross-over trial. Vasa. 1994;23(4):357-62. PMID: 7817618.

24. Giri J, McDermott MM, Greenland P, et al. Statin use and functional decline in patients with and without peripheral arterial disease. Journal of the American College of Cardiology. 2006;47(5):998-1004. PMID: 16516084.

25. Dawson DL, Cutler BS, Hiatt WR, et al. A comparison of cilostazol and pentoxifylline for treating intermittent claudication. Am J Med. 2000;109(7):523-30. PMID: 11063952.

26. McDermott MM, Ades P, Guralnik JM, et al. Treadmill exercise and resistance training in patients with peripheral arterial disease with and without intermittent claudication: a randomized controlled trial. JAMA. 2009;301(2):165-74. PMID: 19141764.

27. Liao JK, Bettmann MA, Sandor T, et al. Differential impairment of vasodilator responsiveness of peripheral resistance and conduit vessels in humans with atherosclerosis. Circ Res. 1991;68(4):1027-34. PMID: 2009605.

28. Fronek A, DiTomasso DG, Allison M. Noninvasive assessment of endothelial activity in patients with peripheral arterial disease and cardiovascular risk factors. Endothelium. 2007;14(4-5):199-205. PMID: 17922336.

29. Yataco AR, Corretti MC, Gardner AW, et al. Endothelial reactivity and cardiac risk factors in older patients with peripheral arterial disease. Am J Cardiol. 1999;83(5):754-8. PMID: 10080432.

30. McDermott MM, Guralnik JM, Ferrucci L, et al. Asymptomatic peripheral arterial disease is associated with more adverse lower extremity characteristics than intermittent claudication. Circulation. 2008;117(19):2484-91. PMID: 18458172.

31. McDermott MM, Hoff F, Ferrucci L, et al. Lower extremity ischemia, calf skeletal muscle characteristics, and functional impairment in peripheral arterial disease. J Am Geriatr Soc. 2007;55(3):400-6. PMID: 17341243.

32. Hiatt WR, Regensteiner JG, Wolfel EE, et al. Effect of exercise training on skeletal muscle histology and metabolism in peripheral arterial disease. J Appl Physiol. 1996;81(2):780-8. PMID: 8872646.

33. Hiatt WR, Wolfel EE, Regensteiner JG, et al. Skeletal muscle carnitine metabolism in patients with unilateral peripheral arterial disease. J Appl Physiol. 1992;73(1):346-53. PMID: 1506390.

34. Pipinos, II, Sharov VG, Shepard AD, et al. Abnormal mitochondrial respiration in skeletal muscle in patients with peripheral arterial disease. J Vasc Surg. 2003;38(4):827-32. PMID: 14560237.

35. Pipinos, II, Judge AR, Zhu Z, et al. Mitochondrial defects and oxidative damage in patients with peripheral arterial disease. Free Radic Biol Med. 2006;41(2):262-9. PMID: 16814106.

36. Schmieder FA, Comerota AJ. Intermittent claudication: magnitude of the problem, patient evaluation, and therapeutic strategies. Am J Cardiol. 2001;87(12A):3D-13D. PMID: 11434894.

37. Jaff MR, Cahill KE, Yu AP, et al. Clinical outcomes and medical care costs among medicare beneficiaries receiving therapy for peripheral arterial disease. Annals of Vascular Surgery. 2010;24(5):577-87. PMID: 20579582.

38. Dosluoglu HH, Lall P, Cherr GS, et al. Role of simple and complex hybrid revascularization procedures for symptomatic lower extremity occlusive disease. J Vasc Surg. 2010;51(6):1425-1435 e1. PMID: 20488323.

39. Adam DJ, Beard JD, Cleveland T, et al. Bypass versus angioplasty in severe ischaemia of the leg (BASIL): multicentre, randomised controlled trial. Lancet. 2005;366(9501):1925-34. PMID: 16325694.

40. Conte MS, Bandyk DF, Clowes AW, et al. Results of PREVENT III: a multicenter, randomized trial of edifoligide for the prevention of vein graft failure in lower extremity bypass surgery. J Vasc Surg. 2006;43(4):742-751; discussion 751. PMID: 16616230.

41. Goodney PP, Schanzer A, Demartino RR, et al. Validation of the Society for Vascular Surgery's objective performance goals for critical limb ischemia in everyday vascular surgery practice. J Vasc Surg. 2011;54(1):100-108 e4. PMID: 21334173.

42. Abou-Zamzam AM, Jr., Gomez NR, Molkara A, et al. A prospective analysis of critical limb ischemia: factors leading to major primary amputation versus revascularization. Ann Vasc Surg. 2007;21(4):458-63. PMID: 17499967.

43. Feinglass J, Sohn MW, Rodriguez H, et al. Perioperative outcomes and amputation-free survival after lower extremity bypass surgery in California hospitals, 1996-1999, with follow-up through 2004. J Vasc Surg. 2009;50(4):776-783 e1. PMID: 19595538.

44. Berger JS, Krantz MJ, Kittelson JM, et al. Aspirin for the prevention of cardiovascular events in patients with peripheral artery disease: a meta-analysis of randomized trials. JAMA. 2009;301(18):1909-19. PMID: 19436018.

45. Agency for Healthcare Research and Quality. Methods Guide for Effectiveness and Comparative Effectiveness Reviews. Rockville, MD: Agency for Healthcare Research and Quality. www.effectivehealthcare.ahrq.gov/index.cfm/search-for-guides-reviews-and-reports/?pageaction=displayproduct&productid=318. Accessed March 16, 2012.

46. Moher D, Liberati A, Tetzlaff J, et al. The PRISMA Group. Preferred reporting items for systematic reviews and meta-analyses: the PRISMA statement. PLoS Med. 2009;6(7):e1000097. PMID: 19621072.

47. Evidence-based Practice Center Systematic Review Protocol. Project Title: Treatment Strategies for Patients With Peripheral Artery Disease. January 31, 2012. http://effectivehealthcare.ahrq.gov/index.cfm/search-for-guides-reviews-and-reports/?productid=948&pageaction=displayproduct. Accessed November 19, 2012.

48. Cohen J. Statistical Power Analysis for the Behavioral Sciences. 2nd ed Hillsdale, N.J.: L. Erlbaum Associates; 1988.

49. Beebe HG, Dawson DL, Cutler BS, et al. A new pharmacological treatment for intermittent claudication: results of a randomized, multicenter trial. Arch Intern Med. 1999;159(17):2041-50. PMID: 10510990.

50. Hasselblad V. Meta-analysis of multitreatment studies. Med Decis Making. 1998;18(1):37-43. PMID: 9456207.

51. Soga Y, Yokoi H, Kawasaki T, et al. Efficacy of cilostazol after endovascular therapy for femoropopliteal artery disease in patients with intermittent claudication. J Am Coll Cardiol. 2009;53(1):48-53. PMID: 19118724.

52. Owens DK, Lohr KN, Atkins D, et al. AHRQ series paper 5: grading the strength of a body of evidence when comparing medical interventions--Agency for Healthcare Research and Quality and the Effective Health-Care Program. J Clin Epidemiol. 2010;63(5):513-23. PMID: 19595577.

53. Atkins D, Chang SM, Gartlehner G, et al. Assessing applicability when comparing medical interventions: AHRQ and the Effective Health Care Program. J Clin Epidemiol. 2011;64(11):1198-207. PMID: 21463926.

54. Belch J, MacCuish A, Campbell I, et al. The prevention of progression of arterial disease and diabetes (POPADAD) trial: factorial randomised placebo controlled trial of aspirin and antioxidants in patients with diabetes and asymptomatic peripheral arterial disease. BMJ. 2008;337:a1840. PMID: 18927173.

55. Catalano M, Born G, Peto R. Prevention of serious vascular events by aspirin amongst patients with peripheral arterial disease: randomized, double-blind trial. J Intern Med. 2007;261(3):276-84. PMID: 17305650.

56. Fowkes FG, Price JF, Stewart MC, et al. Aspirin for prevention of cardiovascular events in a general population screened for a low ankle brachial index: a randomized controlled trial. JAMA. 2010;303(9):841-8. PMID: 20197530.

57. Mahmood A, Sintler M, Edwards AT, et al. The efficacy of aspirin in patients undergoing infra-inguinal bypass and identification of high risk patients. Int Angiol. 2003;22(3):302-7. PMID: 14612858.

58. Minar E, Ahmadi A, Koppensteiner R, et al. Comparison of effects of high-dose and low-dose aspirin on restenosis after femoropopliteal percutaneous transluminal angioplasty. Circulation. 1995;91(8):2167-73. PMID: 7697845.

59. A randomised, blinded trial of clopidogrel versus aspirin in patients at risk of ischaemic events (CAPRIE). Lancet. 1996;348(9038):1329-39. PMID: 8918275.

60. Cacoub PP, Bhatt DL, Steg PG, et al. Patients with peripheral arterial disease in the CHARISMA trial. Eur Heart J. 2009;30(2):192-201. PMID: 19136484.

61. Cassar K, Ford I, Greaves M, et al. Randomized clinical trial of the antiplatelet effects of aspirin-clopidogrel combination versus aspirin alone after lower limb angioplasty. Br J Surg. 2005;92(2):159-65. PMID: 15609386.

62. Horrocks M, Horrocks EH, Murphy P, et al. The effects of platelet inhibitors on platelet uptake and restenosis after femoral angioplasty. Int Angiol. 1997(2):101-6.

63. Belch JJ, Dormandy J, Biasi GM, et al. Results of the randomized, placebo-controlled clopidogrel and acetylsalicylic acid in bypass surgery for peripheral arterial disease (CASPAR) trial. J Vasc Surg. 2010;52(4):825-33, 833 e1-2. PMID: 20678878.

64. Tepe G, Bantleon R, Brechtel K, et al. Management of peripheral arterial interventions with mono or dual antiplatelet therapy-the MIRROR study: a randomised and double-blinded clinical trial. Eur Radiol. 2012;22(9):1998-2006. PMID: 22569995.

65. Bhatt DL, Flather MD, Hacke W, et al. Patients with prior myocardial infarction, stroke, or symptomatic peripheral arterial disease in the CHARISMA trial. J Am Coll Cardiol. 2007;49(19):1982-8. PMID: 17498584.

66. Crowther RG, Spinks WL, Leicht AS, et al. Effects of a long-term exercise program on lower limb mobility, physiological responses, walking performance, and physical activity levels in patients with peripheral arterial disease. J Vasc Surg. 2008;47(2):303-9. PMID: 18241753.

67. Drozdz W, Panek J, Lejman W. Red cell deformability in patients with chronic atheromatous ischemia of the legs. Med Sci Monit. 2001;7(5):933-9. PMID: 11535938.

68. Gardner AW, Katzel LI, Sorkin JD, et al. Effects of long-term exercise rehabilitation on claudication distances in patients with peripheral arterial disease: a randomized controlled trial. J Cardiopulm Rehabil. 2002;22(3):192-8. PMID: 12042688.

69. Gardner AW, Parker DE, Montgomery PS, et al. Efficacy of quantified home-based exercise and supervised exercise in patients with intermittent claudication: a randomized controlled trial. Circulation. 2011;123(5):491-8. PMID: 21262997.

70. Gelin J, Jivegard L, Taft C, et al. Treatment efficacy of intermittent claudication by surgical intervention, supervised physical exercise training compared to no treatment in unselected randomised patients I: one year results of functional and physiological improvements. Eur J Vasc Endovasc Surg. 2001;22(2):107-13. PMID: 11472042.

71. Gibellini R, Fanello M, Bardile AF, et al. Exercise training in intermittent claudication. Int Angiol. 2000;19(1):8-13. PMID: 10853679.

72. Giugliano G, Di Serafino L, Perrino C, et al. Effects of successful percutaneous lower extremity revascularization on cardiovascular outcome in patients with peripheral arterial disease. International Journal of Cardiology. 2012.

73. Hobbs SD, Marshall T, Fegan C, et al. The effect of supervised exercise and cilostazol on coagulation and fibrinolysis in intermittent claudication: a randomized controlled trial. J Vasc Surg. 2007;45(1):65-70; discussion 70. PMID: 17210383.

74. Hobbs SD, Marshall T, Fegan C, et al. The constitutive procoagulant and hypofibrinolytic state in patients with intermittent claudication due to infrainguinal disease significantly improves with percutaneous transluminal balloon angioplasty. J Vasc Surg. 2006;43(1):40-6. PMID: 16414385.

75. Lee HL, Mehta T, Ray B, et al. A non-randomised controlled trial of the clinical and cost effectiveness of a Supervised Exercise Programme for claudication. Eur J Vasc Endovasc Surg. 2007;33(2):202-7. PMID: 17142065.

76. Mori E, Komori K, Kume M, et al. Comparison of the long-term results between surgical and conservative treatment in patients with intermittent claudication. Surgery. 2002;131(1 Suppl):S269-74. PMID: 11821823.

77. Murphy TP, Cutlip DE, Regensteiner JG, et al. Supervised exercise versus primary stenting for claudication resulting from aortoiliac peripheral artery disease: six-month outcomes from the claudication: exercise versus endoluminal revascularization (CLEVER) study. Circulation. 2012;125(1):130-9. PMID: 22090168.

78. Sugimoto I, Ohta T, Ishibashi H, et al. Conservative treatment for patients with intermittent claudication. Int Angiol. 2010;29(2 Suppl):55-60. PMID: 20357750.

79. Tsai JC, Chan P, Wang CH, et al. The effects of exercise training on walking function and perception of health status in elderly patients with peripheral arterial occlusive disease. J Intern Med. 2002;252(5):448-55. PMID: 12528763.

80. Greenhalgh RM, Belch JJ, Brown LC, et al. The adjuvant benefit of angioplasty in patients with mild to moderate intermittent claudication (MIMIC) managed by supervised exercise, smoking cessation advice and best medical therapy: results from two randomised trials for stenotic femoropopliteal and aortoiliac arterial disease. Eur J Vasc Endovasc Surg. 2008;36(6):680-8. PMID: 19022184.

81. Kruidenier LM, Nicolai SP, Rouwet EV, et al. Additional supervised exercise therapy after a percutaneous vascular intervention for peripheral arterial disease: a randomized clinical trial. J Vasc Interv Radiol. 2011;22(7):961-8. PMID: 21571547.

82. Mazari FA, Khan JA, Carradice D, et al. Randomized clinical trial of percutaneous transluminal angioplasty, supervised exercise and combined treatment for intermittent claudication due to femoropopliteal arterial disease. Br J Surg. 2012;99(1):39-48. PMID: 22021102.

83. Nordanstig J, Gelin J, Hensater M, et al. Walking performance and health-related quality of life after surgical or endovascular invasive versus non-invasive treatment for intermittent claudication--a prospective randomised trial. Eur J Vasc Endovasc Surg. 2011;42(2):220-7. PMID: 21397530.

84. Perkins JM, Collin J, Creasy TS, et al. Exercise training versus angioplasty for stable claudication. Long and medium term results of a prospective, randomised trial. Eur J Vasc Endovasc Surg. 1996;11(4):409-13. PMID: 8846172.

85. Belcaro G, Nicolaides AN, Griffin M, et al. Intermittent claudication in diabetics: treatment with exercise and pentoxifylline--a 6-month, controlled, randomized trial. Angiology. 2002;53 Suppl 1:S39-43. PMID: 11865835.

86. Dawson DL, Cutler BS, Meissner MH, et al. Cilostazol has beneficial effects in treatment of intermittent claudication: results from a multicenter, randomized, prospective, double-blind trial. Circulation. 1998;98(7):678-86. PMID: 9715861.

87. De Sanctis MT, Cesarone MR, Belcaro G, et al. Treatment of intermittent claudication with pentoxifylline: a 12-month, randomized trial--walking distance and microcirculation. Angiology. 2002;53 Suppl 1:S7-12. PMID: 11865838.

88. Hiatt WR, Money SR, Brass EP. Long-term safety of cilostazol in patients with peripheral artery disease: the CASTLE study (Cilostazol: A Study in Long-term Effects). J Vasc Surg. 2008;47(2):330-336. PMID: 18155871.

89. Money SR, Herd JA, Isaacsohn JL, et al. Effect of cilostazol on walking distances in patients with intermittent claudication caused by peripheral vascular disease. J Vasc Surg. 1998;27(2):267-74; discussion 274-5. PMID: 9510281.

90. Strandness DE, Jr., Dalman RL, Panian S, et al. Effect of cilostazol in patients with intermittent claudication: a randomized, double-blind, placebo-controlled study. Vasc Endovascular Surg. 2002;36(2):83-91. PMID: 11951094.

91. Feinglass J, McCarthy WJ, Slavensky R, et al. Functional status and walking ability after lower extremity bypass grafting or angioplasty for intermittent claudication: results from a prospective outcomes study. J Vasc Surg. 2000;31(1 Pt 1):93-103. PMID: 10642712.

92. Koivunen K, Lukkarinen H. One-year prospective health-related quality-of-life outcomes in patients treated with conservative method, endovascular treatment or open surgery for symptomatic lower limb atherosclerotic disease. Eur J Cardiovasc Nurs. 2008;7(3):247-56. PMID: 18221916.

93. Nylaende M, Abdelnoor M, Stranden E, et al. The Oslo balloon angioplasty versus conservative treatment study (OBACT)—The 2-years results of a single centre, prospective, randomised study in patients with intermittent claudication. Eur J Vasc Endovasc Surg. 2007;33(1):3-12. PMID: 17055756.

94. Pell JP, Lee AJ. Impact of angioplasty and arterial reconstructive surgery on the quality of life of claudicants. The Scottish Vascular Audit Group. Scott Med J. 1997;42(2):47-8. PMID: 9507581.

95. Whyman MR, Fowkes FG, Kerracher EM, et al. Is intermittent claudication improved by percutaneous transluminal angioplasty? A randomized controlled trial. J Vasc Surg. 1997;26(4):551-7. PMID: 9357454.

96. Treat-Jacobson D, Bronas UG, Leon AS. Efficacy of arm-ergometry versus treadmill exercise training to improve walking distance in patients with claudication. Vasc Med. 2009;14(3):203-13. PMID: 19651669.

97. Stone WM, Demaerschalk BM, Fowl RJ, et al. Type 3 phosphodiesterase inhibitors may be protective against cerebrovascular events in patients with claudication. J Stroke Cerebrovasc Dis. 2008;17(3):129-33. PMID: 18436153.

98. De Sanctis MT, Cesarone MR, Belcaro G, et al. Treatment of long-distance intermittent claudication with pentoxifylline: a 12-month, randomized trial. Angiology. 2002;53 Suppl 1:S13-7. PMID: 11865829.

99. Varty K, Nydahl S, Butterworth P, et al. Changes in the management of critical limb ischaemia. Br J Surg. 1996;83(7):953-6. PMID: 8813785.

100. Ah Chong AK, Tan CB, Wong MW, et al. Bypass surgery or percutaneous transluminal angioplasty to treat critical lower limb ischaemia due to infrainguinal arterial occlusive disease? Hong Kong Med J. 2009;15(4):249-54. PMID: 19652230.

101. Dorigo W, Pulli R, Marek J, et al. A comparison between open and endovascular repair in the treatment of critical limb ischemia. Ital J Vasc Endovasc Surg. 2009;16(1):17-22.

102. Hynes N, Akhtar Y, Manning B, et al. Subintimal angioplasty as a primary modality in the management of critical limb ischemia: comparison to bypass grafting for aortoiliac and femoropopliteal occlusive disease. J Endovasc Ther. 2004;11(4):460-71. PMID: 15298498.

103. Jerabek J, Dvorak M, Vojtisek B. Results of therapy of lower extremity ischemic disease by angiosurgery and radiointervention (PTA) methods. Bratisl Lek Listy. 2003;104(10):314-6. PMID: 15055731.

104. Khan MU, Lall P, Harris LM, et al. Predictors of limb loss despite a patent endovascular-treated arterial segment. J Vasc Surg. 2009;49(6):1440-5; discussion 1445-6. PMID: 19497503.

105. Korhonen M, Biancari F, Soderstrom M, et al. Femoropopliteal balloon angioplasty vs. bypass surgery for CLI: a propensity score analysis. Eur J Vasc Endovasc Surg. 2011;41(3):378-84. PMID: 21195637.

106. Kudo T, Chandra FA, Kwun WH, et al. Changing pattern of surgical revascularization for critical limb ischemia over 12 years: endovascular vs. open bypass surgery. J Vasc Surg. 2006;44(2):304-13. PMID: 16890859.

107. Laurila J, Brommels M, Standertskjold-Nordenstam CG, et al. Cost-effectiveness of Percutaneous Transluminal Angioplasty (PTA) Versus Vascular Surgery in Limb-threatening Ischaemia. Int J Angiol. 2000;9(4):214-219. PMID: 11062310.

108. Loor G, Skelly CL, Wahlgren CM, et al. Is atherectomy the best first-line therapy for limb salvage in patients with critical limb ischemia? Vasc Endovascular Surg. 2009;43(6):542-50. PMID: 19640919.

109. Sultan S, Hynes N. Five-year Irish trial of CLI patients with TASC II type C/D lesions undergoing subintimal angioplasty or bypass surgery based on plaque echolucency. J Endovasc Ther. 2009;16(3):270-83. PMID: 19642779.

110. Soderstrom MI, Arvela EM, Korhonen M, et al. Infrapopliteal percutaneous transluminal angioplasty versus bypass surgery as first-line strategies in critical leg ischemia: a propensity score analysis. Ann Surg. 2010;252(5):765-73. PMID: 21037432.

111. Taylor SM, Kalbaugh CA, Blackhurst DW, et al. Determinants of functional outcome after revascularization for critical limb ischemia: an analysis of 1000 consecutive vascular interventions. J Vasc Surg. 2006;44(4):747-55; discussion 755-6. PMID: 16926083.

112. Taylor SM, Kalbaugh CA, Blackhurst DW, et al. Postoperative outcomes according to preoperative medical and functional status after infrainguinal revascularization for critical limb ischemia in patients 80 years and older. Am Surg. 2005;71(8):640-5; discussion 645-6. PMID: 16217945.

113. Taylor SM, York JW, Cull DL, et al. Clinical success using patient-oriented outcome measures after lower extremity bypass and endovascular intervention for ischemic tissue loss. J Vasc Surg. 2009;50(3):534-41; discussion 541. PMID: 19592193.

114. Varela C, Acin F, De Haro J, et al. Influence of surgical or endovascular distal revascularization of the lower limbs on ischemic ulcer healing. J Cardiovasc Surg (Torino). 2011;52(3):381-9. PMID: 21577193.

115. Venermo M, Biancari F, Arvela E, et al. The role of chronic kidney disease as a predictor of outcome after revascularisation of the ulcerated diabetic foot. Diabetologia. 2011. PMID: 21845468.

116. Wolfle KD, Bruijnen H, Reeps C, et al. Tibioperoneal arterial lesions and critical foot ischaemia: successful management by the use of short vein grafts and percutaneous transluminal angioplasty. Vasa. 2000;29(3):207-14. PMID: 11037720.

117. Zdanowski Z, Troeng T, Norgren L. Outcome and influence of age after infrainguinal revascularisation in critical limb ischaemia. The Swedish Vascular Registry. Eur J Vasc Endovasc Surg. 1998;16(2):137-41. PMID: 9728433.

118. Faglia E, Clerici G, Losa S, et al. Limb revascularization feasibility in diabetic patients with critical limb ischemia: results from a cohort of 344 consecutive unselected diabetic patients evaluated in 2009. Diabetes Res Clin Pract. 2012;95(3):364-71. PMID: 22104261.

119. Dosluoglu HH, Lall P, Harris LM, et al. Long-term limb salvage and survival after endovascular and open revascularization for critical limb ischemia after adoption of endovascular-first approach by vascular surgeons. Journal of Vascular Surgery. 2012.

120. Johnson BF, Singh S, Evans L, et al. A prospective study of the effect of limb-threatening ischaemia and its surgical treatment on the quality of life. Eur J Vasc Endovasc Surg. 1997;13(3):306-14. PMID: 9129605.

121. Hoshino J, Fujimoto Y, Naruse Y, et al. Characteristics of revascularization treatment for arteriosclerosis obliterans in patients with and without hemodialysis. Circ J. 2010;74(11):2426-33. PMID: 20938099.

122. Janne d'Othee B, Morris MF, Powell RJ, et al. Cost determinants of percutaneous and surgical interventions for treatment of intermittent claudication from the perspective of the hospital. Cardiovasc Intervent Radiol. 2008;31(1):56-65. PMID: 17973158.

123. Lepantalo M, Laurila K, Roth WD, et al. PTFE bypass or thrupass for superficial femoral artery occlusion? A randomised controlled trial. Eur J Vasc Endovasc Surg. 2009;37(5):578-84. PMID: 19231250.

124. McQuade K, Gable D, Hohman S, et al. Randomized comparison of ePTFE/nitinol self-expanding stent graft vs prosthetic femoral-popliteal bypass in the treatment of superficial femoral artery occlusive disease. J Vasc Surg. 2009;49(1):109-15, 116 e1-9; discussion 116. PMID: 19028055.

125. Rossi E, Citterio F, Castagneto M, et al. Safety of endovascular treatment in high-cardiac-risk patients with limb-threatening ischemia. Angiology. 1998;49(6):435-40. PMID: 9631888.

126. Sachs T, Pomposelli F, Hamdan A, et al. Trends in the national outcomes and costs for claudication and limb threatening ischemia: Angioplasty vs bypass graft. J Vasc Surg. 2011;54(4):1021-1031 e1. PMID: 21880457.

127. Stoner MC, Defreitas DJ, Manwaring MM, et al. Cost per day of patency: understanding the impact of patency and reintervention in a sustainable model of healthcare. J Vasc Surg. 2008;48(6):1489-96. PMID: 18829227.

128. Timaran CH, Prault TL, Stevens SL, et al. Iliac artery stenting versus surgical reconstruction for TASC (TransAtlantic Inter-Society Consensus) type B and type C iliac lesions. J Vasc Surg. 2003;38(2):272-8. PMID: 12891108.

129. Timaran CH, Ohki T, Gargiulo NJ, 3rd, et al. Iliac artery stenting in patients with poor distal runoff: Influence of concomitant infrainguinal arterial reconstruction. J Vasc Surg. 2003;38(3):479-84; discussion 484-5. PMID: 12947261.

130. Whatling PJ, Gibson M, Torrie EP, et al. Iliac occlusions: stenting or crossover grafting? An examination of patency and cost. Eur J Vasc Endovasc Surg. 2000;20(1):36-40. PMID: 10906295.

131. Kashyap VS, Pavkov ML, Bena JF, et al. The management of severe aortoiliac occlusive disease: endovascular therapy rivals open reconstruction. J Vasc Surg. 2008;48(6):1451-7, 1457 e1-3. PMID: 18804943.

132. Kamiya C, Sakamoto S, Tamori Y, et al. Long-term outcome after percutaneous peripheral intervention vs medical treatment for patients with superficial femoral artery occlusive disease. Circ J. 2008;72(5):734-9. PMID: 18441452.

133. Lawall H, Gorriahn H, Amendt K, et al. Long-term outcomes after medical and interventional therapy of critical limb ischemia. Eur J Intern Med. 2009;20(6):616-21. PMID: 19782924.

134. Adams J, Ogola G, Stafford P, et al. High-intensity interval training for intermittent claudication in a vascular rehabilitation program. J Vasc Nurs. 2006;24(2):46-9. PMID: 16737929.

135. Kedora J, Hohmann S, Garrett W, et al. Randomized comparison of percutaneous Viabahn stent grafts vs prosthetic femoral-popliteal bypass in the treatment of superficial femoral arterial occlusive disease. J Vasc Surg. 2007;45(1):10-6; discussion 16. PMID: 17126520.

136. McQuade K, Gable D, Pearl G, et al. Four-year randomized prospective comparison of percutaneous ePTFE/nitinol self-expanding stent graft versus prosthetic femoral-popliteal bypass in the treatment of superficial femoral artery occlusive disease. J Vasc Surg. 2010;52(3):584-90; discussion 590-1, 591 e1-591 e7. PMID: 20598480.

137. Wong Peng F, Chong Lee Y, Mikhailidis Dimitris P, et al. Antiplatelet agents for intermittent claudication. Cochrane Database of Systematic Reviews. 2011(11). PMID: CD001272.

138. Frans FA, Bipat S, Reekers JA, et al. Systematic review of exercise training or percutaneous transluminal angioplasty for intermittent claudication. Br J Surg. 2011. PMID: 21928409.

139. Leng GC, Fowler B, Ernst E. Exercise for intermittent claudication. Cochrane Database Syst Rev. 2000(2):CD000990. PMID: 10796572.

140. Watson L, Ellis B, Leng GC. Exercise for intermittent claudication. Cochrane Database Syst Rev. 2008(4):CD000990. PMID: 18843614.

141. National Institute for Health and Clinical Excellence. Lower limb peripheral arterial disease: diagnosis and management. NICE Clinical Guideline [draft]. March 2012. www.nice.org.uk/guidance/index.jsp?action=folder&o=58406. Accessed May 22, 2012.

142. Robless P, Mikhailidis DP, Stansby GP. Cilostazol for peripheral arterial disease. Cochrane Database Syst Rev. 2008(1):CD003748. PMID: 18254032.

143. Girolami B, Bernardi E, Prins MH, et al. Treatment of intermittent claudication with physical training, smoking cessation, pentoxifylline, or nafronyl: a meta-analysis. Arch Intern Med. 1999;159(4):337-45. PMID: 10030306.

144. Leng GC, Davis M, Baker D. Bypass surgery for chronic lower limb ischaemia. Cochrane Database Syst Rev. 2000(3):CD002000. PMID: 10908520.

145. Bradbury AW, Adam DJ, Bell J, et al. Bypass versus Angioplasty in Severe Ischaemia of the Leg (BASIL) trial: An intention-to-treat analysis of amputation-free and overall survival in patients randomized to a bypass surgery-first or a balloon angioplasty-first revascularization strategy. J Vasc Surg. 2010;51(5 Suppl):5S-17S. PMID: 20435258.

146. Agency for Healthcare Research and Quality. Horizon Scan of Invasive Interventions for Lower Extremity Peripheral Artery Disease and Systematic Review of Studies Comparing Stent Placement to Other Interventions. Technology Assessment. October 2008. www.cms.gov/Medicare/Coverage/DeterminationProcess/downloads//id63TA.pdf. Accessed May 22, 2012.

147. Robinson KA, Saldanha IJ, Mckoy NA. Frameworks for Determining Research Gaps During Systematic Reviews. Methods Future Research Needs Report No. 2. (Prepared by the Johns Hopkins University Evidence-based Practice Center under Contract No. 290-2007-10061-I.) AHRQ Publication No. 11-EHC043-EF. Rockville, MD: Agency for Healthcare Research and Quality. June 2011. www.effectivehealthcare.ahrq.gov/reports/final.cfm. Accessed May 22, 2012.

Abbreviations

ABI	ankle-brachial index
ACD	absolute claudication distance
AHRQ	Agency for Healthcare Research and Quality
ASA	acetylsalicylic acid (aspirin)
CI	confidence interval
CLI	critical limb ischemia
COT	claudication onset time
CV	cardiovascular
CVA	cerebrovascular accident
DAPT	Dual antiplatelet therapy
EffSE	standard error of effect
ES	effect size
HR	hazard ratio
IC	intermittent claudication
ICD	initial claudication distance
IDDM	insulin-dependent diabetes mellitus
KQ	key question
LDL	low-density lipoprotein
m	meters
MI	myocardial infarction
min	minute
mo	month/months
MWD	maximal walking distance
MWT	maximal walking time
NA	not applicable
NIDDM	noninsulin-dependent diabetes mellitus
NR	not reported
OR	odds ratio
PAD	peripheral artery disease
PAQ	Peripheral Artery Questionnaire
PFWD	pain-free walking distance
PICOTS	population, intervention, comparator, outcome, timing, setting
PTA	percutaneous transluminal angioplasty
PWD	peak walking distance
PWT	peak walking time
QOL	quality of life
RCT	randomized controlled trial
RR	risk ratio
SD	standard deviation
sec	second/seconds
SF-36®	short-form (36) health survey
SFA	superficial femoral artery
SOE	strength of evidence
TEP	Technical Expert Panel

TWD	total walking distance
WIQ	Walking Impairment Questionnaire
wk	week/weeks
yr	year/years

Appendix A. Exact Search Strings

PubMed® Search Strategy (August 13, 2012)

Table A-1. KQ 1: Effectiveness and safety of aspirin and antiplatelets for patients with peripheral artery disease

Set #	Terms
#1	"Peripheral Arterial Disease"[Mesh] OR "Peripheral Vascular Diseases"[Mesh] OR PAD[tiab] OR "peripheral arterial disease"[tiab] OR "peripheral vascular disease"[tiab] OR "arterial occlusive disease"[tiab] OR "intermittent claudication"[MeSH Terms] OR claudication[tiab] OR "rest pain"[tiab] OR (critical[tiab] AND ("extremities"[MeSH Terms] OR "extremities"[tiab] OR "limb"[tiab]) AND ("ischaemia"[tiab] OR "ischemia"[MeSH Terms] OR "ischemia"[tiab])) OR (("ischaemia"[tiab] OR "ischemia"[MeSH Terms] OR "ischemia"[tiab]) AND ("lower extremity"[MeSH Terms] OR ("lower"[tiab] AND "extremity"[tiab]) OR "lower extremity"[tiab])) OR (("extremities"[MeSH Terms] OR "extremities"[tiab] OR "limb"[tiab]) AND ("ischaemia"[tiab] OR "ischemia"[MeSH Terms] OR "ischemia"[tiab])) OR "vascular ulcer"[tiab] OR (vascular[tiab] AND ulcer[tiab]) OR "vascular ulcers"[tiab] OR (vascular[tiab] AND ulcers[tiab]) OR "varicose ulcer"[MeSH] OR "varicose ulcer"[tiab] OR (varicose[tiab] AND ulcer[tiab]) OR "varicose ulcers"[tiab] OR (varicose[tiab] AND ulcers[tiab]) OR "leg ulcer"[MeSH] OR "leg ulcer"[tiab] OR (leg[tiab] AND ulcer[tiab]) OR "leg ulcers"[tiab] OR (leg[tiab] AND ulcers[tiab]) OR gangrene[MeSH] OR gangrene[tiab]
#2	"aspirin"[MeSH Terms] OR "aspirin"[tw] OR ("clopidogrel"[Supplementary Concept] OR "clopidogrel"[tw] OR "plavix"[tw]) OR "prasugrel"[Supplementary Concept] OR "prasugrel"[tw] OR Effient[tw] OR "Ticagrelor"[Supplementary Concept] OR "Ticagrelor"[tw] OR brilinta[tw]
#3	"evaluation studies"[Publication Type] OR "evaluation studies as topic"[MeSH Terms] OR "evaluation study"[tw] OR evaluation studies[tw] OR "intervention studies"[MeSH Terms] OR "intervention study"[tw] OR "intervention studies"[tw] OR "case-control studies"[MeSH Terms] OR "case-control"[tw] OR "cohort studies"[MeSH Terms] OR cohort[tw] OR "longitudinal studies"[MeSH Terms] OR "longitudinal"[tw] OR longitudinally[tw] OR "prospective"[tw] OR prospectively[tw] OR "retrospective studies"[MeSH Terms] OR "retrospective"[tw] OR "follow up"[tw] OR "comparative study"[Publication Type] OR "comparative study"[tw] OR systematic[subset] OR "meta-analysis"[Publication Type] OR "meta-analysis as topic"[MeSH Terms] OR "meta-analysis"[tw] OR "meta-analyses"[tw] OR randomized controlled trial[pt] OR controlled clinical trial[pt] OR randomized[tiab] OR randomised[tiab] OR randomization[tiab] OR randomisation[tiab] OR placebo[tiab] OR "drug therapy"[Subheading] OR randomly[tiab] OR trial[tiab] OR groups[tiab] OR Clinical trial[pt] OR "clinical trial"[tw] OR "clinical trials"[tw] NOT (Editorial[ptyp] OR Letter[ptyp] OR Case Reports[ptyp] OR Comment[ptyp])NOT (Editorial[ptyp] OR Letter[ptyp] OR Case Reports[ptyp] OR Comment[ptyp])
#4	(#1 AND #2 AND #3) not (ANIMALS[MH] not HUMANS[MH])
#5	#4 Limits: English, **Publication Date from 1995 to 2011**

Table A-2. KQ 2: Effectiveness and safety of exercise, medications, endovascular intervention, and surgical revascularization (intermittent claudication)

Set #	Terms
#1	"intermittent claudication"[MeSH Terms] OR claudication[tiab]
#2	("angioplasty"[MeSH Terms] OR "angioplasty"[tiab] OR ("percutaneous"[tiab] AND "transluminal"[tiab] AND "angioplasty"[tiab]) OR "percutaneous transluminal angioplasty"[tiab]) OR PTA[tiab] OR ("stents"[MeSH Terms] OR "stents"[tiab] OR "stent"[tiab]) OR (percutaneous[tiab] AND revascularization[tiab]) OR ("endovascular procedures"[MeSH Terms] OR ("endovascular"[tiab] AND "procedures"[tiab]) OR "endovascular procedures"[tiab]) OR endovascular[tiab] OR ("exercise therapy"[MeSH Terms] OR ("exercise"[tiab] AND "therapy"[tiab]) OR "exercise therapy"[tiab]) OR (("exercise"[MeSH Terms] OR "exercise"[tiab]) AND (program[tiab] OR class[tiab] OR training[tiab] OR prescribed[tiab] OR structure[tiab] OR structured[tiab] OR supervised[tiab])) OR ("aspirin"[MeSH Terms] OR "aspirin"[tiab]) OR ("clopidogrel"[Supplementary Concept] OR "clopidogrel"[tiab]) OR ("cilostazol"[Supplementary Concept] OR "cilostazol"[tiab]) OR ("pentoxifylline"[MeSH Terms] OR "pentoxifylline"[tiab])
#3	"Femoral Artery/surgery"[Mesh] OR "Popliteal Artery/surgery"[Mesh] OR "tibial arteries/surgery"[Mesh Terms] OR "arteries/surgery"[Mesh Terms] OR "transplants"[MeSH Terms] OR transplants[tiab] OR graft[tiab] OR grafts[tiab] OR grafting[tiab] OR bypass[tiab] OR conduit[tiab] OR femoropopliteal[tiab] OR femorotibial[tiab] OR aortobifemoral[tiab] OR ballon[tiab] OR "atherectomy"[MeSH Terms] OR atherectomy[tiab]
#4	"evaluation studies"[Publication Type] OR "evaluation studies as topic"[MeSH Terms] OR "evaluation study"[tw] OR evaluation studies[tw] OR "intervention studies"[MeSH Terms] OR "intervention study"[tw] OR "intervention studies"[tw] OR "case-control studies"[MeSH Terms] OR "case-control"[tw] OR "cohort studies"[MeSH Terms] OR cohort[tw] OR "longitudinal studies"[MeSH Terms] OR "longitudinal"[tw] OR longitudinally[tw] OR "prospective"[tw] OR prospectively[tw] OR "retrospective studies"[MeSH Terms] OR "retrospective"[tw] OR "follow up"[tw] OR "comparative study"[Publication Type] OR "comparative study"[tw] OR systematic[subset] OR "meta-analysis"[Publication Type] OR "meta-analysis as topic"[MeSH Terms] OR "meta-analysis"[tw] OR "meta-analyses"[tw] OR randomized controlled trial[pt] OR controlled clinical trial[pt] OR randomized[tiab] OR randomised[tiab] OR randomization[tiab] OR randomisation[tiab] OR placebo[tiab] OR "drug therapy"[Subheading] OR randomly[tiab] OR trial[tiab] OR groups[tiab] OR Clinical trial[pt] OR "clinical trial"[tw] OR "clinical trials"[tw] NOT (Editorial[ptyp] OR Letter[ptyp] OR Case Reports[ptyp] OR Comment[ptyp])NOT (Editorial[ptyp] OR Letter[ptyp] OR Case Reports[ptyp] OR Comment[ptyp])
#5	#1 AND (#2 OR #3) AND #4 NOT (animals[mh] NOT humans[mh])
#6	#5 AND Limits: English, Publication Date from 1995 to 2011

Table A-3. KQ 3: Effectiveness and safety of endovascular intervention and surgical revascularization (critical limb ischemia)

Set #	Terms
#1	"rest pain"[tiab] OR (critical[tiab] AND ("extremities"[MeSH Terms] OR "extremities"[tiab] OR "limb"[tiab]) AND ("ischaemia"[tiab] OR "ischemia"[MeSH Terms] OR "ischemia"[tiab])) OR (("ischaemia"[tiab] OR "ischemia"[MeSH Terms] OR "ischemia"[tiab]) AND ("lower extremity"[MeSH Terms] OR ("lower"[tiab] AND "extremity"[tiab]) OR "lower extremity"[tiab])) OR (("extremities"[MeSH Terms] OR "extremities"[tiab] OR "limb"[tiab]) AND ("ischaemia"[tiab] OR "ischemia"[MeSH Terms] OR "ischemia"[tiab]))
#2	"angioplasty"[MeSH Terms] OR "angioplasty"[tiab] OR ("percutaneous"[tiab] AND "transluminal"[tiab] AND "angioplasty"[tiab]) OR "percutaneous transluminal angioplasty"[tiab] OR PTA[tiab] OR "stents"[MeSH Terms] OR "stents"[tiab] OR "stent"[tiab] OR (percutaneous[tiab] AND revascularization[tiab]) OR "endovascular procedures"[MeSH Terms] OR endovascular[tiab]
#3	"Femoral Artery/surgery"[Mesh] OR "Popliteal Artery/surgery"[Mesh] OR "tibial arteries/surgery"[Mesh Terms] OR "arteries/surgery"[Mesh Terms] OR "transplants"[MeSH Terms] OR transplants[tiab] OR graft[tiab] OR grafts[tiab] OR grafting[tiab] OR bypass[tiab] OR conduit[tiab] OR femoropopliteal[tiab] OR femorotibial[tiab] OR aortobifemoral[tiab] OR ballon[tiab] OR "atherectomy"[MeSH Terms] OR atherectomy[tiab]
#4	"evaluation studies"[Publication Type] OR "evaluation studies as topic"[MeSH Terms] OR "evaluation study"[tw] OR evaluation studies[tw] OR "intervention studies"[MeSH Terms] OR "intervention study"[tw] OR "intervention studies"[tw] OR "case-control studies"[MeSH Terms] OR "case-control"[tw] OR "cohort studies"[MeSH Terms] OR cohort[tw] OR "longitudinal studies"[MeSH Terms] OR "longitudinal"[tw] OR longitudinally[tw] OR "prospective"[tw] OR prospectively[tw] OR "retrospective studies"[MeSH Terms] OR "retrospective"[tw] OR "follow up"[tw] OR "comparative study"[Publication Type] OR "comparative study"[tw] OR systematic[subset] OR "meta-analysis"[Publication Type] OR "meta-analysis as topic"[MeSH Terms] OR "meta-analysis"[tw] OR "meta-analyses"[tw] OR randomized controlled trial[pt] OR controlled clinical trial[pt] OR randomized[tiab] OR randomised[tiab] OR randomization[tiab] OR randomisation[tiab] OR placebo[tiab] OR "drug therapy"[Subheading] OR randomly[tiab] OR trial[tiab] OR groups[tiab] OR Clinical trial[pt] OR "clinical trial"[tw] OR "clinical trials"[tw] NOT (Editorial[ptyp] OR Letter[ptyp] OR Case Reports[ptyp] OR Comment[ptyp])NOT (Editorial[ptyp] OR Letter[ptyp] OR Case Reports[ptyp] OR Comment[ptyp])
#5	#1 AND (#2 OR #3) AND #4 NOT (animals[mh] NOT humans[mh])
#6	#5 AND Limits: Publication Date from 1995 to 2011

Embase® Search Strategy (August 13, 2012)

Platform: Embase.com

Table A-4. KQ 1: Effectiveness and safety of aspirin and antiplatelets for patients with peripheral artery disease

Set #	Terms
#1	'peripheral arterial disease':ab,ti OR pad:ab,ti OR 'peripheral artery disease':ab,ti OR 'peripheral occlusive artery disease'/de OR 'claudication'/exp OR 'limb ischemia'/exp OR 'leg ischemia'/exp OR 'leg ulcer'/exp OR 'gangrene'/exp OR 'intermittent claudication':ab,ti OR ((extremity:ab,ti OR limb:ab,ti OR leg:ab,ti) AND (ischemia:ab,ti OR iscaemia:ab,ti))
#2	aspirin:ab,ti OR clopidogrel:ab,ti OR plavix:ab,ti OR prasugrel:ab,ti OR effient:ab,ti OR ticagrelor:ab,ti OR brilinta:ab,ti OR 'acetylsalicylic acid'/exp OR 'clopidogrel'/exp OR 'ticagrelor'/exp OR prasugrel/exp
#3	'randomized controlled trial'/exp OR 'crossover procedure'/exp OR 'double blind procedure'/exp OR 'single blind procedure'/exp OR random*:ab,ti OR factorial*:ab,ti OR crossover*:ab,ti OR (cross NEAR/1 over*):ab,ti OR placebo*:ab,ti OR (doubl* NEAR/1 blind*):ab,ti OR (singl* NEAR/1 blind*):ab,ti OR assign*:ab,ti OR allocat*:ab,ti OR volunteer*:ab,ti OR 'clinical study'/exp OR 'clinical trial':ab,ti OR 'clinical trials':ab,ti OR 'controlled study'/exp OR 'evaluation'/exp OR 'evaluation study':ab,ti OR 'evaluation studies':ab,ti OR 'intervention study':ab,ti OR 'intervention studies':ab,ti OR 'case control':ab,ti OR 'cohort analysis'/exp OR cohort:ab,ti ORlongitudinal*:ab,ti OR prospective:ab,ti OR prospectively:ab,ti OR retrospective:ab,ti OR 'follow up'/exp OR 'follow up':ab,ti OR 'comparative effectiveness'/exp OR 'comparative study'/exp OR 'comparative study':ab,ti OR 'comparative studies':ab,ti OR 'evidence based medicine'/exp OR 'systematic review':ab,ti OR 'meta-analysis':ab,ti OR 'meta-analyses':ab,ti NOT ('editorial'/exp OR 'letter'/exp OR 'case report'/exp)
#4	#1 AND #2 AND #3
#5	#4 AND [humans]/lim AND [1995-2012]/py
#6	#5 AND [embase]/lim NOT [medline]/lim AND [1995-2012]/py

Table A-5. KQ 2: Effectiveness and safety of exercise, medications, endovascular intervention, and surgical revascularization (intermittent claudication)

Set #	Terms
#1	'claudication'/exp OR claudication:ab,ti
#2	'angioplasty'/exp OR 'percutaneous transluminal angioplasty'/exp OR 'stent'/exp OR 'endovascular surgery'/de OR angioplasty:ab,ti OR "percutaneous transluminal":ab,ti OR stent:ab,ti OR stents:ab,ti OR endovascular:ab,ti OR revascularization:ab,ti OR percutaneous:ab,ti OR pta:ab,ti OR 'revascularization'/exp OR kinesiotherapy/exp OR ('exercise'/exp AND (therapy:ab,ti OR program:ab,ti OR class:ab,ti OR training:ab,ti OR prescribed:ab,ti OR structure:ab,ti OR structured:ab,ti OR supervised:ab,ti)) OR 'pentoxifylline'/exp OR 'cilostazol'/exp OR pentoxifylline:ab,ti OR cilostazol:ab,ti OR aspirin:ab,ti OR clopidogrel:ab,ti OR 'acetylsalicylic acid'/exp OR clopidogrel/exp
#3	('leg artery'/exp OR femoropopliteal:ab,ti OR femorotibial:ab,ti OR aortobifemoral:ab,ti OR femoral;ab,ti OR popliteal:ab,ti OR tibial:ab,ti) AND (transplant:ab,ti OR graft:ab,ti OR grafts:ab,ti OR grafting:ab,ti OR bypass:ab,ti OR conduit:ab,ti OR ballon:ab,ti OR transplantation:ab,ti) OR 'leg revascularization'/exp
#4	'randomized controlled trial'/exp OR 'crossover procedure'/exp OR 'double blind procedure'/exp OR 'single blind procedure'/exp OR random*:ab,ti OR factorial*:ab,ti OR crossover*:ab,ti OR (cross NEAR/1 over*):ab,ti OR placebo*:ab,ti OR (doubl* NEAR/1 blind*):ab,ti OR (singl* NEAR/1 blind*):ab,ti OR assign*:ab,ti OR allocat*:ab,ti OR volunteer*:ab,ti OR 'clinical study'/exp OR 'clinical trial':ab,ti OR 'clinical trials':ab,ti OR 'controlled study'/exp OR 'evaluation'/exp OR 'evaluation study':ab,ti OR 'evaluation studies':ab,ti OR 'intervention study':ab,ti OR 'intervention studies':ab,ti OR 'case control':ab,ti OR 'cohort analysis'/exp OR cohort:ab,ti ORlongitudinal*:ab,ti OR prospective:ab,ti OR prospectively:ab,ti OR retrospective:ab,ti OR 'follow up'/exp OR 'follow up':ab,ti OR 'comparative effectiveness'/exp OR 'comparative study'/exp OR 'comparative study':ab,ti OR 'comparative studies':ab,ti OR 'evidence based medicine'/exp OR 'systematic review':ab,ti OR 'meta-analysis':ab,ti OR 'meta-analyses':ab,ti NOT ('editorial'/exp OR 'letter'/exp OR 'case report'/exp)
#5	#1 AND (#2 OR #3) AND #4
#6	#5 AND [humans]/lim AND [1995-2012]/py
#7	#6 AND [embase]/lim NOT [medline]/lim

Table A-6. KQ 3: Effectiveness and safety of endovascular intervention and surgical revascularization (critical limb ischemia)

Set #	Terms
#1	"rest pain":ab,ti OR 'limb ischemia'/exp AND 'leg ischemia'/exp OR "critical limb ischemia")OR (critical:ab,ti AND (extremities:ab,ti OR extremity:ab,ti OR limb:ab,ti OR leg:ab,ti) AND ("ischaemia":ab,ti OR "ischemia":ab,ti))
#2	'angioplasty'/exp OR 'percutaneous transluminal angioplasty'/exp OR 'stent'/exp OR 'endovascular surgery'/de OR angioplasty:ab,ti OR 'percutaneous transluminal':ab,ti OR stent:ab,ti OR stents:ab,ti OR endovascular:ab,ti OR revascularization:ab,ti OR percutaneous:ab,ti OR pta:ab,ti OR 'revascularization'/exp
#3	'leg artery'/exp OR femoropopliteal:ab,ti OR femorotibial:ab,ti OR aortobifemoral:ab,ti OR femoral;ab,ti OR popliteal:ab,ti OR tibial:ab,ti AND (transplant:ab,ti OR graft:ab,ti OR grafts:ab,ti OR grafting:ab,ti ORbypass:ab,ti OR conduit:ab,ti OR ballon:ab,ti OR transplantation:ab,ti) OR 'leg revascularization'/exp
#4	'randomized controlled trial'/exp OR 'crossover procedure'/exp OR 'double blind procedure'/exp OR 'single blind procedure'/exp OR random*:ab,ti OR factorial*:ab,ti OR crossover*:ab,ti OR (cross NEAR/1 over*):ab,ti OR placebo*:ab,ti OR (doubl* NEAR/1 blind*):ab,ti OR (singl* NEAR/1 blind*):ab,ti OR assign*:ab,ti OR allocat*:ab,ti OR volunteer*:ab,ti OR 'clinical study'/exp OR 'clinical trial':ab,ti OR 'clinical trials':ab,ti OR 'controlled study'/exp OR 'evaluation'/exp OR 'evaluation study':ab,ti OR 'evaluation studies':ab,ti OR 'intervention study':ab,ti OR 'intervention studies':ab,ti OR 'case control':ab,ti OR 'cohort analysis'/exp OR cohort:ab,ti ORlongitudinal*:ab,ti OR prospective:ab,ti OR prospectively:ab,ti OR retrospective:ab,ti OR 'follow up'/exp OR 'follow up':ab,ti OR 'comparative effectiveness'/exp OR 'comparative study'/exp OR 'comparative study':ab,ti OR 'comparative studies':ab,ti OR 'evidence based medicine'/exp OR 'systematic review':ab,ti OR 'meta-analysis':ab,ti OR 'meta-analyses':ab,ti NOT ('editorial'/exp OR 'letter'/exp OR 'case report'/exp)
#5	#1 AND (#2 OR #3) AND #4
#6	#5 AND [humans]/lim AND [1995-2012]/py
#7	#6 AND [embase]/lim NOT [medline]/lim

Cochrane Search Strategy (August 13, 2012)

Platform: Wiley

Databases searched: Cochrane Central Registry of Controlled Trials and Cochrane Database of Systematic Reviews

Table A-7. KQ 1: Effectiveness and safety of aspirin and antiplatelets for patients with peripheral artery disease

Set #	Terms
#1	MeSH descriptor Peripheral Arterial Disease explode all trees OR MeSH descriptor Intermittent Claudication explode all trees OR MeSH descriptor Leg Ulcer explode all trees OR MeSH descriptor Varicose Ulcer explode all trees OR MeSH descriptor Gangrene explode all trees OR (Peripheral Arterial Disease):ti,ab,kw or (arterial occlusive disease):ti,ab,kw or (intermittent claudication):ti,ab,kw or (rest pain):ti,ab,kw or (pad):ti,ab,kw OR (occlusive artery disease):ti,ab,kw or (leg ischemia):ti,ab,kw or (limb ischemia):ti,ab,kw or (claudication):ti,ab,kw
#2	MeSH descriptor Aspirin explode all trees OR (aspirin):ti,ab,kw or (clopidogrel):ti,ab,kw or (prasugrel):ti,ab,kw or (ticagrelor):ti,ab,kw or (plavix):kw
#3	#1 AND #2 AND (Cochrane Reviews, other reviews, Clinical trials)
#4	#3 AND 1995 - 2012

Table A-8. KQ 2: Effectiveness and safety of exercise, medications, endovascular intervention, and surgical revascularization (intermittent claudication)

Set #	Terms
#1	MeSH descriptor Intermittent Claudication explode all trees OR claudication):ti,ab,kw
#2	MeSH descriptor Angioplasty explode all trees OR MeSH descriptor Stents explode all trees OR MeSH descriptor Endovascular Procedures explode all trees OR percutaneous transluminal):ti,ab,kw OR (pta):ti,ab,kw OR (endovascular):ti,ab,kw OR (revascularization):ti,ab,kw OR (stent OR stents):ti,ab,kw OR MeSH descriptor Exercise Therapy explode all trees OR (exercise):ti,ab,kw OR MeSH descriptor Aspirin explode all trees OR MeSH descriptor Pentoxifylline explode all trees OR (aspirin):ti,ab,kw or (clopidogrel):ti,ab,kw or (cilostazol):ti,ab,kw or (pentoxifylline):ti,ab,kw
#3	MeSH descriptor Femoral Artery explode all trees with qualifier: SU OR MeSH descriptor Popliteal Artery explode all trees with qualifier: SU OR MeSH descriptor Tibial Arteries explode all trees with qualifier: SU OR MeSH descriptor Arteries explode all trees with qualifier: SU OR (graft*):ti,ab,kw or (transplant*):ti,ab,kw or (bypass):ti,ab,kw or (conduit):ti,ab,kw OR (femoropopliteal):ti,ab,kw or (femorotibial):ti,ab,kw or (aortobifermoral):ti,ab,kw or (atherectomy):ti,ab,kw OR (revascularization):ti,ab,kw
#4	#1 AND (#2 OR #3)
#5	#4 AND (Cochrane Reviews, other reviews, Clinical trials)
#6	#5 AND 1995-2012

Table A-9. KQ 3: Effectiveness and safety of endovascular intervention and surgical revascularization (critical limb ischemia)

Set #	Terms
#1	(rest pain):ti,ab,kw or (critical limb ischemia):ti,ab,kw OR (MeSH descriptor Ischemia explode all trees OR (ischemia):ti,ab,kw or (ischaemia):ti,ab,kw) AND ((limb*):ti,ab,kw or (leg*):ti,ab,kw or (extremiti*):ti,ab,kw)
#2	MeSH descriptor Angioplasty explode all trees OR MeSH descriptor Stents explode all trees OR MeSH descriptor Endovascular Procedures explode all trees OR (percutaneous transluminal angioplasty):ti,ab,kw or (stent*):ti,ab,kw or (angioplasty):ti,ab,kw or (revascularization):ti,ab,kw or (endovascular):ti,ab,kw
#3	MeSH descriptor Femoral Artery explode all trees with qualifier: SU OR MeSH descriptor Popliteal Artery explode all trees with qualifier: SU OR MeSH descriptor Tibial Arteries explode all trees with qualifier: SU OR MeSH descriptor Arteries explode all trees with qualifier: SU OR (transplant*):kw or (bypass):ti,ab,kw or (graft*):ti,ab,kw or (conduit*):ti,ab,kw or (ballon):ti,ab,kw OR (femoropopliteal):ti,ab,kw or (femorotibial):ti,ab,kw or (aortobifermoral):ti,ab,kw or (atherectomy):ti,ab,kw
#4	#1 AND (#2 OR #3)
#5	#4 AND (Cochrane Reviews, other reviews, Clinical trials)
#6	#5 AND 1995-2012

Appendix B. Data Abstraction Elements

Study Characteristics
- Study name and acronym
- Other articles used in this abstraction
- Study dates
    - Date enrollment started (MM and YYYY)
    - Date enrollment ended (MM and YYYY)
    - Length of Followup (months or years)
- Enrollment source: Primary care, Cardiology, Radiology, Surgery, NR/NA
- Enrollment approach: consecutive patients, convenience sample, other (specify), unclear/not reported
    - Number of subjects screened/approached for study participation
    - Number eligible for study
    - Number randomized
    - Number completing followup
    - Number included in primary outcome analysis
- Study sites: Single center, Multicenter, Not reported/Unclear
    - Geographic location
        - If single center, enter City and State (if US) or City and Country (if outside US).
        - If multicenter, enter number of sites. Enter NR if not reported.
        - If multicenter, specify applicable geographic regions: US, Canada, UK, Europe, S. America, C. America, Asia, Africa, Australia/NZ, Not reported/Unclear, Other (specify)
- Funding source: Government, Private foundation, Nonprofit Organization, Industry, Not reported, Other (specify)
- Setting: Academic centers, Community hospitals, Outpatient, VA, Not reported/unclear, Other (specify)
- Inclusion and exclusion criteria; Copy/paste criteria as reported in the article.
- Symptom status of population studied: Asymptomatic, Intermittent claudication, Atypical claudication, Critical limb ischemia
- To which key questions and subquestions does this study apply?
    - KQ1: KQ1a, KQ1b, KQ1c
    - KQ2: KQ2a, KQ2b, KQ2c
    - KQ3: KQ3a, KQ3b, KQ3c
- Subgroup Analysis: Yes/No
- Comments (if needed)

Baseline Characteristics
- Number of Subjects
    - Total Population and Treatment Arms 1, 2, 3, 4
        - N
            - Total

- Female
- Male
            - Percentage
                - Female
                - Male
- Total Population – Age in years
    - Total Population and Treatment Arms 1, 2, 3, 4
        - Mean
        - SD
        - SE
        - Median
        - IQR
- Ethnicity
    - Total N and Percentage of Population
        - Hispanic or Latino
        - Not Hispanic or Latino
- Race
    - Total N and Percentage of Population
        - Black/African American
        - American Indian or Alaska Native
        - Asian
        - Native Hawaiian or other Pacific Islander
        - White
        - Multiracial
        - Other (specify)
- Baseline Characteristics
    - Total Population and Treatment Arms 1, 2, 3, 4
        - Diabetes (NR)
        - Tobacco use (NR)
        - Prior MI (NR)
        - Known CAD (NR)
        - Hyperlipidemia (NR)
        - Prior PCI (NR)
        - Prior CABG (NR)
        - Heart failure (NR)
        - Chronic kidney disease (NR)
        - Obesity (NR) – Define
        - Prior stroke (NR)
        - Prior TIA (NR)
        - Prior stroke or TIA (NR)
        - Prior carotid surgery (NR)
        - Claudication (NR)
        - Peripheral vascular disease (NR)
        - Prior lower extremity vascular surgery (NR)
        - Ankle brachial index (NR)
            - Mean/Median

- SD/SE/IQR
        - Fontaine classification
            - Stage I
            - Stage IIa
            - Stage IIb
            - Stage 3
            - Stage 4
        - Rutherford classification
            - Stage 0
            - Stage 1
            - Stage 2
            - Stage 3
            - Stage 4
            - Stage 5
            - Stage 6
        - TASC II classification
            - A
            - B
            - C
            - D
            - A/B
            - C/D
        - Runoff vessels
            - Mean/Median
            - SD/SE/IQR
        - Runoff vessels (N)
            - 1
            - 2
            - 3
- Presentation
    - Total Population and Treatment Arms 1, 2, 3, 4
        - Asymptomatic (NR/NA)
        - Atypical leg pain (NR/NA)
        - Intermittent claudication (NR/NA)
        - Critical limb ischemia (NR/NA)
        - Mixed (specify) (NR/NA)
- Other socioeconomic factors: Yes/No
    - If yes: Specify the factor(s) and categories/units
    - If yes: Enter the characteristics as reported (e.g. range, mean and standard deviation, etc.)
- Comments (if needed)

Intervention Characteristics
- Briefly indicate which population/intervention combination is reflected by the data abstracted

- Treatment Arms 1, 2, 3, 4
  - Population
    - Asymptomatic patients
    - Symptomatic patients with atypical leg symptoms
    - Patients with intermittent claudication
    - Patients with critical limb ischemia
    - Other (specify)
    - NR/NA
  - Intervention
    - Aspirin or antiplatelet agents
    - Cilostazol or pentoxifylline
    - Exercise training
    - Endovascular intervention
    - Surgical revascularization
    - Control/placebo
    - Other
    - NR/NA
- Intervention Characteristics: Describe the intervention received by patients in Treatment Arm 1, Treatment Arm 2, Treatment Arm 3, and Treatment Arm 4 (if applicable)
- Cointerventions
  - Acetylsalicylic acid (ASA); Additional antiplatelet agents (e.g. clopidogrel, prasugrel, ticagrelor); Antithrombin drugs (e.g. LMWH, unfractionated heparin, bivalirudin); Glycoprotein IIb/IIIa inhibitors; Thrombolytic/fibrinolytic drugs; Statins/lipid-lowering drugs; Beta-blockers; ACEIs/ARBs; Calcium channel blockers; Nitrates; Other (specify); NR/NA
- Medical Therapy Intervention(s)
  - Treatment Arm 1, 2, 3, 4 (NA)
    - Clopidogrel
      - Yes/No
      - Loading dose
      - Maintenance dose
      - Timing
      - Duration of treatment
    - Prasugrel
      - Yes/No
      - Loading dose
      - Maintenance dose
      - Timing
      - Duration of treatment
    - Ticagrelor
      - Yes/No
      - Loading dose
      - Maintenance dose
      - Timing

- Duration of treatment
    - Cilostazol
        - Yes/No
        - Loading dose
        - Maintenance dose
        - Timing
        - Duration of treatment
    - Pentoxifylline
        - Yes/No
        - Loading dose
        - Maintenance dose
        - Timing
        - Duration of treatment
    - Aspirin
        - Yes/No
        - Loading dose
        - Maintenance dose
        - Timing
        - Duration of treatment
    - Glycoprotein IIb/IIIa (abciximab, eptifibatide, tirofiban)
        - Yes/No
        - Loading dose
        - Maintenance dose
        - Timing
        - Duration of treatment
    - Dipyridamole
        - Yes/No
        - Loading dose
        - Maintenance dose
        - Timing
        - Duration of treatment
    - Other #1, #2, #3 (specify)
        - Yes/No
        - Loading dose
        - Maintenance dose
        - Timing
        - Duration of treatment
- Exercise Therapy
    - Treatment Arm 1, 2, 3, 4
        - Exercise therapy type
            - Walking
            - Strength
            - Combined
            - Other

- NR/NA
  - Exercise therapy duration
  - Protocol used
  - Supervision status
    - Supervised
    - Home
    - NR/NA
- Endovascular Revascularization Procedural Characteristics
  - Treatment Arm 1, 2, 3, 4
    - Complete revascularization achieved
    - Vessels treated (mean)
      - Mean/median
      - SD/SE/IQR
      - 1
      - 2
      - Unclear/Not specified
    - Interventional approach
      - Balloon
        - N or %
        - Type
          - Drug coated
          - Cutting
          - Cryoplasty
          - Standard
          - Other (specify)
      - Atherectomy
        - N or %
        - Type
          - Laser
          - Orbital
          - Rotational
          - Directional
          - Other (specify)
      - Stents
        - N or %
        - Type
          - Drug-eluting
          - Self-expandable open cell
          - Balloon expandable open cell
          - Closed cell (covered)
          - Other (specify)
          - NR
    - Stents used (mean)
      - Mean/median
      - SD/SE/IQR

- 0
- 1
- 2
- More than 2
- Unclear/not specified
- Surgical Revascularization Procedural Characteristics
  - Treatment Arm 1, 2, 3, 4
    - Type of surgery
      - Axillofem or axillo bifem
      - Aortofem or aorto bifem
      - Fem-fem
      - Fem-pop
      - Fem-distal
      - Other (specify)
    - Type of grafts
      - Vein (native)
      - Synthetic
      - Composite
      - Cadaveric
    - Grafts used (mean)
      - Mean/median
      - SD/SE/IQR
      - 0
      - 1
      - 2
      - Greater than 2

Individual Outcomes
- Select the outcome reported: Total mortality, Cardiovascular mortality, Nonfatal myocardial infarction, Stroke, Repeat revascularization, Hospitalization, Length of hospital stay, Discharge status, Cost of hospital stay, Bleeding, Quality of life, Adverse drug reactions, Vessel patency, Wound healing, Pain, Major Amputation, Minor Amputation, Contrast nephropathy, Radiation, Infection, Exercise-related harms, Periprocedural complications, Maximal Walking distance, Peak Walking Time, Mean or 6-minute walking time, Claudication onset time, Absolute claudication distance, Mean claudication distance, Other 1, 2, 3, 4
  - Additional/alternate outcome name (if applicable)
  - Authors' definition of outcome (if applicable)
  - Was the post-procedure success rate measured? Yes/No/Unknown
    - If yes: Post-procedure success rate
  - Was the outcome reported at the patient level or limb level? Patient level/limb level/Other (specify)/(NR/NA)
  - Complete tables (1-5) to provide data for this outcome/time point(s).
    - Timing of the outcome data reported in the table: Short term ≤ 30 days/ Intermediate term > 30 days and ≤ 1 year/Long-term > 1 year

- If short term: In-hospital/30 days/Other (specify)
- If intermediate term: 6 weeks/6 months/1 year/Other (specify)
- If long term: 2 years/3 years/4 years/5 years/Other (specify)
    - Indicate whether/how the results reported were adjusted (check all that apply): Results are not adjusted, Age, Sex, Race/ethnicity, Comorbidity(ies) (specify), Bodyweight/BMI, Risk factors (smoking), PAD classification, Anatomy-specific factor (disease burden, location/pattern of stenosis, degree of calcification, # of below knee vessel runoff), Hospital characteristics (patient volume, setting, guideline-based treatment protocol), Other (specify all)
    - For each reported group (Antiplatelet therapy, Exercise therapy, Endovascular revascularization, Surgical revascularization, Medication, Other, NR/NA) record the following:
        - N for Analysis
        - Result
            - Mean
            - Median
            - Number of patients with outcome
            - % of patients with outcome
            - Relative risk
            - Relative hazard
            - Odds ratio
            - Risk difference
            - Other (specify)
        - Variability
            - Standard Error (SE)
            - Standard Deviation (SD)
            - Other (specify)
        - Confidence Interval (CI) or Interquartile Range (IQR)
            - 95% CI
                - LL (25% if IQR)
                - UL (75% if IQR)
            - Other %CI
                - LL (25% if IQR)
                - UL (75% if IQR)
            - IQR
                - LL (25% if IQR)
                - UL (75% if IQR)
        - p-value between tx groups
        - Reference group (for comparisons between tx groups)
            - Treatment Arm 1, Treatment Arm 2, Treatment Arm 3, Treatment Arm 4, No Comparison
- Comments (if needed)

Composite Outcomes
- Composite outcome data #1, #2, #3, #4

- Is this a Primary or Secondary composite outcome? Primary/Secondary/Unclear
- Indicate the components that make up this composite outcome (check all that apply): Total mortality, Cardiovascular mortality, Nonfatal myocardial infarction, Stroke, Repeat revascularization, Hospitalization, Length of hospital stay, Discharge status, Cost of hospital stay, Bleeding, Quality of life, Adverse drug reactions, Vessel patency, Wound healing, Pain, Major Amputation, Minor Amputation, Contrast nephropathy, Radiation, Infection, Exercise-related harms, Periprocedural complications, Maximal Walking distance, Peak Walking Time, Mean or 6-minute walking time, Claudication onset time, Absolute claudication distance, Mean claudication distance, Other 1, 2, 3, 4
- Was the outcome reported at the patient level or limb level?
- Complete tables (1-5) to provide data for this outcome/time point(s).
  - Timing of the outcome data reported in the table: Short term ≤ 30 days/ Intermediate term > 30 days and ≤ 1 year/Long-term > 1 year
    - If short term: In-hospital/30 days/Other (specify)
    - If intermediate term: 6 weeks/6 months/1 year/Other (specify)
    - If long term: 2 years/3 years/4 years/5 years/Other (specify)
  - Indicate whether/how the results reported were adjusted (check all that apply): Results are not adjusted, Age, Sex, Race/ethnicity, Comorbidity(ies) (specify), Bodyweight/BMI, Risk factors (smoking), PAD classification, Anatomy-specific factor (disease burden, location/pattern of stenosis, degree of calcification, # of below knee vessel runoff), Hospital characteristics (patient volume, setting, guideline-based treatment protocol), Other (specify all)
  - For each reported group (Antiplatelet therapy, Exercise therapy, Endovascular revascularization, Surgical revascularization, Medication, Other, NR/NA) record the following:
    - N for Analysis
    - Result
      - Mean
      - Median
      - Number of patients with outcome
      - % of patients with outcome
      - Relative risk
      - Relative hazard
      - Odds ratio
      - Risk difference
      - Other (specify)
    - Variability
      - Standard Error (SE)
      - Standard Deviation (SD)
      - Other (specify)
    - Confidence Interval (CI) or Interquartile Range (IQR)
      - 95% CI
        - LL (25% if IQR)
        - UL (75% if IQR)

- Other %CI
  - LL (25% if IQR)
  - UL (75% if IQR)
- IQR
  - LL (25% if IQR)
  - UL (75% if IQR)
- p-value between tx groups
- Reference group (for comparisons between tx groups)
  - Treatment Arm 1, Treatment Arm 2, Treatment Arm 3, Treatment Arm 4, No Comparison
- Comments (if needed)

Quality Assessment
- Was this study randomized? Yes/No
  - If yes:
    - Were study subjects randomized? Yes/No/Unclear
    - Was the randomization process described? Yes/No/Unclear
    - Was the outcome assessor blinded to study assignment? Yes/No/Unclear
    - Were patients blinded to study intervention? Yes/No/Unclear
    - Were results adjusted for clustering? Yes/No/Unclear
    - Were measures of outcomes based on validated procedures or instruments? Yes/No/Unclear
    - Conducted an intent to treat analysis? Yes/No/Unclear
    - Were all outcomes reported (i.e. was there evidence of selective outcome reporting)? Yes/No/Unclear
    - Were incomplete data adequately addressed (i.e. no systematic difference between groups in withdrawals/loss to followup AND no high drop-out or loss to followup rate [>30%])? Yes/No/Unclear
    - Was there adequate power (either based on pre-study or post-hoc power calculations [80% power for primary outcome])? Yes/No/Unclear
    - Were systematic differences observed in baseline characteristics and prognostic factors across the groups compared? Yes/No/Unclear
    - Were comparable groups maintained (Includes crossovers, adherence, and contamination. Consider issues of crossover [e.g. from one intervention to another], adherence [major differences in adherence to the interventions being compared], contamination [e.g. some members of control group get intervention], or other systematic difference in care that was provided.)? Yes/No/Unclear
    - Was there absence of potential important conflict-of-interest (Focus on financial conflicts with for-profit capacities; government or non-profit funding = 'yes')? Yes/No/Unclear
    - Overall Study Rating:
      - A "**Good**" study has the least bias, and results are considered valid. A good study has a clear description of the population, setting, interventions, and comparison groups; uses a valid approach to allocate patients to alternative treatments; has a low dropout rate;

and uses appropriate means to prevent bias, measure outcomes, and analyze and report results.
- A "**Fair**" study is susceptible to some bias but probably not enough to invalidate the results. The study may be missing information, making it difficult to assess limitations and potential problems. As the fair-quality category is broad, studies with this rating vary in their strengths and weaknesses. The results of some fair-quality studies are possibly valid, while others are probably valid.
- A "**Poor**" rating indicates significant bias that may invalidate the results. These studies have serious errors in design, analysis, or reporting; have large amounts of missing information; or have discrepancies in reporting. The results of a poor-quality study are at least as likely to reflect flaws in the study design as to indicate true differences between the compared interventions.

- If no:
  - Basic Design
    - Is the study design prospective, retrospective, or mixed [Prospective design requires that the investigator plans a study before any data are collected. Mixed design includes case-control or cohort studies in which one group is studied prospectively and the other retrospectively.]? Prospective/Mixed/Retrospective/Cannot determine
  - Selection Bias
    - Inclusion/Exclusion Criteria
      - Are the inclusion/exclusion criteria clearly stated (does not require the reader to infer)? Yes/Partially (only some criteria stated or some criteria not stated clearly)/No
      - Did the study apply inclusion/exclusion criteria uniformly to all comparison groups? Yes/Partially (only some criteria stated or some criteria not stated clearly)/No/NA (study does not include comparison groups)
    - Recruitment
      - Did the strategy for recruiting participants into the study differ across study groups? Yes/No/Cannot determine/NA (retrospective study design)
    - Baseline characteristics similar or appropriate adjusted analysis
      - Are key characteristics of study participants similar between intervention and control groups? If not similar, did the analysis appropriately adjust for important differences? Yes (similar or appropriate adjusted analysis)/Partially (only some characteristics described or some characteristics not clearly described; analysis adjusted for some)/No (important baseline differences; unadjusted analysis)/Insufficient reporting to be able to determine
    - Comparison Group

- o Is the selection of the comparison group appropriate? Yes/No/Cannot determine (no description of the derivation of the comparison cohort)/NA (study does not include a comparison cohort – case series, one-arm study)
- Performance Bias
  - Intervention implementation
    - o What is the level of detail in describing the intervention or exposure? High (very clear, all PI-required details provided)/Medium (somewhat clear, majoring of PI-required details provided)/Low (unclear, many PI-required details missing)
  - Concurrent/concomitant interventions
    - o Did researchers isolate the impact from a concurrent intervention or unintended exposure that might bias the results, e.g., through multivariate analysis, stratification, or subgroup analysis? Yes/Partially (only some concurrent interventions eliminated)/Not described
- Attrition Bias
  - Equality of length of followup for participants
    - o In cohort studies, is the length of followup different between groups? Yes/No or cannot determine/not applicable (cross-sectional or only one group followed over time)
  - Completeness of followup
    - o Was there a high rate of differential or overall attrition? Yes/No/Cannot determine
  - Attrition affecting participant composition
    - o Did attrition result in a difference in group characteristics between baseline and followup? Yes/No/Cannot determine
  - Any attempt to balance
    - o Any attempt to balance the allocation between groups (e.g. through stratification, matching, propensity scores)? Yes/No/Cannot determine
  - Intention-to-treat analysis
    - o Is the analysis conducted on an intention-to-treat (ITT) basis, that is, the intervention allocation status rather than the actual intervention received? Yes/No/Cannot determine/NA (retrospective study)
- Detection Bias
  - Source of information re: outcomes
    - o Are <u>procedural outcomes</u> (e.g. vessel patency, wound healing) assessed using valid and reliable measure and implemented consistently across all study participants? Yes/No/Cannot determine (measurement approach not reported)

- Are <u>event outcomes</u> (e.g. mortality, MI, CVA, repeat revascularization, amputation) assessed using valid and reliable measures and implemented consistently across all study participants? Yes/No/Cannot determine (measurement approach not reported)
- Are <u>patient-reported outcomes</u> (e.g. pain scores, quality of life) assessed using valid and reliable measures implemented consistently across all study participants? Yes/No/Cannot determine (measurement approach not reported)
- Are <u>functional capacity outcomes</u> (e.g. walking time/distance, claudication time/distance) assessed using valid and reliable measures, implemented consistently across all study participants? Yes/No/Cannot determine (measurement approach not reported)

- Reporting Bias
  - Are any important primary outcomes missing from the results? Yes/No/Cannot determine/Primary outcomes not pre-specified
- Other risk of bias issues
  - Are the statistical methods used to assess the primary outcomes appropriate to the data? Yes/Partially/No/Cannot determine
  - Power and sample size
    - Did the authors report conducting a power analysis or some other basis for determining the adequacy of study group sizes for the primary outcome(s) being abstracted? Yes/No/NA (primary outcomes statistically significant)
- Overall Rating of the study
  - A "**Low Risk of Bias**" study has the least bias, and results are considered valid. A good study has a clear description of the population, setting, interventions, and comparison groups; uses recruitment and eligibility criteria that minimizes selection bias; has a low attrition rate; and uses appropriate means to prevent bias, measure outcomes, and analyze and report results. These studies will meet the majority of items in each domain.
  - A "**Moderate Risk of Bias**" study is susceptible to some bias but probably not enough to invalidate the results. The study may be missing information, making it difficult to assess limitations and potential problems. As the fair-quality category is broad, studies with this rating vary in their strengths and weaknesses. The results of some fair-quality studies are possibly valid, while others are probably valid. These studies will meet the majority of items in most but not all domains.
  - A "**High Risk of Bias**" rating indicates significant bias that may invalidate the results. These studies have serious errors in design, analysis, or reporting; have large amounts of missing information; or have discrepancies in reporting. The results of a poor-quality

study are at least as likely to reflect flaws in the study design as to indicate true differences between the compared interventions.

Appendix C. Study Characteristics Tables

Table C-1. Study characteristics table for KQ 1: Effectiveness and safety of antiplatelet therapy for adults with peripheral artery disease

Study	Study Details	Intervention (N) and Comparator (N)	Timing and Outcomes Reported	Quality and Limitations to Applicability
Aspirin vs. placebo or no antiplatelet				
		ASYMPTOMATIC OR HIGH-RISK PATIENTS		
Belch, 2008 POPADAD Study	RCT Multicenter UK Funding: Government, Nonprofit Population Diabetics with PAD Total N: 636 Mean Age: 60 N Female: 363 % Female: 57% Race: NR	*Intervention* ASA 100 mg daily (N=318) Concomitant therapy: Standard therapy—statins, beta blockers at discretion of investigator or clinician *Comparator* Placebo (N=318) Concomitant therapy: Standard therapy—statins, beta blockers at discretion of investigator or clinician	Timing: Median 6.7 yr <u>Composite</u> (primary) Cardiovascular mortality Nonfatal MI Stroke Major amputation (secondary) Cardiovascular mortality Fatal stroke <u>Individual</u> Total mortality Cardiovascular mortality Nonfatal MI Stroke Adverse drug reactions Major amputation TIA CLI Intermittent claudication Peripheral revascularization	Good No limitations

C-1

Study	Study Details	Intervention (N) and Comparator (N)	Timing and Outcomes Reported	Quality and Limitations to Applicability
Fowkes, 2010[2]	RCT Multicenter UK Funding: Nonprofit, Industry Population Asymptomatic PAD (low ABI) no previous CAD Total N: 3350 Mean Age: 62 N Female: 2396 % Female: 72% Race: NR	Intervention ASA 100 mg daily (N=1675) Concomitant therapy: Could include diuretic, beta-blocker, nitrate or calcium channel blocker, ACE inhibitor or ARB, or lipid-lowering agent at discretion of physician Comparator Placebo (N=1675) Concomitant therapy: Could include diuretic, beta-blocker, nitrate or calcium channel blocker, ACE inhibitor or ARB, or lipid-lowering agent at discretion of physician	Timing: 5 yr, 10 yr Composite (primary) Cardiovascular mortality Nonfatal MI Stroke Initial peripheral revascularization Coronary revascularization (secondary) Angina IC TIA Individual Total mortality Cardiovascular mortality Nonfatal MI Stroke Bleeding Adverse drug reactions Initial peripheral revascularization TIA Angina IC	Good No limitations

Study	Study Details	Intervention (N) and Comparator (N)	Timing and Outcomes Reported	Quality and Limitations to Applicability
Clopidogrel/aspirin comparisons				
Anonymous, 1996[3] CAPRIE Study	RCT Multicenter US, Canada, Europe Funding: Industry Population PAD subset of high-risk vascular population (prior MI, CVA, PAD) Total N: 6452 Mean Age: 64 N Female: 1806 % Female: 28% Race: 98% white	*Intervention* Clopidogrel 75 mg plus placebo daily (N=3223) Concomitant therapy: None specified *Comparator* ASA 325 mg daily plus placebo (N=3229) Concomitant therapy: None specified	Timing: 1 to 3 yr, Mean 1.9 yr Composite (primary) Cardiovascular mortality Nonfatal MI Stroke Individual Nonfatal MI Nonfatal stroke Fatal stroke Fatal MI Other vascular death	Good No limitations
Cacoub, 2009[4] Bhatt, 2007[5] Bhatt, 2006[6] Berger, 2010[7] CHARISMA Study	RCT Multicenter Location: NR Funding: Industry Population PAD subset of high-risk vascular population (prior MI, CVA, PAD) Total N: 3096 (2838 symptomatic, 258 asymptomatic) Median Age: 66 yr N Female: 930 % Female: 30% Race: 86% White, 9% Hispanic, 3% Black, 1% Asian, and 1% Other	*Intervention* Clopidogrel 75 mg plus ASA 75-162 mg daily (N=1575) Concomitant therapy: Could include diuretic, beta-blocker, nitrate or calcium channel blocker, ACE inhibitor or ARB, or lipid-lowering agent at discretion of physician *Comparator* Placebo plus ASA 75-162 mg daily (N=1551) Concomitant therapy: Could include diuretic, beta-blocker, nitrate or calcium channel blocker, ACE inhibitor or ARB, or lipid-lowering agent at discretion of physician	Timing: 28 mo Composite (primary) Cardiovascular mortality Nonfatal MI Stroke Individual Total mortality Cardiovascular mortality Stroke Hospitalization Bleeding MI (fatal + nonfatal) Ischemic stroke	Good No limitations

Study	Study Details	Intervention (N) and Comparator (N)	Timing and Outcomes Reported	Quality and Limitations to Applicability
PATIENTS WITH INTERMITTENT CLAUDICATION				
Aspirin vs. placebo or no antiplatelet				
Catalano, 2007[8] CLIPS Study	RCT Multicenter Europe Funding: Industry Population Asymptomatic PAD or IC Total N: 181 (Claudication= 142 Asymptomatic=39) Mean Age: 64 to 66 N Female: 40 % Female: 22% Race: NR	*Intervention* ASA 100 mg daily (N=91) Concomitant therapy: Antioxidants (600 mg vitamin E, 250 mg vitamin C and 20 mg beta-carotene) daily *Comparator* Placebo (N=90) Concomitant therapy: Antioxidants (600 mg vitamin E, 250 mg vitamin C and 20 mg beta-carotene) daily	Timing: 2 yr <u>Composite</u> Stroke MI Vascular death <u>Individual</u> Cardiovascular mortality Nonfatal MI Stroke Bleeding Nonvascular death Hemorrhagic stroke Ischemic stroke	Fair No limitations
Clopidogrel/aspirin comparisons				
Cassar, 2005[9]	RCT Single center UK Funding: Nonprofit, Industry Population IC for endovascular procedure Total N: 132 Mean Age: 65 to 66 N Female: 30 % Female: 23% Race: NR	*Intervention* Loading dose clopidogrel 300 mg then clopidogrel 75 mg plus ASA 75 mg daily (N=67) Concomitant therapy: None specified *Comparator* Loading dose of placebo then placebo plus ASA 75 mg daily (N=65) Concomitant therapy: None specified	Timing: 30 days <u>Individual</u> Adverse drug reactions	Good Study did not use a clinically relevant surrogate outcome where applicable

Study	Study Details	Intervention (N) and Comparator (N)	Timing and Outcomes Reported	Quality and Limitations to Applicability
PATIENTS WITH CRITICAL LIMB ISCHEMIA			
Aspirin vs. placebo or no antiplatelet			
Mahmood, 2003[10]	Observational Single center UK Funding: NR Population CLI for infrainguinal bypass Total N: 113 Mean Age: 72 yr N Female: NR % Female: NR Race: NR	*Intervention* ASA (N=79; 47 preoperative, 32 postoperative) Concomitant therapy: None specified *Comparator* No ASA (N=34) Concomitant therapy: None specified	Timing: 2 yr Individual Cardiovascular mortality Nonfatal MI Stroke Vessel patency	Poor Study did not report participants' baseline characteristics

Study	Study Details	Intervention (N) and Comparator (N)	Timing and Outcomes Reported	Quality and Limitations to Applicability
PATIENTS WITH IC or CLI				
Clopidogrel/aspirin comparisons				
Belch, 2010[11] CASPAR Study	RCT Multicenter Europe, Australia/NZ Funding: Industry Population IC-CLI (undergoing unilateral below the knee bypass) Total N: 851 Mean Age: 66 to 67 N Female: 207 % Female: 24% Race: NR	*Intervention* Clopidogrel 75 mg plus ASA 75-100 mg daily (N=425) Concomitant therapy High-dose UFH or LMWH was used during surgery and was permitted for use for prevention of DVT when indicated *Comparator* Placebo plus ASA 75-100 mg daily (N=426) Concomitant therapy: High-dose UFH or LMWH was used during surgery and was permitted for use for prevention of DVT when indicated	Timing: 1 yr, 2 yr Composite (primary) Total mortality Repeat revascularization Major amputation Occlusion of index bypass graft (secondary) Repeat revascularization Major amputation Occlusion of graft (secondary) Cardiovascular mortality Nonfatal MI Stroke Individual Total mortality Cardiovascular mortality Nonfatal MI Stroke Bleeding Major amputation Occlusion of index bypass graft	Good No limitations

Study	Study Details	Intervention (N) and Comparator (N)	Timing and Outcomes Reported	Quality and Limitations to Applicability
Tepe, 2012[12]	RCT Single center Europe Funding: Industry Population PAD patients with IC or CLI Total N: 80 Mean Age: 70 N Female: 38 % Female: 48% Race: NR	*Intervention* Clopidogrel 75mg plus ASA 100mg daily for 6 mo (N=40) Concomitant therapy: Clopidogrel 300mg plus ASA 500mg 6-12 h before the intervention as a bolus *Comparator* Placebo plus ASA 500mg daily for 6 mo (N=40) Concomitant therapy: Clopidogrel 300mg plus ASA 500mg 6-12 h before the intervention as a bolus	Timing: 6 mo Individual Total mortality Repeat revascularization Bleeding Vessel patency Major amputation Cardiovascular event Change in ABI Embolic event	Good No limitations
Other antiplatelet comparisons				
Horrocks, 1997[13]	RCT Multicenter UK Funding: NR Population IC or CLI after femoral PTA Total N: 38 Mean Age: 63 to 66 N Female: 12 % Female: 32% Race: NR	*Intervention* ASA 300 mg daily (N=13) Iloprost 2.0 ng/kg/min x 3 days, then ASA 300 mg daily (N=11) Concomitant therapy: None specified *Comparator* No antiplatelet (N=14) Concomitant therapy: None specified	Timing: 3 mo, 1 yr Individual Restenosis Reocclusion	Fair Study interventions (active arm) were not similar to interventions used in routine clinical practice Duration of participant followup was inadequate

C-7

Study	Study Details	Intervention (N) and Comparator (N)	Timing and Outcomes Reported	Quality and Limitations to Applicability
Minar, 1995[14]	RCT Single center Europe Funding: NR Population IC or CLI for femoropopliteal PTA Total N: 216 Median Age: 66 N Female: 95 % Female: 44% Race: NR	Intervention ASA 1000 mg daily (N=107) Concomitant therapy: 500 mg aspirin IV at least 1 hr before the planned procedure, and the same dosage was applied for 2 additional days. During the intervention 5000 IU heparin was administered and the patients also received heparin intravenously for 3 days starting at a dosage of 1000 IU/h and was adjusted twice daily according to the thrombin time (prolongation to at least three times the normal value). Comparator ASA 100 mg daily (N=109) Concomitant therapy: 500 mg aspirin IV at least 1 hr before the planned procedure, and the same dosage was applied for 2 additional days. During the intervention 5000 IU heparin was administered and the patients also received heparin intravenously for 3 days starting at a dosage of 1000 IU/h and was adjusted twice daily according to the thrombin time (prolongation to at least three times the normal value).	Timing: 24 mo <u>Individual</u> Total mortality Vessel patency	Fair Study interventions (active arm) were not similar to interventions used in routine clinical practice Study was conducted only at a single site

Abbreviations: ABI=ankle brachial index; ASA=acetylsalicylic acid (aspirin); CI=confidence interval; CLI=critical limb ischemia; CV=cardiovascular; DVT=deep vein thrombosis; GI=gastrointestinal; HR=hazard ratio; IC=intermittent claudication; IU=international units; LMWH=low molecular weight heparin; MI=myocardial infarction; mo=month/months; N=number of patients; NR=not reported; NS=not significant; PAD=peripheral artery disease; PTA=percutaneous transluminal angiography; RCT=randomized controlled trial; SD=standard deviation; TIA=transient ischemic attack; UFH=unfractionated heparin; wk=week/weeks; yr=year/years

Table C-2. Study characteristics table for KQ 2: Effectiveness and safety of exercise, medications, and endovascular and surgical revascularization for intermittent claudication

Study	Study Details	Intervention (N) and Comparator (N)	Timing and Outcomes Reported	Quality and Limitations to Applicability
Medical therapy vs. usual care				
Beebe, 1999[15]	RCT Multicenter US Funding: industry <u>Population</u> PAD patients with IC Total N: 516 Mean Age: 64 to 65 N Female: 124 % Female: 24% Race: 9.1% African American, 0.4% Asian, 88.6% White, 1.9% Other	*Intervention* Cilostazol 100 mg twice daily (N=175) 50 mg twice daily (N=171) Concomitant therapy: None specified *Comparator* Placebo (N=170) Concomitant therapy: None specified	Timing: 6 mo <u>Individual</u> Mortality MI Stroke QOL Amputation MWD PFWD	Good No limitations
Belcaro, 2002[16]	RCT Multicenter Europe Funding: NR <u>Population</u> PAD patients with IC Total N: 60 Mean Age: 55 to 56 N Female: 29 % Female: 54.7% Race: NR	*Intervention* Pentoxifylline 400 mg four times daily (N=27) Concomitant therapy: Antiplatelet treatment 300 mg daily *Comparator* Placebo (N=26) Concomitant therapy: Antiplatelet treatment 300 mg daily	Timing: 2 wk, 3 mo, 6 mo <u>Individual</u> MWD	Fair Study interventions (active arm) were not similar to interventions used in routine clinical practice Study's cointerventions did not adequately reflect routine clinical practice (e.g., use of medical therapy for secondary prevention – antiplatelet agents, HTN/DM/lipid control) Study conducted solely outside the US

C-9

Study	Study Details	Intervention (N) and Comparator (N)	Timing and Outcomes Reported	Quality and Limitations to Applicability
Dawson, 1998[17]	RCT Multicenter US Funding: NR Population PAD patients with IC Total N: 81 Mean Age: 66 to 67 N Female: 19 % Female: 23.4% Race: 1% African American, 99% White	Intervention Cilostazol 100 mg twice daily (N=54) Concomitant therapy: Could include ACE inhibitors, beta-blockers, or calcium channel blockers Comparator Placebo (N=27) Concomitant therapy: Could include ACE inhibitors, beta-blockers, or calcium channel blockers	Timing: 2 wk, 4 wk, 8 wk, 12 wk Individual ACD ICD Adverse events	Good No limitations
Dawson, 2000[18]	RCT Multicenter US Funding: Otsuka America Pharmaceuticals Population PAD patients with IC Total N: 698 Mean Age: 66 N Female: 169 % Female: 24.2% Race: 89% White, 9% Black, 2% Hispanic	Intervention Cilostazol 100 mg twice daily (N=227), pentoxifylline 400 mg three times daily (232 patients) Concomitant therapy: None specified Comparator Placebo (N=239) Concomitant therapy: None specified	Timing: 4 wk, 8 wk, 12 wk, 16 wk, 24 wk Individual MWD PFWD Change in ABI	Fair No limitations

Study	Study Details	Intervention (N) and Comparator (N)	Timing and Outcomes Reported	Quality and Limitations to Applicability
De Sanctis, 2002[19,20] Cesarone, 2002[21]	RCT Multicenter Europe Funding: independent Population PAD patients with IC Total N: 194 Mean Age: 62 to 63 N Female: 51 % Female: 37.8% Race: NR	Intervention Pentoxifylline 600 mg three times daily (N=75) Concomitant therapy: None specified Comparator Placebo (N=60) Concomitant therapy: None specified	Timing: 6 mo, 12 mo Individual Total Walking Distance	Fair Study did not report participants' comorbid conditions Participant diagnosis and identification for eligibility screening before random allocation was not appropriate/Cohort selection was not appropriate Study interventions (active arm) were not similar to interventions used in routine clinical practice Study conducted solely outside the US
Hiatt, 2008[22] Stone, 2008[23] CASTLE Study	RCT Multicenter US Funding: industry Population PAD patients with IC Total N: 1435 Mean Age: 66 N Female: 495 % Female: 34% Race: 79% White, 4% Hispanic, 16% African American, 1% Other	Intervention Cilostazol 100 mg twice daily (N=717) Concomitant therapy: Could include aspirin, clopidogrel, statin or warfarin Comparator Placebo (N=718) Concomitant therapy: Could include aspirin, clopidogrel, statin or warfarin	Timing: 36 mo Composite (primary) Stroke TIA Carotid revascularization Individual Mortality Stroke Adverse events	Good No limitations

Study	Study Details	Intervention (N) and Comparator (N)	Timing and Outcomes Reported	Quality and Limitations to Applicability
Hobbs, 2007[24] INEXACT Study	RCT Single center UK Funding: NR Population PAD patients with IC Total N: 38 Median Age: 67 N Female: 7 % Female: 20.6% Race: NR	*Intervention* Cilostazol 100 mg twice daily + best medical therapy (N=9) Best medical therapy: Smoking cessation via repeated advice and/or nicotine replacement/bupropion/smoking cessation classes; statin therapy for 25% reduction in cholesterol; aspirin 75 mg daily or clopidogrel 75 mg daily if intolerant of aspirin; treat/screen for diabetes; blood pressure <140/85; ACE-I considered for all patients; and written advice regarding exercise *Comparator* Best medical therapy (N=9) Best medical therapy: Smoking cessation via repeated advice and/or nicotine replacement/bupropion/smoking cessation classes; statin therapy for 25% reduction in cholesterol; aspirin 75 mg daily or clopidogrel 75 mg daily if intolerant of aspirin; treat/screen for diabetes; blood pressure <140/85; ACE-I considered for all patients; and written advice regarding exercise	Timing: 3 mo, 6 mo <u>Individual</u> Adverse drug reaction Change in ABI ACD ICD	Good Study conducted solely outside the US Study was conducted only at a single site
Money, 1998[25]	RCT Multicenter US Funding: NR Population PAD patients with IC Total N: 239 Mean Age: 65 N Female: 59 % Female: 24.7% Race: 9% African American, 0.4% Asian, 87% White, 3.6% Other	*Intervention* Cilostazol 100 mg twice daily (N=119) Concomitant therapy: None specified *Comparator* Placebo (N=120) Concomitant therapy: None specified	Timing: 8 wk, 12 wk, 16 wk <u>Individual</u> Mortality QOL Adverse events ACD	Fair Study did not report participants' comorbid conditions

Study	Study Details	Intervention (N) and Comparator (N)	Timing and Outcomes Reported	Quality and Limitations to Applicability
Soga, 2009[26]	RCT Multicenter Asia Funding: NR Population PAD patients with IC Total N: 78 Mean Age: 71 N Female: 13 % Female: 16.7% Race: NR	*Intervention* Cilostazol 100 mg twice daily (N=39) Concomitant therapy: Percutaneous transluminal angioplasty ± stent ASA 81-100 mg daily ± ticlopidine 200 mg daily (in some stent patients) Also could include statin, beta-blocker, ACE inhibitor or ARB *Comparator* Placebo (N=39) Concomitant therapy: Percutaneous transluminal angioplasty ± stent ASA 81-100 mg daily ± ticlopidine 200 mg daily (in some stent patients) Also could include statin, beta-blocker, ACE inhibitor or ARB	Timing: 24 mo Composite (secondary) Total mortality Cardiovascular mortality Nonfatal MI Stroke Repeat revascularization Major amputation Minor amputation Individual Mortality MI Stroke Repeat revascularization Bleeding Amputation	Good No limitations
Strandness, 2002[27]	RCT Multicenter US Funding: industry Population PAD patients with IC Total N: 394 Mean Age: 63 to 64 N Female: 94 % Female: 24% Race: 86.3% White, 11.2% Black, 1.5% Hispanic, .5% Asian, .5% Other	*Intervention* Cilostazol 100 mg twice daily (N=133) 50 mg twice daily (N=132) Concomitant therapy: None specified *Comparator* Placebo (N=129) Concomitant therapy: None specified	Timing: 6 mo Composite (secondary) Total mortality Cardiovascular mortality Individual MWD Adverse drug reactions	Fair No limitations

Study	Study Details	Intervention (N) and Comparator (N)	Timing and Outcomes Reported	Quality and Limitations to Applicability
Exercise training vs. usual care				
Crowther, 2008[28]	RCT Single center Australia Funding: NR Population PAD patients with IC Total N: 21 Mean Age: 67 to 71 N Female: 11 % Female: 52% Race: NR	*Intervention* Supervised Exercise (N=10) Treadmill walking group: 3 times per wk for 12 mo Concomitant therapy: Could include beta-blocker *Comparator* Control (N=11) No specific instructions given Concomitant therapy: Could include beta-blocker	Timing: 12 mo Individual PFWT	Fair Study selectively recruited participants who demonstrated a history of favorable or unfavorable response to drug or other interventions for the condition Study conducted solely outside the US Study was conducted only at a single site
Gardner, 2002[29]	RCT Multicenter US Funding: Government Population PAD patients with IC Total N: 61 Mean Age: 71 ro 72 N Female: NR % Female: NR Race: NR	*Intervention* Exercise training (N=28) Supervised treadmill walking 3 times per wk Concomitant therapy: None specified *Comparator* Usual care (N=24) Concomitant therapy: None specified	Timing: 6 mo, 18 mo Individual Total mortality QOL - Walking impairment questionnaire Major amputation Exercise-related harms Mean or 6-minute walking time Absolute claudication distance QOL - SF36 Initial Claudication Distance	Fair No limitations

C-14

Study	Study Details	Intervention (N) and Comparator (N)	Timing and Outcomes Reported	Quality and Limitations to Applicability
Gardner, 2011[30]	RCT Single center US Funding: Government Population PAD patients with IC Total N: 119 Mean Age: 65 to 66 N Female: 62 % Female: 52% Race: 57% White	*Intervention* Supervised exercise (N=40); Home exercise (N=40) Supervised treadmill walking group: 3 times per wk at specified pace for specified duration of time for 12 wk Home treadmill walking group: 3 times per wk at self-selected pace for specified duration of time for 12 wk Concomitant therapy: None specified *Comparator* Control (N=39) Encouraged to walk more on their own but did not receive specific recommendations about an exercise program during the study. Concomitant therapy: None specified	Timing: 12 wk Individual MI Stroke QOL PWT COT	Good Study was conducted only at a single site
Gelin, 2001[31] Taft, 2001[32]	RCT Single center Europe Funding: Government Population PAD patients with IC Total N: 264 Mean Age: 66 to 67 N Female: 90 % Female: 34.1% Race: NR	*Intervention* Supervised exercise (N=88) Treadmill walking training 3 times per wk for 6 mo, then 2 times per wk Concomitant therapy: None specified *Comparator* Control (N=89) Received no other specific advice or treatment apart from the general advice given to the two treatment groups Concomitant therapy: None specified	Timing: 12 mo Individual Mortality QOL Vessel patency Amputation MWD	Fair Study conducted solely outside the US Study was conducted only at a single site

Study	Study Details	Intervention (N) and Comparator (N)	Timing and Outcomes Reported	Quality and Limitations to Applicability
Gibellini, 2000[33]	RCT Study centers: NR Location: NR Funding: NR Population PAD patients with IC Total N: 40 Mean Age: 67 N Female: 4 % Female: 10% Race: NR	Intervention Supervised exercise (N=20) Treadmill walking training 5 times per wk for 4 wk Concomitant therapy: ASA 325 mg daily Comparator Control (N=20) No specific instructions given Concomitant therapy: ASA 325 mg daily	Timing: 1 mo, 6 mo Individual ACD ICD	Fair Participant diagnosis and identification for eligibility screening before random allocation was not appropriate/Cohort selection was not appropriate Study eligibility criteria were poorly described or not appropriate Study conducted solely outside the US Study was conducted only at a single site
Hobbs, 2006[34] EXACT Study	RCT Multicenter UK Funding: Government Population PAD patients with IC Total N: 23 Median Age: 67 N Female: 7 % Female: 30.4% Race: NR	Intervention Supervised Exercise + best medical therapy(N=7) Circuit of moderate intensity exercises 2 times per wk for 12 wk Concomitant therapy: Could include antiplatelet agents, statin, ACE inhibitor or other antihypertensive agent Comparator Best medical therapy (N=7) Best medical therapy: Not defined but could include antiplatelet agents, statin, ACE inhibitor or other antihypertensive agent	Timing: 3 mo, 6 mo Individual Adverse drug reaction ACD ICD	Fair Study interventions (active arm) were not similar to interventions used in routine clinical practice Study conducted solely outside the US Study was conducted only at a single site

Study	Study Details	Intervention (N) and Comparator (N)	Timing and Outcomes Reported	Quality and Limitations to Applicability
Hobbs, 2007[24] INEXACT Study	RCT Single center UK Funding: NR Population PAD patients with IC Total N: 38 Median Age: 67 N Female: 7 % Female: 30.4% Race: NR	*Intervention* Supervised exercise + best medical therapy (N=9) Circuit of moderate intensity exercises 2 times per wk for 12 wk Best medical therapy: Smoking cessation via repeated advice and/or nicotine replacement / bupropion/smoking cessation classes; statin therapy for 25% reduction in cholesterol; aspirin 75 mg daily or clopidogrel 75 mg daily if intolerant of aspirin; treatment/screen for diabetes; blood pressure < 140/85; ACE-I considered for all patients; and written advice regarding exercise *Comparator* Best medical therapy (N=9) Best medical therapy: Smoking cessation via repeated advice and/or nicotine replacement / bupropion/smoking cessation classes; statin therapy for 25% reduction in cholesterol; aspirin 75 mg daily or clopidogrel 75 mg daily if intolerant of aspirin; treatment/screen for diabetes; blood pressure <140/85; ACE-I considered for all patients; and written advice regarding exercise	Timing: 3 mo, 6 mo *Individual* Adverse drug reaction Change in ABI ACD ICD	Good Study conducted solely outside the US Study was conducted only at a single site

Study	Study Details	Intervention (N) and Comparator (N)	Timing and Outcomes Reported	Quality and Limitations to Applicability
Lee, 2007[35]	Observational Single center UK Funding: NR *Population* PAD patients with IC Total N: 70 Median Age: 67 to 69 N Female: 22 % Female: 31.4% Race: NR	*Intervention* Supervised exercise (N=33) Circuit of exercises 3 times per wk for 12 wk Concomitant therapy: Prescribed an antiplatelet, received smoking cessation advice and support (including nicotine replacement therapy), and risk factor modification (appropriate management of hypertension, hypercholesterolemia and diabetes. All patients also received an advice leaflet regarding exercise. *Comparator* Conservative medical therapy (N=37) Prescribed an antiplatelet, received smoking cessation advice and support (including nicotine replacement therapy), and risk factor modification (appropriate management of hypertension, hypercholesterolemia and diabetes. All patients also received an advice leaflet regarding exercise.	Timing: 6 mo <u>Individual</u> MWD ICD QOL	Poor Study did not report participants' baseline characteristics Study did not report participants' comorbid conditions Study conducted solely outside the US Study was conducted only at a single site
Murphy, 2012[36] CLEVER Study	RCT Multicenter US, Canada Funding: Government *Population* PAD patients with IC Total N: 111 Mean Age: 62 to 65 N Female: 42 % Female: 37.8% Race: NR	*Intervention* Supervised Exercise + optimal medical therapy (N=43) Exercises 3 times per wk for 26 wk Concomitant therapy: Could include ASA, thienopyridine, and statin *Comparator* Optimal medical therapy (N=22) Optimal medical therapy: Cilostazol 10 0 mg twice daily; advice about home exercise and diet Concomitant therapy: Could include ASA, thienopyridine, and statin	Timing: 30 days, 6 mo <u>Individual</u> PWT COT QOL Change in ABI Safety	Good Study selectively recruited participants who demonstrated a history of favorable or unfavorable response to drug or other interventions for the condition

C-18

Study	Study Details	Intervention (N) and Comparator (N)	Timing and Outcomes Reported	Quality and Limitations to Applicability
Sugimoto, 2010[37]	Observational Single center Asia Funding: NR Population PAD patients with IC Total N: 100 Mean Age: 67 N Female: 5 % Female: 5% Race: NR	*Intervention* Supervised exercise + medical therapy (N=61) Treadmill walking 2 times per day for 3 wk plus medical therapy which could include the following medications or combinations: Cilostazol alone or with beraprost, warfarin, or aspirin; beraprost alone or with aspirin or ticlopidine; limaprost alone or with aspirin + ticlopidine; sarpogrelate alone or with ethyl icosapentate or aspirin; aspirin alone or with ticlopidine; warfarin alone *Comparator* Medical therapy (N=39) Could include the following medications or combinations: Cilostazol alone or with beraprost, warfarin, or aspirin; beraprost alone or with aspirin or ticlopidine; limaprost alone or with aspirin + ticlopidine; sarpogrelate alone or with ethyl icosapentate or aspirin; aspirin alone or with ticlopidine; warfarin alone	Timing: 6 mo <u>Individual</u> ACD Change in ABI	Poor Study selectively recruited participants who demonstrated a history of favorable or unfavorable response to drug or other interventions for the condition Comparator(s) not well described Study conducted solely outside the US Study was conducted only at a single site

Study	Study Details	Intervention (N) and Comparator (N)	Timing and Outcomes Reported	Quality and Limitations to Applicability
Treat-Jacobson, 2009[38] Bronas, 2011[39]	RCT Single center US Funding: American Heart Association Population PAD patients with IC Total N: 41 Mean Age: 68 N Female: 12 % Female: 29% Race: 85% White	*Intervention* Supervised exercise (N=20) Treadmill walking group: 3 times per wk for 12 wk Arm-ergometry cycle training group: 3 times per wk for 12 wk Concomitant therapy: Could be on cilostazol, antiplatelet agent, lipid-lowering agent, beta-blocker or ACE inhibitor at discretion of physician *Comparator* Control (N=8) Instructed to follow care given by their physician, received written instructions on how to exercise independently if they chose to do so and were asked to keep a daily record of any exercise Concomitant therapy: Could be on cilostazol, antiplatelet agent, lipid-lowering agent, beta-blocker or ACE inhibitor at discretion of physician	Timing: 12 wk, 24 wk Individual MWD PFWD	Good No limitations
Tsai, 2002[40]	RCT Multicenter Asia Funding: NR Population PAD patients with IC Total N: 64 Mean Age: 76 N Female: 9 % Female: 17% Race: NR	*Intervention* Supervised exercise (N=27) Treadmill walking 3 times per wk for 12 wk Concomitant therapy: None specified *Comparator* Control (N=26) No specific instructions noted Concomitant therapy: None specified	Timing: 3 mo Individual PWT COT QOL	Poor Study did not report participants' comorbid conditions Study conducted solely outside the US Study was conducted only at a single site

C-20

Study	Study Details	Intervention (N) and Comparator (N)	Timing and Outcomes Reported	Quality and Limitations to Applicability
Endovascular intervention vs. usual care				
Feinglass, 2000[41]	Observational Multicenter US Funding: Government Population PAD patients with IC Total N: 526 Mean Age: 69 N Female: 105 % Female: 20% Race: 16% African American	*Intervention* Endovascular revascularization (N=44) Angioplasty Concomitant therapy: Could include ASA, statin, pentoxifylline, warfarin, diuretics, ACE inhibitors, vasodilators, nitrates, calcium channel blockers and beta-blockers *Comparator* Medical therapy (N=277) Not defined Concomitant therapy: Could include ASA, statin, pentoxifylline, warfarin, diuretics, ACE inhibitors, vasodilators, nitrates, calcium channel blockers and beta-blockers	Timing: 18 mo Individual Cardiovascular mortality Stroke QOL Major amputation Change in ABI	Fair Study exclusion criteria were poorly described or not appropriate Study selectively recruited participants who demonstrated a history of favorable or unfavorable response to drug or other interventions for the condition Diagnostic or therapeutic advances have been made in routine practice since the study was conducted Comparator(s) not well described
Gelin, 2001[31] Taft, 2001[32]	RCT Single center Europe Funding: Government Population PAD patients with IC Total N: 264 Mean Age: 66 to 67 N Female: 90 % Female: 34.1% Race: NR	*Intervention* Endovascular revascularization (N=87) No description of endovascular procedures Concomitant therapy: Not specified *Comparator* Control (N=89) No specific information given Concomitant therapy: Not specified	Timing: 12 mo Individual Mortality QOL Vessel patency Amputation MWD	Fair Study conducted solely outside the US Study was conducted only at a single site

C-21

Study	Study Details	Intervention (N) and Comparator (N)	Timing and Outcomes Reported	Quality and Limitations to Applicability
Giugliano, 2012[42]	Observational Single center Europe Funding: NR Population PAD patients with IC Total N: 479 Mean Age: 64 to 66 N Female: 89 % Female: 18.6% Race: NR	Intervention Endovascular revascularization (N=264) Percutaneous transluminal angioplasty Concomitant therapy: None specified Comparator Conservative medical therapy (N=215) Concomitant therapy: None specified	Timing: 21 mo (median followup) Composite (total events) Cardiovascular mortality Nonfatal MI Nonfatal stroke PTCA CABG Carotid PTA Composite (total cardiovascular mortality) Sudden death Fatal MI Fatal stroke Individual Fatal MI Nonfatal MI Fatal stroke Nonfatal stroke PTCA CABG Carotid PTA	Fair Study selectively recruited participants who demonstrated a history of favorable or unfavorable response to drug or other interventions for the condition Comparator(s) not well described Study was conducted solely outside the US Study was conducted only at a single site
Hobbs, 2006[34] EXACT Study	RCT Multicenter UK Funding: Government Population PAD patients with IC Total N: 23 Median Age: 67 N Female: 7 % Female: 30.4% Race: NR	Intervention Endovascular revascularization + best medical therapy (N=9) Percutaneous transluminal angioplasty Best medical therapy: Not defined Concomitant therapy: None specified Comparator Best medical therapy (N=7) Best medical therapy: Not defined Concomitant therapy: None specified	Timing: 6 mo Individual ACD ICD	Fair Study interventions (active arm) were not similar to interventions used in routine clinical practice Study conducted solely outside the US Study was conducted only at a single site

Study	Study Details	Intervention (N) and Comparator (N)	Timing and Outcomes Reported	Quality and Limitations to Applicability
Koivunen, 2008[43]	Observational Single center Europe Funding: Academy of Finland Population PAD patients with IC Total N: 180 Mean Age: 67 N Female: 62 % Female: 34.4% Race: NR	*Intervention* Endovascular revascularization (N=85) Percutaneous transluminal angioplasty Concomitant therapy: None specified *Comparator* Conservative treatment (N=64) Lifestyle modification and medication Concomitant therapy: None specified	Timing: 12 mo Individual QOL PFWD	Poor Comparator(s) not well described Study did not use a clinically relevant surrogate outcome where applicable Study conducted solely outside the US Study was conducted only at a single site
Murphy, 2012[36] CLEVER Study	RCT Multicenter US, Canada Funding: Government Population PAD patients with IC Total N: 111 Mean Age: 62 to 65 N Female: 42 % Female: 37.8% Race: NR	*Intervention* Endovascular revascularization + optimal medical therapy (N=46) Revascularization with stent (not otherwise specified) Optimal medical therapy: Cilostazol 100 mg bid; advice about home exercise and diet Concomitant therapy: Could include ASA, thienopyridine, and statin *Comparator* Optimal medical therapy (N=22) Optimal medical therapy: Cilostazol 100 mg twice daily; advice about home exercise and diet Concomitant therapy: Could include ASA, thienopyridine, and statin	Timing: 30 days, 6 mo Individual PWT COT QOL Change in ABI Safety	Good Study selectively recruited participants who demonstrated a history of favorable or unfavorable response to drug or other interventions for the condition

Study	Study Details	Intervention (N) and Comparator (N)	Timing and Outcomes Reported	Quality and Limitations to Applicability
Nylaende, 2007[44] OBACT Study	RCT Single center Europe Funding: industry Population PAD patients with IC Total N: 56 Mean Age: 68 to 69 N Female: 25 % Female: 44.6% Race: NR	Intervention Endovascular revascularization + optimal medical therapy (N=28) Percutaneous transluminal angioplasty ± stent Optimal medical therapy: Nicotine plaster and bupropion prescribed to smokers if not contraindicated; instructions for a home-based exercise training program; nutritional advice given; ASA 160 mg daily (or Plavix in patients with history of peptic ulcer); statins for patients with hypercholesterolemia; individualized hypertension treatment Comparator Optimal medical therapy (N=28) Optimal medical therapy: Nicotine plaster and bupropion prescribed to smokers if not contraindicated; instructions for a home-based exercise training program; nutritional advice given; ASA 160 mg daily (or Plavix in patients with history of peptic ulcer); statins for patients with hypercholesterolemia; individualized hypertension treatment	Timing: 3 mo, 12 mo, 24 mo Individual Mortality QOL MWD PFWD	Good Study conducted solely outside the US Study was conducted only at a single site

C-24

Study	Study Details	Intervention (N) and Comparator (N)	Timing and Outcomes Reported	Quality and Limitations to Applicability
Pell, 1997[45]	Observational Multicenter Europe Funding: Government Population PAD patients with IC Total N: 201 Mean Age: 67 N Female: 78 % Female: 38.8% Race: NR	Intervention Endovascular revascularization (N=19) Percutaneous transluminal angioplasty Concomitant therapy: None specified Comparator Conservative treatment (N=119) No description provided Concomitant therapy: None specified	Timing: 6 mo Individual Mortality QOL	Fair Study did not report participants' baseline characteristics Study did not report participants' comorbid conditions Study exclusion criteria were poorly described or not appropriate Comparator(s) not well described Study conducted solely outside the US
Whyman, 1997[46] Whyman, 1996[47]	RCT Single center UK Funding: Government Population PAD patients with IC Total N: 62 Mean Age: 61 to 63 N Female: 11 % Female: 17.7% Race: NR	Intervention Endovascular revascularization + conventional medical therapy (N=30) Percutaneous transluminal angioplasty Conventional medical therapy: Low dose aspirin plus advice on smoking and exercise Comparator conventional medical therapy (N=32) Conventional medical therapy: Low dose aspirin plus advice on smoking and exercise	Timing: 6 mo, 24 mo Individual MWD ICD Change in ABI	Fair Study conducted solely outside the US Study was conducted only at a single site

C-25

Study	Study Details	Intervention (N) and Comparator (N)	Timing and Outcomes Reported	Quality and Limitations to Applicability
Surgical revascularization vs. usual care				
Mori, 2002[48]	Observational Single center Asia Funding: NR <u>Population</u> PAD patients with IC Total N: 427 Mean Age: 64 to 66 N Female: 54 % Female: 13% Race: NR	*Intervention* Surgical Revascularization (N=259) Surgical bypass, percutaneous transluminal angioplasty or stent Concomitant therapy: None specified *Comparator* Usual Care (N=168) Concomitant therapy: None specified	Timing: 3 yr, 5 yr <u>Individual</u> Total mortality Vessel patency Symptom improvement	Low Study eligibility/exclusion criteria were poorly described or not appropriate Study's cointerventions did not adequately reflect routine clinical practice Diagnostic or therapeutic advances have been made in routine practice since the study was conducted Comparator(s) not well described Study conducted solely outside the US Study was conducted only at a single site

Study	Study Details	Intervention (N) and Comparator (N)	Timing and Outcomes Reported	Quality and Limitations to Applicability
Endovascular intervention vs. exercise training				
Gelin, 2001[31] Taft, 2001[32]	RCT Single center Europe Funding: Government Population PAD patients with IC Total N: 264 Mean Age: 66 to 67 N Female: 90 % Female: 34.1% Race: NR	*Intervention* Endovascular revascularization (N=87) A variety of procedures were performed. Concomitant therapy: None specified *Comparator* Supervised exercise (N=88) Treadmill walking training 3 times per wk for 6 mo Concomitant therapy: None specified	Timing: 12 mo Individual Mortality QOL Vessel patency Amputation MWD	Fair Study conducted solely outside the US Study was conducted only at a single site
Greenhalgh, 2008[49] MIMIC Study	RCT Multicenter UK Funding: Government Population PAD patients with IC; 93 patients with femoropopliteal disease, 34 patients with aortoiliac disease Total N: 127 Mean Age: 63 to 69 N Female: 46 % Female: 36.2% Race: NR	*Intervention* Endovascular revascularization (N=67) Percutaneous transluminal angioplasty ± stent Concomitant therapy: Counseling regarding smoking cessation and nicotine replacement therapy was prescribed where necessary. Optimal medical management of hypertension, hyperlipidemia, diabetes, and medication management including antiplatelet therapy was coordinated through the patient's primary physician. *Comparator* Supervised exercise (N=60) Walking circuit interspersed with seven lower limb training stations at least 1 times per wk for 6 mo. Concomitant therapy: Counseling regarding smoking cessation and nicotine replacement therapy was prescribed where necessary. Optimal medical management of hypertension, hyperlipidemia, diabetes, and medication management including antiplatelet therapy was coordinated through the patient's primary physician.	Timing: 6 mo, 12 mo, 24 mo Individual Mortality MI Stroke Repeat revascularization QOL MWD ICD	Fair No limitations

Study	Study Details	Intervention (N) and Comparator (N)	Timing and Outcomes Reported	Quality and Limitations to Applicability
Hobbs, 2006[34] EXACT Study	RCT Multicenter UK Funding: Government *Population* PAD patients with IC Total N: 23 Median Age: 67 N Female: 7 % Female: 30.4% Race: NR	*Intervention* Supervised Exercise + best medical therapy (N=7) Circuit of moderate intensity exercises 2 times per wk for 12 wk Best medical therapy: Could include antiplatelet agents, statin, ACE inhibitor or other antihypertensive agent *Comparator* Endovascular revascularization + best medical therapy (N=9) Percutaneous transluminal angioplasty Best medical therapy: Could include antiplatelet agents, statin, ACE inhibitor or other antihypertensive agent	Timing: 6 mo *Individual* ACD ICD	Fair Study interventions (active arm) were not similar to interventions used in routine clinical practice Study conducted solely outside the US Study was conducted only at a single site
Kruidenier, 2011[50]	RCT Single center Europe Funding: NR *Population* PAD patients with IC Total N: 70 Mean Age: 62 N Female: 27 % Female: 38.6% Race: NR	*Intervention* Endovascular revascularization (N=35) Consisted of iliac angioplasty with selective stent placement for iliac stenoses, angioplasty with primary stent placement for superficial femoral artery stenoses, or recanalization with primary stent placement for iliac and femoral occlusions Concomitant therapy: None specified *Comparator* Endovascular revascularization + supervised exercise (N=35) Endovascular intervention as per intervention plus a nonspecified exercise program 2 times per wk for 6 mo Concomitant therapy: None specified	Timing: within 3 wk of procedure, 3 mo, 6 mo *Individual* ACD QOL Change in ABI Vessel patency Repeat revascularization	Good Study conducted solely outside the US Study was conducted only at a single site

C-28

Study	Study Details	Intervention (N) and Comparator (N)	Timing and Outcomes Reported	Quality and Limitations to Applicability
Mazari, 2012[51] Mazari, 2010[52]	RCT Single center UK Funding: European Society of Vascular Surgery Population PAD patients with IC Total N: 178 Median Age: 70 N Female: 71 % Female: 39.9% Race: NR	Intervention Endovascular revascularization (N=60), Endovascular revascularization + supervised exercise (N=58) Endovascular therapy: Percutaneous transluminal angioplasty Supervised exercise therapy: Circuit of exercises 3 times per wk for 12 wk Concomitant therapy: All patients were prescribed antiplatelet therapy (aspirin and/or clopidogrel), received smoking cessation advice and support (including nicotine replacement therapy and NHS smoking cessation program), and risk factor modification (target oriented management of hypertension, hypercholesterolemia, and diabetes. All patients also received an advice leaflet regarding exercise. Comparator Supervised exercise (N=60) Supervised exercise therapy: Circuit of exercises 3 times per wk for 12 wk Concomitant therapy: All patients were prescribed antiplatelet therapy (aspirin and/or clopidogrel), received smoking cessation advice and support (including nicotine replacement therapy and NHS smoking cessation program), and risk factor modification (target oriented management of hypertension, hypercholesterolemia, and diabetes. All patients also received an advice leaflet regarding exercise.	Timing: 3 mo, 6 mo, 12 mo Individual Repeat revascularization Periprocedural complications QOL Vessel patency MWD ICD	Good Comparator(s) not well described Study conducted solely outside the US Study was conducted only at a single site

C-29

Study	Study Details	Intervention (N) and Comparator (N)	Timing and Outcomes Reported	Quality and Limitations to Applicability
Murphy, 2012[36] CLEVER Study	RCT Multicenter US, Canada Funding: Government Population PAD patients with IC Total N:111 Mean Age: 62 to 65 N Female: 42 % Female: 37.8% Race: NR	Intervention Supervised exercise + optimal medical therapy (N=43) Exercises 3 times per wk for 26 wk Optimal medical therapy: Cilostazol 100 mg bid; advice about home exercise and diet Concomitant therapy: Could include ASA, thienopyridine, and statin Comparator Endovascular revascularization + optimal medical therapy (N=46) Revascularization with stent (not otherwise specified) Optimal medical therapy: Cilostazol 100 mg bid; advice about home exercise and diet Concomitant therapy: Could include ASA, thienopyridine, and statin	Timing: 30 days, 6 mo Individual PWT COT QOL Change in ABI Safety	Good Study selectively recruited participants who demonstrated a history of favorable or unfavorable response to drug or other interventions for the condition

Study	Study Details	Intervention (N) and Comparator (N)	Timing and Outcomes Reported	Quality and Limitations to Applicability
Nordanstig, 2011[53]	RCT Multicenter Europe Funding: Government Population PAD patients with IC Total N: 201 Mean Age: 68 N Female: 74 % Female: 37% Race: NR	*Intervention* Revascularization (surgical or endovascular) + optimal medical therapy (N=100) Revascularization: In general, aorto-iliac TASC A and B lesions were treated endovascularly and TASC C and D lesions with surgery. Femoropopliteal TASC A lesions were offered angioplasty, whereas TASC BeD lesions usually were treated surgically. For lesions in the common femoral artery, endarterectomy with or without patch angioplasty was used. Optimal medical therapy: ASA 75 mg daily (or ticlopidine if contraindication to aspirin). Smokers were offered participation in a smoking cessation support programme and received verbal and written information with smoking cessation advice. Hypertension, diabetes and hyperlipidemia were managed according to national guidelines. Verbal training advice and a written training programme for IC. Instructed to walk at least 1 h/day and to walk up to their maximal claudication distance as often as possible and to perform an additional exercise programme at home several times a day. *Comparator* Optimal medical therapy (N=100) Optimal medical therapy: ASA 75 mg daily (or ticlopidine if contraindication to aspirin). Smokers were offered participation in a smoking cessation support programme and received verbal and written information with smoking cessation advice. Hypertension, diabetes and hyperlipidemia were managed according to national guidelines. Verbal training advice and a written training programme for IC. Instructed to walk at least 1 h/day and to walk up to their maximal claudication distance as often as possible and to perform an additional exercise programme at home several times a day.	Timing: 24 mo <u>Individual</u> Mortality Repeat revascularization QOL Vessel patency Major amputation MWD	Good Study conducted solely outside the US

Study	Study Details	Intervention (N) and Comparator (N)	Timing and Outcomes Reported	Quality and Limitations to Applicability
Perkins, 1996[54]	RCT Single center UK Funding: Oxford Direct Research Committee Population PAD patients with IC Total N: 56 Mean Age: 63 N Female: 6 % Female: 10.7% Race: NR	Intervention Endovascular revascularization (N=30) Percutaneous transluminal angioplasty Concomitant therapy: None specified Comparator Supervised exercise (N=26) Dynamic leg exercises 2 times per wk for 6 mo Concomitant therapy: None specified	Timing: 3 mo, 6 mo, 9 mo, 12 mo, 15 mo, 6 yr Individual Mortality Repeat revascularization MWD Periprocedural complications	Fair Study exclusion criteria were poorly described or not appropriate Diagnostic or therapeutic advances have been made in routine practice since the study was conducted Study conducted solely outside the US Study was conducted only at a single site
Spronk, 2009[55] Spronk, 2008[56]	RCT Single center Europe Funding: NR Population PAD patients with IC Total N: 151 Median Age: 65 to 66 N Female: 67 % Female: 44.4% Race: NR	Intervention Endovascular revascularization (N=75) Percutaneous transluminal angioplasty ± stent Concomitant therapy: ASA 100 mg daily Comparator Supervised exercise (N=75) Hospital based treadmill exercise 2 times per wk for 24 wk Concomitant therapy: ASA 100 mg daily	Timing: 6 mo, 12 mo Individual Mortality QOL MWD PFWD Change in ABI	Fair Study conducted solely outside the US Study was conducted only at a single site

Study	Study Details	Intervention (N) and Comparator (N)	Timing and Outcomes Reported	Quality and Limitations to Applicability
Surgical revascularization vs. exercise + medical therapy				
Drozdz, 2001[57]	Observational Single center Europe Funding: NR Population PAD patients with IC Total N: 127 Mean Age: 58 N Female: 28 % Female: 22% Race: NR	*Intervention* Exercise training (N=83) Treadmill 3 times a week for 12 weeks Concomitant therapy: 600mg pentoxifylline orally twice daily *Comparator* Surgical revascularization (N=44) Vascular bypass prostheses Concomitant therapy: None specified	Timing: 6 wk, 12 wk <u>Individual</u> MWD COT ABI	Fair Study eligibility/exclusion criteria were poorly described or not appropriate Study's cointerventions did not adequately reflect routine clinical practice Study conducted solely outside the US Study was conducted only at a single site

Study	Study Details	Intervention (N) and Comparator (N)	Timing and Outcomes Reported	Quality and Limitations to Applicability
Endovascular intervention vs. surgical revascularization				
Feinglass, 2000[41]	Observational Multicenter US Funding: Government Population PAD patients with IC Total N: 526 Mean Age: 69 N Female: 105 % Female: 20% Race: 16% African American	*Intervention* Endovascular revascularization (N=44) Percutaneous transluminal angioplasty Concomitant therapy: None specified *Comparator* Surgical revascularization (N=60) Bypass grafting ± angioplasty Concomitant therapy: None specified	Timing: 18 mo Individual Cardiovascular mortality Stroke QOL Major amputation Change in ABI	Fair Study exclusion criteria were poorly described or not appropriate Study selectively recruited participants who demonstrated a history of favorable or unfavorable response to drug or other interventions for the condition Diagnostic or therapeutic advances have been made in routine practice since the study was conducted Comparator(s) not well described
Koivunen, 2008[43]	Observational Single center Europe Funding: Academy of Finland Population PAD patients with IC Total N: 180 Mean Age: 67 to 68 N Female: 62 % Female: 34.4% Race: NR	*Intervention* Endovascular revascularization (N=85) Percutaneous transluminal angioplasty ± stent Concomitant therapy: None specified *Comparator* Surgical revascularization (N=31) Surgical bypass or endarterectomy Concomitant therapy: None specified	Timing: 12 mo Individual QOL PFWD	Poor Comparator(s) not well described Study did not use a clinically relevant surrogate outcome where applicable Study conducted solely outside the US Study was conducted only at a single site

Study	Study Details	Intervention (N) and Comparator (N)	Timing and Outcomes Reported	Quality and Limitations to Applicability
Pell, 1997[45]	Observational Multicenter Europe Funding: Government Population PAD patients with IC Total N: 201 Mean Age: 67 N Female: 78 % Female: 38.8% Race: NR	*Intervention* Endovascular revascularization (N=19) Percutaneous transluminal angioplasty Concomitant therapy: None specified *Comparator* Surgical revascularization (N=19) Arterial reconstruction Concomitant therapy: None specified	Timing: 6 mo Individual Mortality QOL	Fair Study did not report participants' baseline characteristics Study did not report participants' comorbid conditions Study exclusion criteria were poorly described or not appropriate. Comparator(s) not well described Study conducted solely outside the US

Abbreviations: ABI=ankle brachial index; ACE=angiotensin converting enzyme; ASA=acetylsalicylic acid (aspirin); CI=confidence interval; CLI=critical limb ischemia; COT=claudication onset time; CV=cardiovascular; DVT=deep vein thrombosis; GI=gastrointestinal; HR=hazard ratio; IC=intermittent claudication; ICD=initial claudication distance; IU=international units; LMWH=low molecular weight heparin; MI=myocardial infarction; mo=month/months; MWD=maximal walking distance; MWT=maximal walking time; N=number of patients; NR=not reported; NS=not significant; PAD=peripheral artery disease; PFWD=pain-free walking distance; PTA=percutaneous transluminal angiography; PUD=peptic ulcer disease; PWD=peak walking distance; PWT=peak walking time; QOL=quality of life; RCT=randomized controlled trial; SD=standard deviation; TIA=transient ischemic attack; UFH=unfractionated heparin; wk=week/weeks; yr=year/years

Table C-3. Study characteristics table for KQ 3: Effectiveness and safety of endovascular and surgical revascularization for critical limb ischemia and mixed IC-CLI population

Study	Study Details	Intervention (N) and Comparator (N)	Timing and Outcomes Reported	Quality and Limitations to Applicability
Endovascular intervention vs. usual care				
Faglia, 2012[58]	Observational Single center US Funding: NR Population PAD patients with CLI Total N: 344 Mean Age: 73 to 76 N Female: 119 % Female: 35% Race: NR	*Intervention* Endovascular intervention (N=292) Percutaneous transluminal angioplasty Concomitant therapy: Aspirin and/or other antiplatelet agents *Comparator* Usual care (N=12) Concomitant therapy: None specified	Timing: 30 days, 6 mo, 16mo, 18 mo Individual Total mortality Repeat revascularization Length of stay Major amputation Periprocedural complications Restenosis	Fair Study did not report participants' baseline characteristics Study eligibility/exclusion criteria were poorly described or not appropriate Study conducted solely outside the US
Kamiya, 2008[59]	Observational Single center Asia Funding: Government Population: IC: 3 patients CLI: 55 patients Total N: 107 Mean Age: 71 to 72 N Female: 15 % Female: 14% Race: NR	*Intervention* Endovascular revascularization (N=55) Percutaneous balloon angioplasty ± stent Concomitant therapy: Could include aspirin, cilostazol, ticlopidine, beraprost, sarpogrelate, limaprost, and warfarin *Comparator* Usual care (N=52) Not defined Concomitant therapy: Could include aspirin, cilostazol, ticlopidine, beraprost, sarpogrelate, limaprost, and warfarin	Timing: Average followup 30.6 mo Individual Mortality MI Stroke Repeat revascularization Length of stay Major amputation	Fair Use of substandard alternative therapy (e.g., standard of treatment not from current practice) Study conducted solely outside the US Study was conducted only at a single site

C-36

Study	Study Details	Intervention (N) and Comparator (N)	Timing and Outcomes Reported	Quality and Limitations to Applicability
Lawall, 2009[60]	Observational Multicenter Europe Funding: Industry Population PAD patients with CLI Total N: 155 Mean Age: 72 N Female: 58 % Female: 37% Race: NR	Intervention Endovascular intervention (N=56) Percutaneous transluminal angioplasty with locoregional lysis and stent Concomitant therapy: Could include antibiotics Comparator Usual care (N=17) Received analgesics and antibiotics	Timing: 18 mo Individual Mortality Hospitalization Major amputation Amputation-free survival	Poor Study did not report participants' severity of disease Study selectively recruited participants who demonstrated a history of favorable or unfavorable response to drug or other interventions for the condition Study interventions (active arm) were not similar to interventions used in routine clinical practice Use of substandard alternative therapy (e.g., standard of treatment not from current practice) Study centers and/or clinicians were not selected on the basis of their skill or experience Study conducted solely outside the US
Varty, 1996[61] Varty, 1998[62]	Observational Single center UK Funding: NR Population PAD patients with CLI Total N: 188 Mean Age: 74 N Female: 81 % Female: 43% Race: NR	Intervention Endovascular intervention (N=108) Percutaneous transluminal angioplasty Concomitant therapy: None specified Comparator Conservative management (N=38) Sympathectomy, analgesia, antibiotics, ulcer dressings or rehabilitation Concomitant therapy: None specified	Timing: 12 mo Individual Mortality Major amputation Limb salvage	Fair Study exclusion criteria were poorly described or not appropriate Study conducted solely outside the US Study was conducted only at a single site

C-37

Study	Study Details	Intervention (N) and Comparator (N)	Timing and Outcomes Reported	Quality and Limitations to Applicability
Endovascular intervention vs. surgical revascularization				
Adam, 2005[63] Bradbury, 2010[64-68] Forbes, 2010[69] BASIL Study	RCT Multicenter Europe Funding: Government Population PAD patients with CLI Total N: 452 Mean Age: NR N Female: 183 % Female: 40% Race: NR	*Intervention* Endovascular intervention (N=224) Percutaneous transluminal angioplasty Concomitant therapy: Could include antiplatelet agent, statin, or warfarin *Comparator* Surgical revascularization (N=228) Surgical bypass Concomitant therapy: Could include antiplatelet agent, statin, or warfarin	Timing: 36 mo <u>Individual</u> Mortality Amputation-free survival MI Stroke Length of stay QOL	Good No limitations
Ah Chong, 2009[70]	Observational Single center Asia Funding: NR Population PAD patients with CLI Total N: 405 Median Age: 74 N Female: 196 % Female: 48% Race: NR	*Intervention* Endovascular intervention (N=92) Percutaneous transluminal angioplasty Concomitant therapy: None specified *Comparator* Surgical revascularization (N=364) Surgical bypass Concomitant therapy: None specified	Timing: 24 mo <u>Individual</u> Mortality Length of stay Vessel patency Limb salvage	Poor Study conducted solely outside the US Study was conducted only at a single site

Study	Study Details	Intervention (N) and Comparator (N)	Timing and Outcomes Reported	Quality and Limitations to Applicability
Dorigo, 2009[71]	Observational Single center Europe Funding: NR Population PAD patients with CLI Total N: 73 Mean Age: 73 to 75 N Female: 21 % Female: 29% Race: NR	Intervention Endovascular intervention (N=34) Percutaneous transluminal angioplasty ± stent Concomitant therapy (postprocedure): Could include oral anticoagulant, antiplatelet drug(s), or LMWH Comparator Surgical revascularization (N=39) Surgical bypass Concomitant therapy (postoperative): Could include oral anticoagulant, antiplatelet drug(s), or LMWH	Timing: 13 mo Individual Mortality Repeat revascularization Length of stay Major amputation QOL	Fair Study did not report participants' baseline characteristics Study did not report participants' comorbid condition Study centers and/or clinicians were not selected on the basis of their skill or experience Study conducted solely outside the US Study was conducted only at a single site
Dosluoglu, 2012[72]	Observational Single center US Funding: NR Population PAD patients with CLI Total N: 433 Mean Age: 69 to 73 N Female: NR % Female: NR Race: NR	Intervention Endovascular intervention (N=295) Percutaneous transluminal angioplasty ± stent Concomitant therapy: Aspirin and/or other antiplatelet agents Comparator Surgical revascularization (N=138) Surgical bypass Concomitant therapy: Aspirin and/or other antiplatelet agents	Timing: 30 days, 1 yr, 2 yr, 3 yr, 4 yr, 5 yr Individual Total mortality Repeat revascularization Vessel patency Amputation-free survival Limb salvage ABI Composite Total mortality Cardiovascular mortality Nonfatal MI Stroke Limb ischemia	Fair No limitations

C-39

Study	Study Details	Intervention (N) and Comparator (N)	Timing and Outcomes Reported	Quality and Limitations to Applicability
Dosluoglu, 2010[73]	Observational Single center US Funding: NR Population: IC: 38% in endovascular arm, 25% in surgical and hybrid arms CLI: 62% in endovascular arm, 75% in surgical and hybrid arms Total N: 654 Mean Age: 66 to 70 N Female: 7 % Female: 1% Race: NR	*Intervention* Endovascular revascularization (N=356) Not defined Concomitant therapy: Clopidogrel 75 mg daily for at least 30 days, lifelong aspirin 81 mg daily *Comparator* Surgical revascularization (N=207); hybrid revascularization (N=91) Included a variety of procedures Concomitant therapy: Clopidogrel 75 mg daily for at least 30 days, lifelong aspirin 81 mg daily	Timing: 30 days, 1 yr, 3 yr <u>Individual</u> Mortality MI Stroke Length of stay Bleeding Major amputation Limb salvage	Poor Study selectively recruited participants who demonstrated a history of favorable or unfavorable response to drug or other interventions for the condition Study was conducted only at a single site
Faglia, 2012[58]	Observational Single center US Funding: NR Population PAD patients with CLI Total N: 344 Mean Age: 73 to 76 N Female: 119 % Female: 35% Race: NR	*Intervention* Endovascular intervention (N=292) Percutaneous transluminal angioplasty Concomitant therapy: Aspirin and/or other antiplatelet agents *Comparator* Surgical revascularization (N=40) Proximal or distal bypass grafting Concomitant therapy: Aspirin and/or other antiplatelet agents	Timing: 30 days, 6 mo, 16 mo, 18 mo <u>Individual</u> Total mortality Repeat revascularization Length of stay Major amputation Periprocedural complications Restenosis	Fair Study did not report participants' baseline characteristics Study eligibility/exclusion criteria were poorly described or not appropriate Study conducted solely outside the US

Study	Study Details	Intervention (N) and Comparator (N)	Timing and Outcomes Reported	Quality and Limitations to Applicability
Hoshino, 2010[74]	Observational Single center Asia Funding: Private foundation Population: IC: 148 patients CLI: 32 patients Total N: 180 Mean Age: 63 to 69 N Female: 21 % Female: 12% Race: NR	*Intervention* Endovascular revascularization (N not reported) Percutaneous transluminal angioplasty Concomitant therapy: Anticoagulants and/or aspirin; may include statin *Comparator* Surgical revascularization (N not reported) Surgical bypass Concomitant therapy: Anticoagulants and/or aspirin; may include statin	Timing: 1 yr, 3 yr, 5 yr <u>Individual</u> Mortality Vessel patency Amputation-free survival	Fair Study did not report participants' baseline characteristics Study did not report participants' comorbid conditions Study conducted solely outside the US Study was conducted only at a single site
Hynes, 2004[75]	Observational Single center Europe Funding: NR Population: PAD patients with CLI; 28 patients with femoropopliteal disease and 35 patients with aortoiliac disease Total N: 137 Mean Age: 70 N Female: 74 % Female: 54% Race: NR	*Intervention* Endovascular intervention (N=88) Subintimal angioplasty Concomitant therapy: Aspirin, pravastatin, and cardioselective beta-blockers during and after treatment; postoperatively, clopidogrel was added for 1 yr *Comparator* Surgical revascularization (49) Surgical bypass Concomitant therapy: Aspirin, pravastatin, and cardioselective beta-blockers during and after treatment; postoperatively, clopidogrel was added for 1 yr	Timing: 15 mo <u>Individual</u> Mortality MI Length of stay Limb salvage Vessel patency Change in ABI	Fair Study conducted solely outside the US Study was conducted only at a single site

Study	Study Details	Intervention (N) and Comparator (N)	Timing and Outcomes Reported	Quality and Limitations to Applicability
Janne d'Othee, 2008[76]	Observational Single center Location: NR Funding: Nonprofit organization Population: IC: 97 patients CLI: NR Total N: 97 Mean Age: 63 to 64 N Female: 33 % Female: 34% Race: NR	*Intervention* Endovascular revascularization (N=64) Included a variety of percutaneous procedures (mainly percutaneous transluminal angioplasty ± stent) Concomitant therapy: None specified *Comparator* Surgical revascularization (N=33) Included a variety of surgical procedures (mainly bypass and endarterectomy) Concomitant therapy: None specified	Timing: 30 days, 1 yr, 2 yr <u>Individual</u> Mortality Vessel patency Periprocedural complications	Fair Study selectively recruited participants who demonstrated a history of favorable or unfavorable response to drug or other interventions for the condition Study was conducted only at a single site
Jerabek, 2003[77]	Observational Single center Europe Funding: NR Population PAD patients with CLI Total N: 131 Mean Age: 61 to 62 N Female: 30 % Female: 23% Race: NR	*Intervention* Endovascular intervention (N=36) Percutaneous transluminal angioplasty ±stent Concomitant therapy: None specified *Comparator* Surgical revascularization (N=95) Surgical bypass Concomitant therapy: None specified	Timing: 2 to 105 days <u>Individual</u> Length of stay	Poor Study selectively recruited participants who demonstrated a history of favorable or unfavorable response to drug or other interventions for the condition Study was conducted only at a single site

Study	Study Details	Intervention (N) and Comparator (N)	Timing and Outcomes Reported	Quality and Limitations to Applicability
Johnson, 1997[78]	Observational Single center UK Funding: NR Population PAD patients with CLI Total N: 150 Mean Age: 71 N Female: 58 % Female: 39% Race: NR	*Intervention* Endovascular intervention (N=26) Angioplasty Concomitant therapy: None specified *Comparator* Surgical revascularization (N=44) Surgical bypass Concomitant therapy: None specified	Timing: 6 mo, 1 yr <u>Individual</u> Total mortality QOL Pain Anxiety Depression ADL index Mobility score	Fair Study did not report participants' comorbid conditions Study eligibility/exclusion criteria were poorly described or not appropriate Study conducted solely outside the US Study was conducted only at a single site
Kashyap, 2008[79]	Observational Single center US Funding: NR Population: IC: 54% in endovascular arm, 51% in surgical arm CLI: 46% in endovascular arm, 49% in surgical arm Total N: 169 Mean Age: 60 to 65 N Female: 66 % Female: 39% Race: NR	*Intervention* Endovascular revascularization (N=83) Recanalization, percutaneous transluminal angioplasty and stent Concomitant therapy: None specified *Comparator* Surgical revascularization (N=86) Surgical bypass Concomitant therapy: None specified	Timing: 30 days, 1 yr, 2 yr, 3 yr <u>Individual</u> Mortality MI Vessel patency Contrast nephropathy Periprocedural complications Limb salvage	Fair Study conducted solely outside the US Study was conducted only at a single site

Study	Study Details	Intervention (N) and Comparator (N)	Timing and Outcomes Reported	Quality and Limitations to Applicability
Khan, 2009[80]	Observational Single center US Funding: NR Population PAD patients with CLI Total N: 358 patients, 412 limbs Mean Age: 69 to 72 N Female: 3 % Female: 1% Race: NR	*Intervention* Endovascular intervention (N=197 patients, 236 limbs) Successful endovascular (not otherwise specified) Concomitant therapy: None specified *Comparator* Surgical revascularization (N=161 patients, 176 limbs) Successful surgical bypass Concomitant therapy: None specified	Timing: 36 mo <u>Individual</u> Limb salvage	Poor Study did not report participants' baseline characteristics Study exclusion criteria were poorly described or not appropriate Comparator(s) not well described Study centers and/or clinicians were not selected on the basis of their skill or experience Study was conducted only at a single site
Korhonen, 2011[81]	Observational Single center Europe Funding: NR Population PAD patients with CLI Total N: 858 Mean Age: 72 to 75 N Female: 374 % Female: 44% Race: NR	*Intervention* Endovascular intervention (N=517) Percutaneous transluminal angioplasty ± stent Concomitant therapy (postprocedure): Clopidogrel 300 mg once, then 75 mg daily x at least 1 mo (unless already on anticoagulation); ASA 100 mg daily *Comparator* Surgical revascularization (N=341) Surgical bypass Concomitant therapy (postoperative): LMWH during hospital; ASA 100 mg daily	Timing: 2.6 yr <u>Individual</u> Mortality Limb salvage Amputation-free survival Freedom from repeat revascularization	Good Study did not report participants' severity of disease Study eligibility criteria were poorly described or not appropriate Study exclusion criteria were poorly described or not appropriate Study centers and/or clinicians were not selected on the basis of their skill or experience Study conducted solely outside the US Study was conducted only at a single site

Study	Study Details	Intervention (N) and Comparator (N)	Timing and Outcomes Reported	Quality and Limitations to Applicability
Kudo, 2006[82]	Observational Single center US Funding: NR <u>Population</u> PAD patients with CLI Total N: 192 patients, 237 limbs Mean Age: 70 N Female: NR % Female: NR Race: NR	*Intervention* Endovascular intervention (N=153 limbs) Angioplasty ± stent Concomitant therapy: None specified *Comparator* Surgical revascularization (N=84 limbs) Surgical bypass Concomitant therapy: None specified	Timing: 23 mo <u>Individual</u> Mortality Length of stay Vessel patency Limb salvage Clinical improvement	Poor Participant diagnosis and identification for eligibility screening before random allocation was not appropriate/Cohort selection was not appropriate Study exclusion criteria were poorly described or not appropriate Study centers and/or clinicians were not selected on the basis of their skill or experience Study was conducted only at a single site
Laurila, 2000[83]	Observational Multicenter Europe Funding: NR <u>Population</u> PAD patients with CLI Total N: 118 patients, 124 limbs Mean Age: 70 to 74 N Female: NR % Female: NR Race: NR	*Intervention* Endovascular intervention (N=86) Percutaneous transluminal angioplasty Concomitant therapy: ASA 50-100 mg daily *Comparator* Surgical revascularization (N=38) Surgical bypass Concomitant therapy: None specified	Timing: 20 mo <u>Individual</u> Mortality	Poor No limitations

Study	Study Details	Intervention (N) and Comparator (N)	Timing and Outcomes Reported	Quality and Limitations to Applicability
Lepantalo, 2009[84]	RCT Multicenter Europe Funding: NR Population: IC: 87% in endovascular arm, 90% in surgical arm CLI: 13% in endovascular arm, 10% in surgical arm Total N: 44 Mean Age: 64 to 66 N Female: 19 % Female: 43% Race: NR	*Intervention* Endovascular revascularization (N=23) Endoluminal thrupass Concomitant therapy: Aspirin and/or clopidogrel; postoperative LMWH for 2 days; may include prophylactic antibiotic *Comparator* Surgical revascularization (N=21) Surgical bypass Concomitant therapy: Aspirin and/or clopidogrel; postoperative LMWH for 2 days; may include prophylactic antibiotic	Timing: 30 days, 12 mo, 17 mo, 18 mo Individual Mortality Repeat revascularization Length of stay Vessel patency Major amputation Periprocedural complications	Fair Study conducted solely outside the US
Loor, 2009[85]	Observational Single center US Funding: NR Population PAD patients with CLI Total N: 92 patients, 99 procedures Mean Age: 64 to 69 N Female: NR % Female: NR Race: NR	*Intervention* Endovascular intervention (N=33 patients, 34 procedures) Atherectomy Concomitant therapy (postprocedure): Antiplatelet agents (ASA or clopidogrel or anticoagulants (warfarin, heparin or enoxaparin) *Comparator* Surgical revascularization (N=59 patients, 65 procedures) Surgical bypass Concomitant therapy (postoperative) Antiplatelet agents (ASA or clopidogrel) or anticoagulants (warfarin, heparin or enoxaparin)	Timing: 17 mo Individual Mortality Length of stay Vessel patency Limb salvage	Fair Study exclusion criteria were poorly described or not appropriate Study was conducted only at a single site

C-46

Study	Study Details	Intervention (N) and Comparator (N)	Timing and Outcomes Reported	Quality and Limitations to Applicability
McQuade, 2009[86] McQuade, 2010[87] Kedora, 2007[88]	RCT Single center US Funding: Industry Population: IC: 82% in endovascular arm, 62% in surgical arm CLI: 18% in endovascular arm, 38% in surgical arm Total N: 86 Mean Age: 67 to 72 N Female: NR % Female: NR Race: NR	*Intervention* Endovascular revascularization (N=40) Percutaneous angioplasty with stent Concomitant therapy: Aspirin 81-325 mg daily and clopidogrel 75 mg daily for at least 3 mo (unless previously on warfarin which was continued in place of clopidogrel) *Comparator* Surgical revascularization (N=46) Surgical bypass Concomitant therapy: Aspirin 81-325 mg daily and clopidogrel 75 mg daily for at least 3 mo (unless previously on warfarin which was continued in place of clopidogrel)	Timing: 1 yr, 18 mo, 2 yr, 3 yr, 4 yr Individual Mortality Repeat revascularization Length of stay Vessel patency Major amputation Periprocedural complications Graft failure Change in ABI	Fair Participant diagnosis and identification for eligibility screening before random allocation was not appropriate/Cohort selection was not appropriate Study exclusion criteria were poorly described or not appropriate Study was conducted only at a single site
Rossi, 1998[89]	Observational Single center Europe Funding: CNR grant Population: IC: 24% in endovascular arm, 0% in surgical arm CLI: 76% in endovascular arm, 100% in surgical arm Total N: 48 Mean Age: 68 to 70 N Female: NR % Female: NR Race: NR	*Intervention* Endovascular revascularization (N=37) Percutaneous balloon angioplasty or atherectomy Concomitant therapy: None specified *Comparator* Surgical revascularization (N=11) Surgical bypass Concomitant therapy: None specified	Timing: 12 mo, 18 mo Individual Mortality MI Periprocedural complications Limb salvage	Poor Study eligibility criteria were poorly described or not appropriate Study exclusion criteria were poorly described or not appropriate Study conducted solely outside the US Study was conducted only at a single site

Study	Study Details	Intervention (N) and Comparator (N)	Timing and Outcomes Reported	Quality and Limitations to Applicability
Sachs, 2011[90]	Observational Multicenter US Funding: NR Population: IC: NR CLI: NR Total N: 563,143 Mean Age: 60 to 69 N Female: 66,363 % Female: 43% Race: 8.7% African American; 83.7% White	*Intervention* Endovascular revascularization (N=128,937) Percutaneous transluminal angioplasty ± stent Concomitant therapy: None specified *Comparator* Surgical revascularization (24,033 aorto-femoral bypass; 102,604 peripheral bypass) Surgical bypass Concomitant therapy: None specified	Timing: In-hospital <u>Individual</u> Mortality Length of stay Discharge status Major amputation Amputation-free survival	Poor Study did not report participants' severity of disease Study centers and/or clinicians were not selected on the basis of their skill or experience Duration of participant followup was inadequate
Soderstrom, 2010[91]	Observational Single center Europe Funding: NR Population PAD patients with CLI Total N: 1023 Mean Age: 74 to 75 N Female: 589 % Female: 58% Race: NR	*Intervention* Endovascular intervention (N=262) Percutaneous transluminal angioplasty Concomitant therapy: None specified *Comparator* Surgical revascularization (N=761) Surgical bypass Concomitant therapy: None specified	Timing: 2.4 yr <u>Individual</u> Mortality Repeat revascularization Limb salvage Amputation-free survival Freedom from repeat revascularization	Fair No limitations

Study	Study Details	Intervention (N) and Comparator (N)	Timing and Outcomes Reported	Quality and Limitations to Applicability
Stoner, 2008[92]	Observational Single center US Funding: Not complete Population: IC: 57% in endovascular arm, 44% in surgical arm CLI: 43% in endovascular arm, 56% in surgical arm Total N: 359 patients, 381 lesions Mean Age: 64 to 66 N Female: NR % Female: NR Race: NR	*Intervention* Endovascular revascularization (198 procedures) Included a variety of procedures (percutaneous transluminal angioplasty ± stent, subintimal angioplasty, atherectomy) Concomitant therapy: Could include aspirin, clopidogrel, warfarin and lipid-lowering medications *Comparator* Surgical revascularization (183 procedures) Surgical bypass Concomitant therapy: Could include aspirin, clopidogrel, warfarin and lipid-lowering medications	Timing: 1 yr Individual: Vessel patency	Poor Study did not report participants' baseline characteristics Study did not report participants' comorbid conditions Study exclusion criteria were poorly described or not appropriate Study centers and/or clinicians were not selected on the basis of their skill or experience Study was conducted only at a single site
Sultan, 2009[93] Sultan, 2011[94]	Observational Single center Europe Funding: NR Population PAD patients with CLI Total N: 309 Mean Age: 70 to 73 N Female: 146 % Female: 47% Race: NR	*Intervention* Endovascular intervention (N=190) Subintimal angioplasty Concomitant therapy: Preprocedure, ASA, pravastatin, cardioselective beta-blocker and/or calcium channel blocker; postprocedure, clopidogrel *Comparator* Surgical revascularization (N=119) Surgical bypass Concomitant therapy: Preoperative, ASA, pravastatin, cardioselective beta-blocker and/or calcium channel blocker; postoperative, clopidogrel	Timing: 5 yr Composite Total mortality Nonfatal MI Stroke Major amputation Individual Mortality Length of stay Major amputation Amputation-free survival Clinical improvement Repeat revascularization	Fair Participant diagnosis and identification for eligibility screening before random allocation was not appropriate/Cohort selection was not appropriate Study eligibility criteria were poorly described or not appropriate Study exclusion criteria were poorly described or not appropriate Study conducted solely outside the US Study was conducted only at a single site

Study	Study Details	Intervention (N) and Comparator (N)	Timing and Outcomes Reported	Quality and Limitations to Applicability
Taylor, 2005[95]	Observational Single center US Funding: NR Population PAD patients with CLI Total N: 122 Mean Age: 83 N Female: 49 % Female: 40% Race: 80% White	Intervention Endovascular intervention (N=65) Percutaneous transluminal angioplasty ± stent Concomitant therapy: None specified Comparator Surgical revascularization (N=57) Surgical bypass Concomitant therapy: None specified	Timing: 36 mo Individual Vessel patency Wound healing Mortality Limb salvage Amputation-free survival Maintenance of ambulation	Fair No limitations
Taylor, 2006[96]	Observational Single center US Funding: NR Population PAD patients with CLI Total N: 841 Mean Age: 68 N Female: 362 % Female: 43% Race: 76.1% White, 23.1% Black, 0.8% Other	Intervention Endovascular intervention (N=299) Not further specified Concomitant therapy: None specified Comparator Surgical revascularization (N=519) Surgical bypass Concomitant therapy: None specified	Timing: 24 mo, 60 mo Individual Vessel patency Limb salvage Maintenance of ambulation	Poor Study did not report participants' baseline characteristics Study did not report participants' severity of disease Study did not report participants' comorbid conditions Study eligibility criteria were poorly described or not appropriate Study exclusion criteria were poorly described or not appropriate Study interventions (active arm) were not similar to interventions used in routine clinical practice Study was conducted only at a single site

Study	Study Details	Intervention (N) and Comparator (N)	Timing and Outcomes Reported	Quality and Limitations to Applicability
Taylor, 2009[97]	Observational Single center US Funding: NR <u>Population</u> PAD patients with CLI Total N: 677 Mean Age: 69 N Female: 297 % Female: 44% Race: 72% white	*Intervention* Endovascular revascularization (N=316) PTA Concomitant therapy: None specified *Comparator* Surgical revascularization (N=361) Open surgery Concomitant therapy: None specified	Timing: 6 mo, 1 yr <u>Individual</u> Vessel patency Wound healing Limb salvage Survival	Poor No limitations
Timaran, 2003[98]	Observational Multicenter US Funding: NR <u>Population</u> PAD patients with CLI Total N: 62 Median Age: 64 N Female: 22 % Female: 35% Race: NR	*Intervention* Iliac angioplasty and stenting with concomitant infrainguinal arterial reconstruction (N=27) Concomitant therapy: None specified *Comparator* Iliac angioplasty and stenting (N=35) Concomitant therapy: None specified	Timing: 1 yr, 3 yr, 5 yr <u>Individual</u> Primary patency Limb salvage	Poor Study selectively recruited participants who demonstrated a history of favorable or unfavorable response to drug or other interventions for the condition Study's cointerventions did not adequately reflect routine clinical practice Study centers and/or clinicians were not selected on the bases of their skill of experience

C-51

Study	Study Details	Intervention (N) and Comparator (N)	Timing and Outcomes Reported	Quality and Limitations to Applicability
Timaran, 2003[99]	Observational Single center US Funding: NR Population: IC: 61% of endovascular arm, 84% of surgical arm CLI: 39% of endovascular arm, 16% of surgical arm Total N: 188 Mean Age: 59 N Female: 85 % Female: 45% Race: NR	*Intervention* Endovascular revascularization (N=136) Angioplasty with stent Concomitant therapy: None specified *Comparator* Surgical revascularization (N=52) Surgical bypass Concomitant therapy: None specified	Timing: 1 yr, 3 yr, 5 yr <u>Individual</u> Vessel patency	Fair Study centers and/or clinicians were not selected on the basis of their skill or experience Study was conducted only at a single site
Varela, 2011[100]	Observational Single center Europe Funding: NR Population PAD patients with CLI Total N: 88 patients, 91 limbs Mean Age: NR N Female: NR % Female: NR Race: NR	*Intervention* Endovascular intervention (N=42 limbs) Not further specified Concomitant therapy: None specified *Comparator* Surgical revascularization (N=49 limbs) Surgical bypass Concomitant therapy: None specified	Timing: 310 days <u>Individual</u> Mortality Hospitalization Vessel patency Wound healing Major amputation Limb salvage Amputation-free survival	Fair Study centers and/or clinicians were not selected on the basis of their skill or experience Study was conducted only at a single site

Study	Study Details	Intervention (N) and Comparator (N)	Timing and Outcomes Reported	Quality and Limitations to Applicability
Varty, 1996[61] Varty, 1998[62]	Observational Single center UK Funding: NR *Population* PAD patients with CLI Total N: 188 Mean Age: 74 N Female: 81 % Female: 43% Race: NR	*Intervention* Endovascular intervention (N=108 procedures) Percutaneous transluminal angioplasty Concomitant therapy: None specified *Comparator* Surgical revascularization (N=68 procedures) Surgical bypass Concomitant therapy: None specified	Timing: 12 mo <u>Individual</u> Mortality Major amputation Limb salvage	Fair Study exclusion criteria were poorly described or not appropriate Study conducted solely outside the US Study was conducted only at a single site
Venermo, 2011[101]	Observational Single center Europe Funding: NR *Population* PAD patients with CLI Total N: 597 patients, 732 procedures Mean Age: 72 N Female: NR % Female: NR Race: NR	*Intervention* Endovascular intervention (N=377 procedures) Percutaneous transluminal angioplasty Concomitant therapy: None specified *Comparator* Surgical revascularization (N=355 procedures) Surgical bypass Concomitant therapy: None specified	Timing: 2.8 yr <u>Individual</u> Limb salvage	Poor Study exclusion criteria were poorly described or not appropriate Comparator(s) not well described Study conducted solely outside the US Study was conducted only at a single site

C-53

Study	Study Details	Intervention (N) and Comparator (N)	Timing and Outcomes Reported	Quality and Limitations to Applicability
Whatling, 2000[102]	Observational Single center UK Funding: NR Population: IC: 121 patients of total population CLI: 17 patients of total population Total N: 138 Mean Age: 62 to 68 N Female: 45 % Female: 33% Race: NR	*Intervention* Endovascular revascularization (N=51) Percutaneous transluminal angioplasty with stent Concomitant therapy: Aspirin 75 mg daily *Comparator* Surgical revascularization (N=87) Surgical crossover grafting Concomitant therapy: None specified	Timing: 6 mo Individual Length of stay Vessel patency	Poor Study did not report participants' baseline characteristics Study did not report participants' comorbid conditions Study eligibility criteria were poorly described or not appropriate Study exclusion criteria were poorly described or not appropriate Study conducted solely outside the US Study was conducted only at a single site
Wolfle, 2000[103]	Observational Single center Location: Germany Funding: Government Population PAD patients with CLI Total N: 209 Mean Age: 68 to 70 N Female: NR % Female: NR Race: NR	*Intervention* Endovascular intervention (N=84) Percutaneous transluminal angioplasty Concomitant therapy (postprocedure): ASA 100 mg daily *Comparator* Surgical revascularization (N=125) Surgical bypass Concomitant therapy (postoperative): ASA 100 mg daily	Timing: 84 mo Individual Mortality Limb salvage	Poor Study did not report participants' baseline characteristics Study eligibility criteria were poorly described or not appropriate Study conducted solely outside the US Study was conducted only at a single site

Study	Study Details	Intervention (N) and Comparator (N)	Timing and Outcomes Reported	Quality and Limitations to Applicability
Zdanowski, 1998[104]	Observational Single center Europe Funding: NR Population PAD patients with CLI Total N: 4929 Mean Age: 76 N Female: 2612 % Female: 53% Race: NR	*Intervention* Endovascular intervention (N=1199) Percutaneous transluminal angioplasty Concomitant therapy: None specified *Comparator* Surgical revascularization (N=3730) Surgical bypass Concomitant therapy: None specified	Timing: 12 mo <u>Individual</u> Mortality Amputation-free survival	Poor Study did not report participants' baseline characteristics Study eligibility criteria were poorly described or not appropriate Comparator(s) not well described Study conducted solely outside the US Study was conducted only at a single site

Abbreviations: ABI=ankle-brachial index; ASA=acetylsalicylic acid (aspirin); CLI=critical limb ischemia; IC=intermittent claudication; MI=myocardial infarction; mg=milligrams; min=minute/minutes; mo=month/months; N=number of patients; NR=not reported; PAD=peripheral artery disease; QOL=quality of life; RCT=randomized controlled trial; SD=standard deviation; sec=second/seconds; wk=week/weeks; yr=year/years

References Cited in Appendix C

1. Belch J, MacCuish A, Campbell I, et al. The prevention of progression of arterial disease and diabetes (POPADAD) trial: factorial randomised placebo controlled trial of aspirin and antioxidants in patients with diabetes and asymptomatic peripheral arterial disease. BMJ. 2008;337:a1840. PMID: 18927173.

2. Fowkes FG, Price JF, Stewart MC, et al. Aspirin for prevention of cardiovascular events in a general population screened for a low ankle brachial index: a randomized controlled trial. JAMA. 2010;303(9):841-8. PMID: 20197530.

3. Anonymous. A randomised, blinded, trial of clopidogrel versus aspirin in patients at risk of ischaemic events (CAPRIE). Lancet. 1996;348(9038):1329-39. PMID: 8918275.

4. Cacoub PP, Bhatt DL, Steg PG, et al. Patients with peripheral arterial disease in the CHARISMA trial. Eur Heart J. 2009;30(2):192-201. PMID: 19136484.

5. Bhatt DL, Flather MD, Hacke W, et al. Patients with prior myocardial infarction, stroke, or symptomatic peripheral arterial disease in the CHARISMA trial. J Am Coll Cardiol. 2007;49(19):1982-8. PMID: 17498584.

6. Bhatt DL, Fox KA, Hacke W, et al. Clopidogrel and aspirin versus aspirin alone for the prevention of atherothrombotic events. N Engl J Med. 2006;354(16):1706-17. PMID: 16531616.

7. Berger PB, Bhatt DL, Fuster V, et al. Bleeding complications with dual antiplatelet therapy among patients with stable vascular disease or risk factors for vascular disease: results from the Clopidogrel for High Atherothrombotic Risk and Ischemic Stabilization, Management, and Avoidance (CHARISMA) trial. Circulation. 2010;121(23):2575-83. PMID: 20516378.

8. Catalano M, Born G, Peto R. Prevention of serious vascular events by aspirin amongst patients with peripheral arterial disease: randomized, double-blind trial. J Intern Med. 2007;261(3):276-84. PMID: 17305650.

9. Cassar K, Ford I, Greaves M, et al. Randomized clinical trial of the antiplatelet effects of aspirin-clopidogrel combination versus aspirin alone after lower limb angioplasty. Br J Surg. 2005;92(2):159-65. PMID: 15609386.

10. Mahmood A, Sintler M, Edwards AT, et al. The efficacy of aspirin in patients undergoing infra-inguinal bypass and identification of high risk patients. Int Angiol. 2003;22(3):302-7. PMID: 14612858.

11. Belch JJ, Dormandy J, Biasi GM, et al. Results of the randomized, placebo-controlled clopidogrel and acetylsalicylic acid in bypass surgery for peripheral arterial disease (CASPAR) trial. J Vasc Surg. 2010;52(4):825-33, 833 e1-2. PMID: 20678878.

12. Tepe G, Bantleon R, Brechtel K, et al. Management of peripheral arterial interventions with mono or dual antiplatelet therapy-the MIRROR study: a randomised and double-blinded clinical trial. Eur Radiol. 2012;22(9):1998-2006. PMID: 22569995.

13. Horrocks M, Horrocks EH, Murphy P, et al. The effects of platelet inhibitors on platelet uptake and restenosis after femoral angioplasty. Int Angiol. 1997(2):101-6. PMID:

14. Minar E, Ahmadi A, Koppensteiner R, et al. Comparison of effects of high-dose and low-dose aspirin on restenosis after femoropopliteal percutaneous transluminal angioplasty. Circulation. 1995;91(8):2167-73. PMID: 7697845.

15. Beebe HG, Dawson DL, Cutler BS, et al. A new pharmacological treatment for intermittent claudication: results of a randomized, multicenter trial. Arch Intern Med. 1999;159(17):2041-50. PMID: 10510990.

16. Belcaro G, Nicolaides AN, Griffin M, et al. Intermittent claudication in diabetics: treatment with exercise and pentoxifylline--a 6-month, controlled, randomized trial. Angiology. 2002;53 Suppl 1:S39-43. PMID: 11865835.

17. Dawson DL, Cutler BS, Meissner MH, et al. Cilostazol has beneficial effects in treatment of intermittent claudication: results from a multicenter, randomized, prospective, double-blind trial. Circulation. 1998;98(7):678-86. PMID: 9715861.

18. Dawson DL, Cutler BS, Hiatt WR, et al. A comparison of cilostazol and pentoxifylline for treating intermittent claudication. Am J Med. 2000;109(7):523-30. PMID: 11063952.

19. De Sanctis MT, Cesarone MR, Belcaro G, et al. Treatment of intermittent claudication with pentoxifylline: a 12-month, randomized trial--walking distance and microcirculation. Angiology. 2002;53 Suppl 1:S7-12. PMID: 11865838.

20. De Sanctis MT, Cesarone MR, Belcaro G, et al. Treatment of long-distance intermittent claudication with pentoxifylline: a 12-month, randomized trial. Angiology. 2002;53 Suppl 1:S13-7. PMID: 11865829.

21. Cesarone MR, Belcaro G, Nicolaides AN, et al. Treatment of severe intermittent claudication with pentoxifylline: a 40-week, controlled, randomized trial. Angiology. 2002;53 Suppl 1:S1-5. PMID: 11865828.

22. Hiatt WR, Money SR, Brass EP. Long-term safety of cilostazol in patients with peripheral artery disease: the CASTLE study (Cilostazol: A Study in Long-term Effects). J Vasc Surg. 2008;47(2):330-336. PMID: 18155871.

23. Stone WM, Demaerschalk BM, Fowl RJ, et al. Type 3 phosphodiesterase inhibitors may be protective against cerebrovascular events in patients with claudication. J Stroke Cerebrovasc Dis. 2008;17(3):129-33. PMID: 18436153.

24. Hobbs SD, Marshall T, Fegan C, et al. The effect of supervised exercise and cilostazol on coagulation and fibrinolysis in intermittent claudication: a randomized controlled trial. J Vasc Surg. 2007;45(1):65-70; discussion 70. PMID: 17210383.

25. Money SR, Herd JA, Isaacsohn JL, et al. Effect of cilostazol on walking distances in patients with intermittent claudication caused by peripheral vascular disease. J Vasc Surg. 1998;27(2):267-74; discussion 274-5. PMID: 9510281.

26. Soga Y, Yokoi H, Kawasaki T, et al. Efficacy of cilostazol after endovascular therapy for femoropopliteal artery disease in patients with intermittent claudication. J Am Coll Cardiol. 2009;53(1):48-53. PMID: 19118724.

27. Strandness DE, Jr., Dalman RL, Panian S, et al. Effect of cilostazol in patients with intermittent claudication: a randomized, double-blind, placebo-controlled study. Vasc Endovascular Surg. 2002;36(2):83-91. PMID: 11951094.

28. Crowther RG, Spinks WL, Leicht AS, et al. Effects of a long-term exercise program on lower limb mobility, physiological responses, walking performance, and physical activity levels in patients with peripheral arterial disease. J Vasc Surg. 2008;47(2):303-9. PMID: 18241753.

29. Gardner AW, Katzel LI, Sorkin JD, et al. Effects of long-term exercise rehabilitation on claudication distances in patients with peripheral arterial disease: a randomized controlled trial. J Cardiopulm Rehabil. 2002;22(3):192-8. PMID: 12042688.

30. Gardner AW, Parker DE, Montgomery PS, et al. Efficacy of quantified home-based exercise and supervised exercise in patients with intermittent claudication: a randomized controlled trial. Circulation. 2011;123(5):491-8. PMID: 21262997.

31. Gelin J, Jivegard L, Taft C, et al. Treatment efficacy of intermittent claudication by surgical intervention, supervised physical exercise training compared to no treatment in unselected randomised patients I: one year results of functional and physiological improvements. Eur J Vasc Endovasc Surg. 2001;22(2):107-13. PMID: 11472042.

32. Taft C, Karlsson J, Gelin J, et al. Treatment efficacy of intermittent claudication by invasive therapy, supervised physical exercise training compared to no treatment in unselected randomised patients II: one-year results of health-related quality of life. Eur J Vasc Endovasc Surg. 2001;22(2):114-23. PMID: 11472043.

33. Gibellini R, Fanello M, Bardile AF, et al. Exercise training in intermittent claudication. Int Angiol. 2000;19(1):8-13. PMID: 10853679.

34. Hobbs SD, Marshall T, Fegan C, et al. The constitutive procoagulant and hypofibrinolytic state in patients with intermittent claudication due to infrainguinal disease significantly improves with percutaneous transluminal balloon angioplasty. J Vasc Surg. 2006;43(1):40-6. PMID: 16414385.

35. Lee HL, Mehta T, Ray B, et al. A non-randomised controlled trial of the clinical and cost effectiveness of a Supervised Exercise Programme for claudication. Eur J Vasc Endovasc Surg. 2007;33(2):202-7. PMID: 17142065.

36. Murphy TP, Cutlip DE, Regensteiner JG, et al. Supervised exercise versus primary stenting for claudication resulting from aortoiliac peripheral artery disease: six-month outcomes from the claudication: exercise versus endoluminal revascularization (CLEVER) study. Circulation. 2012;125(1):130-9. PMID: 22090168.

37. Sugimoto I, Ohta T, Ishibashi H, et al. Conservative treatment for patients with intermittent claudication. Int Angiol. 2010;29(2 Suppl):55-60. PMID: 20357750.

38. Treat-Jacobson D, Bronas UG, Leon AS. Efficacy of arm-ergometry versus treadmill exercise training to improve walking distance in patients with claudication. Vasc Med. 2009;14(3):203-13. PMID: 19651669.

39. Bronas UG, Treat-Jacobson D, Leon AS. Comparison of the effect of upper body-ergometry aerobic training vs treadmill training on central cardiorespiratory improvement and walking distance in patients with claudication. J Vasc Surg. 2011;53(6):1557-64. PMID: 21515017.

40. Tsai JC, Chan P, Wang CH, et al. The effects of exercise training on walking function and perception of health status in elderly patients with peripheral arterial occlusive disease. J Intern Med. 2002;252(5):448-55. PMID: 12528763.

41. Feinglass J, McCarthy WJ, Slavensky R, et al. Functional status and walking ability after lower extremity bypass grafting or angioplasty for intermittent claudication: results from a prospective outcomes study. J Vasc Surg. 2000;31(1 Pt 1):93-103. PMID: 10642712.

42. Giugliano G, Di Serafino L, Perrino C, et al. Effects of successful percutaneous lower extremity revascularization on cardiovascular outcome in patients with peripheral arterial disease. International Journal of Cardiology. 2012. PMID:

43. Koivunen K, Lukkarinen H. One-year prospective health-related quality-of-life outcomes in patients treated with conservative method, endovascular treatment or open surgery for symptomatic lower limb atherosclerotic disease. Eur J Cardiovasc Nurs. 2008;7(3):247-56. PMID: 18221916.

44. Nylaende M, Abdelnoor M, Stranden E, et al. The Oslo balloon angioplasty versus conservative treatment study (OBACT)—The 2-years results of a single centre, prospective, randomised study in patients with intermittent claudication. Eur J Vasc Endovasc Surg. 2007;33(1):3-12. PMID: 17055756.

45. Pell JP, Lee AJ. Impact of angioplasty and arterial reconstructive surgery on the quality of life of claudicants. The Scottish Vascular Audit Group. Scott Med J. 1997;42(2):47-8. PMID: 9507581.

46. Whyman MR, Fowkes FG, Kerracher EM, et al. Is intermittent claudication improved by percutaneous transluminal angioplasty? A randomized controlled trial. J Vasc Surg. 1997;26(4):551-7. PMID: 9357454.

47. Whyman MR, Fowkes FG, Kerracher EM, et al. Randomised controlled trial of percutaneous transluminal angioplasty for intermittent claudication. Eur J Vasc Endovasc Surg. 1996;12(2):167-72. PMID: 8760978.

48. Mori E, Komori K, Kume M, et al. Comparison of the long-term results between surgical and conservative treatment in patients with intermittent claudication. Surgery. 2002;131(1 Suppl):S269-74. PMID: 11821823.

49. Greenhalgh RM, Belch JJ, Brown LC, et al. The adjuvant benefit of angioplasty in patients with mild to moderate intermittent claudication (MIMIC) managed by supervised exercise, smoking cessation advice and best medical therapy: results from two randomised trials for stenotic femoropopliteal and aortoiliac arterial disease. Eur J Vasc Endovasc Surg. 2008;36(6):680-8. PMID: 19022184.

50. Kruidenier LM, Nicolai SP, Rouwet EV, et al. Additional supervised exercise therapy after a percutaneous vascular intervention for peripheral arterial disease: a randomized clinical trial. J Vasc Interv Radiol. 2011;22(7):961-8. PMID: 21571547.

51. Mazari FA, Khan JA, Carradice D, et al. Randomized clinical trial of percutaneous transluminal angioplasty, supervised exercise and combined treatment for intermittent claudication due to femoropopliteal arterial disease. Br J Surg. 2012;99(1):39-48. PMID: 22021102.

52. Mazari FA, Gulati S, Rahman MN, et al. Early outcomes from a randomized, controlled trial of supervised exercise, angioplasty, and combined therapy in intermittent claudication. Ann Vasc Surg. 2010;24(1):69-79. PMID: 19762206.

53. Nordanstig J, Gelin J, Hensater M, et al. Walking performance and health-related quality of life after surgical or endovascular invasive versus non-invasive treatment for intermittent claudication--a prospective randomised trial. Eur J Vasc Endovasc Surg. 2011;42(2):220-7. PMID: 21397530.

54. Perkins JM, Collin J, Creasy TS, et al. Exercise training versus angioplasty for stable claudication. Long and medium term results of a prospective, randomised trial. Eur J Vasc Endovasc Surg. 1996;11(4):409-13. PMID: 8846172.

55. Spronk S, Bosch JL, den Hoed PT, et al. Intermittent claudication: clinical effectiveness of endovascular revascularization versus supervised hospital-based exercise training--randomized controlled trial. Radiology. 2009;250(2):586-95. PMID: 19188327.

56. Spronk S, Bosch JL, den Hoed PT, et al. Cost-effectiveness of endovascular revascularization compared to supervised hospital-based exercise training in patients with intermittent claudication: a randomized controlled trial. J Vasc Surg. 2008;48(6):1472-80. PMID: 18771879.

57. Drozdz W, Panek J, Lejman W. Red cell deformability in patients with chronic atheromatous ischemia of the legs. Med Sci Monit. 2001;7(5):933-9. PMID: 11535938.

58. Faglia E, Clerici G, Losa S, et al. Limb revascularization feasibility in diabetic patients with critical limb ischemia: results from a cohort of 344 consecutive unselected diabetic patients evaluated in 2009. Diabetes Res Clin Pract. 2012;95(3):364-71. PMID: 22104261.

59. Kamiya C, Sakamoto S, Tamori Y, et al. Long-term outcome after percutaneous peripheral intervention vs medical treatment for patients with superficial femoral artery occlusive disease. Circ J. 2008;72(5):734-9. PMID: 18441452.

60. Lawall H, Gorriahn H, Amendt K, et al. Long-term outcomes after medical and interventional therapy of critical limb ischemia. Eur J Intern Med. 2009;20(6):616-21. PMID: 19782924.

61. Varty K, Nydahl S, Butterworth P, et al. Changes in the management of critical limb ischaemia. Br J Surg. 1996;83(7):953-6. PMID: 8813785.

62. Varty K, Nydahl S, Nasim A, et al. Results of surgery and angioplasty for the treatment of chronic severe lower limb ischaemia. Eur J Vasc Endovasc Surg. 1998;16(2):159-63. PMID: 9728437.

63. Adam DJ, Beard JD, Cleveland T, et al. Bypass versus angioplasty in severe ischaemia of the leg (BASIL): multicentre, randomised controlled trial. Lancet. 2005;366(9501):1925-34. PMID: 16325694.

64. Bradbury AW, Adam DJ, Bell J, et al. Bypass versus Angioplasty in Severe Ischaemia of the Leg (BASIL) trial: A survival prediction model to facilitate clinical decision making. J Vasc Surg. 2010;51(5 Suppl):52S-68S. PMID: 20435262.

65. Bradbury AW, Adam DJ, Bell J, et al. Bypass versus Angioplasty in Severe Ischaemia of the Leg (BASIL) trial: A description of the severity and extent of disease using the Bollinger angiogram scoring method and the TransAtlantic Inter-Society Consensus II classification. J Vasc Surg. 2010;51(5 Suppl):32S-42S. PMID: 20435260.

66. Bradbury AW, Adam DJ, Bell J, et al. Bypass versus Angioplasty in Severe Ischaemia of the Leg (BASIL) trial: An intention-to-treat analysis of amputation-free and overall survival in patients randomized to a bypass surgery-first or a balloon angioplasty-first revascularization strategy. J Vasc Surg. 2010;51(5 Suppl):5S-17S. PMID: 20435258.

67. Bradbury AW, Adam DJ, Bell J, et al. Bypass versus Angioplasty in Severe Ischaemia of the Leg (BASIL) trial: Analysis of amputation free and overall survival by treatment received. J Vasc Surg. 2010;51(5 Suppl):18S-31S. PMID: 20435259.

68. Bradbury AW, Adam DJ, Bell J, et al. Multicentre randomised controlled trial of the clinical and cost-effectiveness of a bypass-surgery-first versus a balloon-angioplasty-first revascularisation strategy for severe limb ischaemia due to infrainguinal disease. The Bypass versus Angioplasty in Severe Ischaemia of the Leg (BASIL) trial. Health Technol Assess. 2010;14(14):1-210, iii-iv. PMID: 20307380.

69. Forbes JF, Adam DJ, Bell J, et al. Bypass versus Angioplasty in Severe Ischaemia of the Leg (BASIL) trial: Health-related quality of life outcomes, resource utilization, and cost-effectiveness analysis. J Vasc Surg. 2010;51(5 Suppl):43S-51S. PMID: 20435261.

70. Ah Chong AK, Tan CB, Wong MW, et al. Bypass surgery or percutaneous transluminal angioplasty to treat critical lower limb ischaemia due to infrainguinal arterial occlusive disease? Hong Kong Med J. 2009;15(4):249-54. PMID: 19652230.

71. Dorigo W, Pulli R, Marek J, et al. A comparison between open and endovascular repair in the treatment of critical limb ischemia. Ital J Vasc Endovasc Surg. 2009;16(1):17-22. PMID:

72. Dosluoglu HH, Lall P, Harris LM, et al. Long-term limb salvage and survival after endovascular and open revascularization for critical limb ischemia after adoption of endovascular-first approach by vascular surgeons. Journal of Vascular Surgery. 2012. PMID:

73. Dosluoglu HH, Lall P, Cherr GS, et al. Role of simple and complex hybrid revascularization procedures for symptomatic lower extremity occlusive disease. J Vasc Surg. 2010;51(6):1425-1435 e1. PMID: 20488323.

74. Hoshino J, Fujimoto Y, Naruse Y, et al. Characteristics of revascularization treatment for arteriosclerosis obliterans in patients with and without hemodialysis. Circ J. 2010;74(11):2426-33. PMID: 20938099.

75. Hynes N, Akhtar Y, Manning B, et al. Subintimal angioplasty as a primary modality in the management of critical limb ischemia: comparison to bypass grafting for aortoiliac and femoropopliteal occlusive disease. J Endovasc Ther. 2004;11(4):460-71. PMID: 15298498.

76. Janne d'Othee B, Morris MF, Powell RJ, et al. Cost determinants of percutaneous and surgical interventions for treatment of intermittent claudication from the perspective of the hospital. Cardiovasc Intervent Radiol. 2008;31(1):56-65. PMID: 17973158.

77. Jerabek J, Dvorak M, Vojtisek B. Results of therapy of lower extremity ischemic disease by angiosurgery and radiointervention (PTA) methods. Bratisl Lek Listy. 2003;104(10):314-6. PMID: 15055731.

78. Johnson BF, Singh S, Evans L, et al. A prospective study of the effect of limb-threatening ischaemia and its surgical treatment on the quality of life. Eur J Vasc Endovasc Surg. 1997;13(3):306-14. PMID: 9129605.

79. Kashyap VS, Pavkov ML, Bena JF, et al. The management of severe aortoiliac occlusive disease: endovascular therapy rivals open reconstruction. J Vasc Surg. 2008;48(6):1451-7, 1457 e1-3. PMID: 18804943.

80. Khan MU, Lall P, Harris LM, et al. Predictors of limb loss despite a patent endovascular-treated arterial segment. J Vasc Surg. 2009;49(6):1440-5; discussion 1445-6. PMID: 19497503.

81. Korhonen M, Biancari F, Soderstrom M, et al. Femoropopliteal balloon angioplasty vs. bypass surgery for CLI: a propensity score analysis. Eur J Vasc Endovasc Surg. 2011;41(3):378-84. PMID: 21195637.

82. Kudo T, Chandra FA, Kwun WH, et al. Changing pattern of surgical revascularization for critical limb ischemia over 12 years: endovascular vs. open bypass surgery. J Vasc Surg. 2006;44(2):304-13. PMID: 16890859.

83. Laurila J, Brommels M, Standertskjold-Nordenstam CG, et al. Cost-effectiveness of Percutaneous Transluminal Angioplasty (PTA) Versus Vascular Surgery in Limb-threatening Ischaemia. Int J Angiol. 2000;9(4):214-219. PMID: 11062310.

84. Lepantalo M, Laurila K, Roth WD, et al. PTFE bypass or thrupass for superficial femoral artery occlusion? A randomised controlled trial. Eur J Vasc Endovasc Surg. 2009;37(5):578-84. PMID: 19231250.

85. Loor G, Skelly CL, Wahlgren CM, et al. Is atherectomy the best first-line therapy for limb salvage in patients with critical limb ischemia? Vasc Endovascular Surg. 2009;43(6):542-50. PMID: 19640919.

86. McQuade K, Gable D, Hohman S, et al. Randomized comparison of ePTFE/nitinol self-expanding stent graft vs prosthetic femoral-popliteal bypass in the treatment of superficial femoral artery occlusive disease. J Vasc Surg. 2009;49(1):109-15, 116 e1-9; discussion 116. PMID: 19028055.

87. McQuade K, Gable D, Pearl G, et al. Four-year randomized prospective comparison of percutaneous ePTFE/nitinol self-expanding stent graft versus prosthetic femoral-popliteal bypass in the treatment of superficial femoral artery occlusive disease. J Vasc Surg. 2010;52(3):584-90; discussion 590-1, 591 e1-591 e7. PMID: 20598480.

88. Kedora J, Hohmann S, Garrett W, et al. Randomized comparison of percutaneous Viabahn stent grafts vs prosthetic femoral-popliteal bypass in the treatment of superficial femoral arterial occlusive disease. J Vasc Surg. 2007;45(1):10-6; discussion 16. PMID: 17126520.

89. Rossi E, Citterio F, Castagneto M, et al. Safety of endovascular treatment in high-cardiac-risk patients with limb-threatening ischemia. Angiology. 1998;49(6):435-40. PMID: 9631888.

90. Sachs T, Pomposelli F, Hamdan A, et al. Trends in the national outcomes and costs for claudication and limb threatening ischemia: Angioplasty vs bypass graft. J Vasc Surg. 2011;54(4):1021-1031 e1. PMID: 21880457.

91. Soderstrom MI, Arvela EM, Korhonen M, et al. Infrapopliteal percutaneous transluminal angioplasty versus bypass surgery as first-line strategies in critical leg ischemia: a propensity score analysis. Ann Surg. 2010;252(5):765-73. PMID: 21037432.

92. Stoner MC, Defreitas DJ, Manwaring MM, et al. Cost per day of patency: understanding the impact of patency and reintervention in a sustainable model of healthcare. J Vasc Surg. 2008;48(6):1489-96. PMID: 18829227.

93. Sultan S, Hynes N. Five-year Irish trial of CLI patients with TASC II type C/D lesions undergoing subintimal angioplasty or bypass surgery based on plaque echolucency. J Endovasc Ther. 2009;16(3):270-83. PMID: 19642779.

94. Sultan S, Hynes N. Mid-term results of subintimal angioplasty for critical limb ischemia 5-year outcomes. Vasc Dis Manage. 2011;8(9):E155-E163. PMID:

95. Taylor SM, Kalbaugh CA, Blackhurst DW, et al. Postoperative outcomes according to preoperative medical and functional status after infrainguinal revascularization for critical limb ischemia in patients 80 years and older. Am Surg. 2005;71(8):640-5; discussion 645-6. PMID: 16217945.

96. Taylor SM, Kalbaugh CA, Blackhurst DW, et al. Determinants of functional outcome after revascularization for critical limb ischemia: an analysis of 1000 consecutive vascular interventions. J Vasc Surg. 2006;44(4):747-55; discussion 755-6. PMID: 16926083.

97. Taylor SM, York JW, Cull DL, et al. Clinical success using patient-oriented outcome measures after lower extremity bypass and endovascular intervention for ischemic tissue loss. J Vasc Surg. 2009;50(3):534-41; discussion 541. PMID: 19592193.

98. Timaran CH, Ohki T, Gargiulo NJ, 3rd, et al. Iliac artery stenting in patients with poor distal runoff: Influence of concomitant infrainguinal arterial reconstruction. J Vasc Surg. 2003;38(3):479-84; discussion 484-5. PMID: 12947261.

99. Timaran CH, Prault TL, Stevens SL, et al. Iliac artery stenting versus surgical reconstruction for TASC (TransAtlantic Inter-Society Consensus) type B and type C iliac lesions. J Vasc Surg. 2003;38(2):272-8. PMID: 12891108.

100. Varela C, Acin F, De Haro J, et al. Influence of surgical or endovascular distal revascularization of the lower limbs on ischemic ulcer healing. J Cardiovasc Surg (Torino). 2011;52(3):381-9. PMID: 21577193.

101. Venermo M, Biancari F, Arvela E, et al. The role of chronic kidney disease as a predictor of outcome after revascularisation of the ulcerated diabetic foot. Diabetologia. 2011. PMID: 21845468.

102. Whatling PJ, Gibson M, Torrie EP, et al. Iliac occlusions: stenting or crossover grafting? An examination of patency and cost. Eur J Vasc Endovasc Surg. 2000;20(1):36-40. PMID: 10906295.

103. Wolfle KD, Bruijnen H, Reeps C, et al. Tibioperoneal arterial lesions and critical foot ischaemia: successful management by the use of short vein grafts and percutaneous transluminal angioplasty. Vasa. 2000;29(3):207-14. PMID: 11037720.

104. Zdanowski Z, Troeng T, Norgren L. Outcome and influence of age after infrainguinal revascularisation in critical limb ischaemia. The Swedish Vascular Registry. Eur J Vasc Endovasc Surg. 1998;16(2):137-41. PMID: 9728433.

Appendix D. Included Studies

Adam DJ, Beard JD, Cleveland T, et al. Bypass versus angioplasty in severe ischaemia of the leg (BASIL): multicentre, randomised controlled trial. Lancet. 2005;366(9501):1925-34. PMID: 16325694.

Ah Chong AK, Tan CB, Wong MW, et al. Bypass surgery or percutaneous transluminal angioplasty to treat critical lower limb ischaemia due to infrainguinal arterial occlusive disease? Hong Kong Med J. 2009;15(4):249-54. PMID: 19652230.

Anonymous. A randomised, blinded, trial of clopidogrel versus aspirin in patients at risk of ischaemic events (CAPRIE). CAPRIE Steering Committee. Lancet. 1996;348(9038):1329-39. PMID: 8918275.

Beebe HG, Dawson DL, Cutler BS, et al. A new pharmacological treatment for intermittent claudication: results of a randomized, multicenter trial. Arch Intern Med. 1999;159(17):2041-50. PMID: 10510990.

Belcaro G, Nicolaides AN, Griffin M, et al. Intermittent claudication in diabetics: treatment with exercise and pentoxifylline--a 6-month, controlled, randomized trial. Angiology. 2002;53(Suppl 1):S39-43. PMID: 11865835.

Belch J, Maccuish A, Campbell I, et al. The prevention of progression of arterial disease and diabetes (POPADAD) trial: factorial randomised placebo controlled trial of aspirin and antioxidants in patients with diabetes and asymptomatic peripheral arterial disease. BMJ. 2008;337:a1840. PMID: 18927173.

Belch JJ, Dormandy J, Biasi GM, et al. Results of the randomized, placebo-controlled clopidogrel and acetylsalicylic acid in bypass surgery for peripheral arterial disease (CASPAR) trial. J Vasc Surg. 2010;52(4):825-33, 833.e1-2. PMID: 20678878.

Berger PB, Bhatt DL, Fuster V, et al. Bleeding complications with dual antiplatelet therapy among patients with stable vascular disease or risk factors for vascular disease: results from the Clopidogrel for High Atherothrombotic Risk and Ischemic Stabilization, Management, and Avoidance (CHARISMA) trial. Circulation. 2010;121(23):2575-83. PMID: 20516378.

Bhatt DL, Flather MD, Hacke W, et al. Patients with prior myocardial infarction, stroke, or symptomatic peripheral arterial disease in the CHARISMA trial. J Am Coll Cardiol. 2007;49(19):1982-8. PMID: 17498584.

Bhatt DL, Fox KA, Hacke W, et al. Clopidogrel and aspirin versus aspirin alone for the prevention of atherothrombotic events. N Engl J Med. 2006;354(16):1706-17. PMID: 16531616.

Bradbury AW, Adam DJ, Bell J, et al. Bypass versus Angioplasty in Severe Ischaemia of the Leg (BASIL) trial: A description of the severity and extent of disease using the Bollinger angiogram scoring method and the TransAtlantic Inter-Society Consensus II classification. J Vasc Surg. 2010;51(5 Suppl):32S-42S. PMID: 20435260.

Bradbury AW, Adam DJ, Bell J, et al. Bypass versus Angioplasty in Severe Ischaemia of the Leg (BASIL) trial: A survival prediction model to facilitate clinical decision making. J Vasc Surg. 2010;51(5 Suppl):52S-68S. PMID: 20435262.

Bradbury AW, Adam DJ, Bell J, et al. Bypass versus Angioplasty in Severe Ischaemia of the Leg (BASIL) trial: An intention-to-treat analysis of amputation-free and overall survival in patients randomized to a bypass surgery-first or a balloon angioplasty-first revascularization strategy. J Vasc Surg. 2010;51(5 Suppl):5S-17S. PMID: 20435258.

Bradbury AW, Adam DJ, Bell J, et al. Bypass versus Angioplasty in Severe Ischaemia of the Leg (BASIL) trial: Analysis of amputation free and overall survival by treatment received. J Vasc Surg. 2010;51(5 Suppl):18S-31S. PMID: 20435259.

Bradbury AW, Adam DJ, Bell J, et al. Multicentre randomised controlled trial of the clinical and cost-effectiveness of a bypass-surgery-first versus a balloon-angioplasty-first revascularisation strategy for severe limb ischaemia due to infrainguinal disease. The Bypass versus Angioplasty in Severe Ischaemia of the Leg (BASIL) trial. Health Technol Assess. 2010;14(14):1-210, iii-iv. PMID: 20307380.

Bronas UG, Treat-Jacobson D, Leon AS. Comparison of the effect of upper body-ergometry aerobic training vs treadmill training on central cardiorespiratory improvement and walking distance in patients with claudication. J Vasc Surg. 2011;53(6):1557-64. PMID: 21515017.

Cacoub PP, Bhatt DL, Steg PG, et al. Patients with peripheral arterial disease in the CHARISMA trial. Eur Heart J. 2009;30(2):192-201. PMID: 19136484.

Cassar K, Ford I, Greaves M, et al. Randomized clinical trial of the antiplatelet effects of aspirin-clopidogrel combination versus aspirin alone after lower limb angioplasty. Br J Surg. 2005;92(2):159-65. PMID: 15609386.

Catalano M, Born G, Peto R. Prevention of serious vascular events by aspirin amongst patients with peripheral arterial disease: randomized, double-blind trial. J Intern Med. 2007;261(3):276-84. PMID: 17305650.

Cesarone MR, Belcaro G, Nicolaides AN, et al. Treatment of severe intermittent claudication with pentoxifylline: a 40-week, controlled, randomized trial. Angiology. 2002;53(Suppl 1):S1-5. PMID: 11865828.

Crowther RG, Spinks WL, Leicht AS, et al. Effects of a long-term exercise program on lower limb mobility, physiological responses, walking performance, and physical activity levels in patients with peripheral arterial disease. J Vasc Surg. 2008;47(2):303-9. PMID: 18241753.

Dawson DL, Cutler BS, Hiatt WR, et al. A comparison of cilostazol and pentoxifylline for treating intermittent claudication. Am J Med. 2000;109(7):523-30. PMID: 11063952.

Dawson DL, Cutler BS, Meissner MH, et al. Cilostazol has beneficial effects in treatment of intermittent claudication: results from a multicenter, randomized, prospective, double-blind trial. Circulation. 1998;98(7):678-86. PMID: 9715861.

De Sanctis MT, Cesarone MR, Belcaro G, et al. Treatment of intermittent claudication with pentoxifylline: a 12-month, randomized trial--walking distance and microcirculation. Angiology. 2002;53(Suppl 1):S7-12. PMID: 11865838.

De Sanctis MT, Cesarone MR, Belcaro G, et al. Treatment of long-distance intermittent claudication with pentoxifylline: a 12-month, randomized trial. Angiology. 2002;53(Suppl 1):S13-7. PMID: 11865829.

Dorigo W, Pulli R, Marek J, et al. A comparison between open and endovascular repair in the treatment of critical limb ischemia. Ital J Vasc Endovasc Surg. 2009;16(1):17-22.

Dosluoglu HH, Lall P, Cherr GS, et al. Role of simple and complex hybrid revascularization procedures for symptomatic lower extremity occlusive disease. J Vasc Surg. 2010;51(6):1425-35.e1. PMID: 20488323.

Dosluoglu HH, Lall P, Harris LM, et al. Long-term limb salvage and survival after endovascular and open revascularization for critical limb ischemia after adoption of endovascular-first approach by vascular surgeons. J Vasc Surg. 2012;56(2):361-71. PMID: 22560307.

Drozdz W, Panek J, Lejman W. Red cell deformability in patients with chronic atheromatous ischemia of the legs. Med Sci Monit. 2001;7(5):933-9. PMID: 11535938.

Faglia E, Clerici G, Losa S, et al. Limb revascularization feasibility in diabetic patients with critical limb ischemia: results from a cohort of 344 consecutive unselected diabetic patients evaluated in 2009. Diabetes Res Clin Pract. 2012;95(3):364-71. PMID: 22104261.

Feinglass J, Mccarthy WJ, Slavensky R, et al. Functional status and walking ability after lower extremity bypass grafting or angioplasty for intermittent claudication: results from a prospective outcomes study. J Vasc Surg. 2000;31(1 Pt 1):93-103. PMID: 10642712.

Forbes JF, Adam DJ, Bell J, et al. Bypass versus Angioplasty in Severe Ischaemia of the Leg (BASIL) trial: Health-related quality of life outcomes, resource utilization, and cost-effectiveness analysis. J Vasc Surg. 2010;51(5 Suppl):43S-51S. PMID: 20435261.

Fowkes FG, Price JF, Stewart MC, et al. Aspirin for prevention of cardiovascular events in a general population screened for a low ankle brachial index: a randomized controlled trial. JAMA. 2010;303(9):841-8. PMID: 20197530.

Gardner AW, Katzel LI, Sorkin JD, et al. Effects of long-term exercise rehabilitation on claudication distances in patients with peripheral arterial disease: a randomized controlled trial. J Cardiopulm Rehabil. 2002;22(3):192-8. PMID: 12042688.

Gardner AW, Parker DE, Montgomery PS, et al. Efficacy of quantified home-based exercise and supervised exercise in patients with intermittent claudication: a randomized controlled trial. Circulation. 2011;123(5):491-8. PMID: 21262997.

Gelin J, Jivegard L, Taft C, et al. Treatment efficacy of intermittent claudication by surgical intervention, supervised physical exercise training compared to no treatment in unselected randomised patients I: one year results of functional and physiological improvements. Eur J Vasc Endovasc Surg. 2001;22(2):107-13. PMID: 11472042.

Gibellini R, Fanello M, Bardile AF, et al. Exercise training in intermittent claudication. Int Angiol. 2000;19(1):8-13. PMID: 10853679.

Giugliano G, Di Serafino L, Perrino C, et al. Effects of successful percutaneous lower extremity revascularization on cardiovascular outcome in patients with peripheral arterial disease. Int J Cardiol. 2012. PMID: 22790191.

Greenhalgh RM, Belch JJ, Brown LC, et al. The adjuvant benefit of angioplasty in patients with mild to moderate intermittent claudication (MIMIC) managed by supervised exercise, smoking cessation advice and best medical therapy: results from two randomised trials for stenotic femoropopliteal and aortoiliac arterial disease. Eur J Vasc Endovasc Surg. 2008;36(6):680-8. PMID: 19022184.

Hiatt WR, Money SR, Brass EP. Long-term safety of cilostazol in patients with peripheral artery disease: the CASTLE study (Cilostazol: A Study in Long-term Effects). J Vasc Surg. 2008;47(2):330-6. PMID: 18155871.

Hobbs SD, Marshall T, Fegan C, et al. The constitutive procoagulant and hypofibrinolytic state in patients with intermittent claudication due to infrainguinal disease significantly improves with percutaneous transluminal balloon angioplasty. J Vasc Surg. 2006;43(1):40-6. PMID: 16414385.

Hobbs SD, Marshall T, Fegan C, et al. The effect of supervised exercise and cilostazol on coagulation and fibrinolysis in intermittent claudication: a randomized controlled trial. J Vasc Surg. 2007;45(1):65-70; discussion 70. PMID: 17210383.

Horrocks M, Horrocks EH, Murphy P, et al. The effects of platelet inhibitors on platelet uptake and restenosis after femoral angioplasty. Int Angiol. 1997;16(2):101-6. PMID: 9257670.

Hoshino J, Fujimoto Y, Naruse Y, et al. Characteristics of revascularization treatment for arteriosclerosis obliterans in patients with and without hemodialysis. Circ J. 2010;74(11):2426-33. PMID: 20938099.

Hynes N, Akhtar Y, Manning B, et al. Subintimal angioplasty as a primary modality in the management of critical limb ischemia: comparison to bypass grafting for aortoiliac and femoropopliteal occlusive disease. J Endovasc Ther. 2004;11(4):460-71. PMID: 15298498.

Janne D'othee B, Morris MF, Powell RJ, et al. Cost determinants of percutaneous and surgical interventions for treatment of intermittent claudication from the perspective of the hospital. Cardiovasc Intervent Radiol. 2008;31(1):56-65. PMID: 17973158.

Jerabek J, Dvorak M, Vojtisek B. Results of therapy of lower extremity ischemic disease by angiosurgery and radiointervention (PTA) methods. Bratisl Lek Listy. 2003;104(10):314-6. PMID: 15055731.

Johnson BF, Singh S, Evans L, et al. A prospective study of the effect of limb-threatening ischaemia and its surgical treatment on the quality of life. Eur J Vasc Endovasc Surg. 1997;13(3):306-14. PMID: 9129605.

Kamiya C, Sakamoto S, Tamori Y, et al. Long-term outcome after percutaneous peripheral intervention vs medical treatment for patients with superficial femoral artery occlusive disease. Circ J. 2008;72(5):734-9. PMID: 18441452.

Kashyap VS, Pavkov ML, Bena JF, et al. The management of severe aortoiliac occlusive disease: endovascular therapy rivals open reconstruction. J Vasc Surg. 2008;48(6):1451-7, 1457.e1-3. PMID: 18804943.

Kedora J, Hohmann S, Garrett W, et al. Randomized comparison of percutaneous Viabahn stent grafts vs prosthetic femoral-popliteal bypass in the treatment of superficial femoral arterial occlusive disease. J Vasc Surg. 2007;45(1):10-6; discussion 16. PMID: 17126520.

Khan MU, Lall P, Harris LM, et al. Predictors of limb loss despite a patent endovascular-treated arterial segment. J Vasc Surg. 2009;49(6):1440-5; discussion 1445-6. PMID: 19497503.

Koivunen K, Lukkarinen H. One-year prospective health-related quality-of-life outcomes in patients treated with conservative method, endovascular treatment or open surgery for symptomatic lower limb atherosclerotic disease. Eur J Cardiovasc Nurs. 2008;7(3):247-56. PMID: 18221916.

Korhonen M, Biancari F, Soderstrom M, et al. Femoropopliteal balloon angioplasty vs. bypass surgery for CLI: a propensity score analysis. Eur J Vasc Endovasc Surg. 2011;41(3):378-84. PMID: 21195637.

Kruidenier LM, Nicolai SP, Rouwet EV, et al. Additional supervised exercise therapy after a percutaneous vascular intervention for peripheral arterial disease: a randomized clinical trial. J Vasc Interv Radiol. 2011;22(7):961-8. PMID: 21571547.

Kudo T, Chandra FA, Kwun WH, et al. Changing pattern of surgical revascularization for critical limb ischemia over 12 years: endovascular vs. open bypass surgery. J Vasc Surg. 2006;44(2):304-13. PMID: 16890859.

Laurila J, Brommels M, Standertskjold-Nordenstam CG, et al. Cost-effectiveness of Percutaneous Transluminal Angioplasty (PTA) Versus Vascular Surgery in Limb-threatening Ischaemia. Int J Angiol. 2000;9(4):214-9. PMID: 11062310.

Lawall H, Gorriahn H, Amendt K, et al. Long-term outcomes after medical and interventional therapy of critical limb ischemia. Eur J Intern Med. 2009;20(6):616-21. PMID: 19782924.

Lee HL, Mehta T, Ray B, et al. A non-randomised controlled trial of the clinical and cost effectiveness of a Supervised Exercise Programme for claudication. Eur J Vasc Endovasc Surg. 2007;33(2):202-7. PMID: 17142065.

Lepantalo M, Laurila K, Roth WD, et al. PTFE bypass or thrupass for superficial femoral artery occlusion? A randomised controlled trial. Eur J Vasc Endovasc Surg. 2009;37(5):578-84. PMID: 19231250.

Loor G, Skelly CL, Wahlgren CM, et al. Is atherectomy the best first-line therapy for limb salvage in patients with critical limb ischemia? Vasc Endovascular Surg. 2009;43(6):542-50. PMID: 19640919.

Mahmood A, Sintler M, Edwards AT, et al. The efficacy of aspirin in patients undergoing infra-inguinal bypass and identification of high risk patients. Int Angiol. 2003;22(3):302-7. PMID: 14612858.

Mazari FA, Gulati S, Rahman MN, et al. Early outcomes from a randomized, controlled trial of supervised exercise, angioplasty, and combined therapy in intermittent claudication. Ann Vasc Surg. 2010;24(1):69-79. PMID: 19762206.

Mazari FA, Khan JA, Carradice D, et al. Randomized clinical trial of percutaneous transluminal angioplasty, supervised exercise and combined treatment for intermittent claudication due to femoropopliteal arterial disease. Br J Surg. 2012;99(1):39-48. PMID: 22021102.

McQuade K, Gable D, Hohman S, et al. Randomized comparison of ePTFE/nitinol self-expanding stent graft vs prosthetic femoral-popliteal bypass in the treatment of superficial femoral artery occlusive disease. J Vasc Surg. 2009;49(1):109-15, 116.e1-9; discussion 116. PMID: 19028055.

McQuade K, Gable D, Pearl G, et al. Four-year randomized prospective comparison of percutaneous ePTFE/nitinol self-expanding stent graft versus prosthetic femoral-popliteal bypass in the treatment of superficial femoral artery occlusive disease. J Vasc Surg. 2010;52(3):584-90; discussion 590-1, 591.e1-591.e7. PMID: 20598480.

Minar E, Ahmadi A, Koppensteiner R, et al. Comparison of effects of high-dose and low-dose aspirin on restenosis after femoropopliteal percutaneous transluminal angioplasty. Circulation. 1995;91(8):2167-73. PMID: 7697845.

Money SR, Herd JA, Isaacsohn JL, et al. Effect of cilostazol on walking distances in patients with intermittent claudication caused by peripheral vascular disease. J Vasc Surg. 1998;27(2):267-74; discussion 274-5. PMID: 9510281.

Mori E, Komori K, Kume M, et al. Comparison of the long-term results between surgical and conservative treatment in patients with intermittent claudication. Surgery. 2002. 131(1 Suppl):S269-74. PMID: 11821823.

Murphy TP, Cutlip DE, Regensteiner JG, et al. Supervised exercise versus primary stenting for claudication resulting from aortoiliac peripheral artery disease: six-month outcomes from the claudication: exercise versus endoluminal revascularization (CLEVER) study. Circulation. 2012;125(1):130-9. PMID: 22090168.

Nordanstig J, Gelin J, Hensater M, et al. Walking performance and health-related quality of life after surgical or endovascular invasive versus non-invasive treatment for intermittent claudication--a prospective randomised trial. Eur J Vasc Endovasc Surg. 2011;42(2):220-7. PMID: 21397530.

Nylaende M, Abdelnoor M, Stranden E, et al. The Oslo balloon angioplasty versus conservative treatment study (OBACT)--the 2-years results of a single centre, prospective, randomised study in patients with intermittent claudication. Eur J Vasc Endovasc Surg. 2007;33(1):3-12. PMID: 17055756.

Nylaende M, Kroese AJ, Morken B, et al. Beneficial effects of 1-year optimal medical treatment with and without additional PTA on inflammatory markers of atherosclerosis in patients with PAD. Results from the Oslo Balloon Angioplasty versus Conservative Treatment (OBACT) study. Vasc Med. 2007;12(4):275-83. PMID: 18048463.

Pell JP, Lee AJ. Impact of angioplasty and arterial reconstructive surgery on the quality of life of claudicants. The Scottish Vascular Audit Group. Scott Med J. 1997;42(2):47-8. PMID: 9507581.

Perkins JM, Collin J, Creasy TS, et al. Exercise training versus angioplasty for stable claudication. Long and medium term results of a prospective, randomised trial. Eur J Vasc Endovasc Surg. 1996;11(4):409-13. PMID: 8846172.

Rossi E, Citterio F, Castagneto M, et al. Safety of endovascular treatment in high-cardiac-risk patients with limb-threatening ischemia. Angiology. 1998;49(6):435-40. PMID: 9631888.

Sachs T, Pomposelli F, Hamdan A, et al. Trends in the national outcomes and costs for claudication and limb threatening ischemia: Angioplasty vs bypass graft. J Vasc Surg. 2011;54(4):1021-31.e1. PMID: 21880457.

Soderstrom MI, Arvela EM, Korhonen M, et al. Infrapopliteal percutaneous transluminal angioplasty versus bypass surgery as first-line strategies in critical leg ischemia: a propensity score analysis. Ann Surg. 2010;252(5):765-73. PMID: 21037432.

Soga Y, Yokoi H, Kawasaki T, et al. Efficacy of cilostazol after endovascular therapy for femoropopliteal artery disease in patients with intermittent claudication. J Am Coll Cardiol. 2009;53(1):48-53. PMID: 19118724.

Spronk S, Bosch JL, Den Hoed PT, et al. Cost-effectiveness of endovascular revascularization compared to supervised hospital-based exercise training in patients with intermittent claudication: a randomized controlled trial. J Vasc Surg. 2008;48(6):1472-80. PMID: 18771879.

Spronk S, Bosch JL, Den Hoed PT, et al. Intermittent claudication: clinical effectiveness of endovascular revascularization versus supervised hospital-based exercise training--randomized controlled trial. Radiology. 2009;250(2):586-95. PMID: 19188327.

Stone WM, Demaerschalk BM, Fowl RJ, et al. Type 3 phosphodiesterase inhibitors may be protective against cerebrovascular events in patients with claudication. J Stroke Cerebrovasc Dis. 2008;17(3):129-33. PMID: 18436153.

Stoner MC, Defreitas DJ, Manwaring MM, et al. Cost per day of patency: understanding the impact of patency and reintervention in a sustainable model of healthcare. J Vasc Surg. 2008;48(6):1489-96. PMID: 18829227.

Strandness DE, Jr., Dalman RL, Panian S, et al. Effect of cilostazol in patients with intermittent claudication: a randomized, double-blind, placebo-controlled study. Vasc Endovascular Surg. 2002;36(2):83-91. PMID: 11951094.

Sugimoto I, Ohta T, Ishibashi H, et al. Conservative treatment for patients with intermittent claudication. Int Angiol. 2010;29(2 Suppl):55-60. PMID: 20357750.

Sultan S, Hynes N. Five-year Irish trial of CLI patients with TASC II type C/D lesions undergoing subintimal angioplasty or bypass surgery based on plaque echolucency. J Endovasc Ther. 2009;16(3):270-83. PMID: 19642779.

Sultan S, Hynes N. Mid-term results of subintimal angioplasty for critical limb ischemia 5-year outcomes. Vasc Dis Manage. 2011;8(9):E155-63.

Taft C, Karlsson J, Gelin J, et al. Treatment efficacy of intermittent claudication by invasive therapy, supervised physical exercise training compared to no treatment in unselected randomised patients II: one-year results of health-related quality of life. Eur J Vasc Endovasc Surg. 2001;22(2):114-23. PMID: 11472043.

Taylor SM, Kalbaugh CA, Blackhurst DW, et al. Determinants of functional outcome after revascularization for critical limb ischemia: an analysis of 1000 consecutive vascular interventions. J Vasc Surg. 2006;44(4):747-55; discussion 755-6. PMID: 16926083.

Taylor SM, Kalbaugh CA, Blackhurst DW, et al. Postoperative outcomes according to preoperative medical and functional status after infrainguinal revascularization for critical limb ischemia in patients 80 years and older. Am Surg. 2005;71(8):640-5; discussion 645-6. PMID: 16217945.

Taylor SM, York JW, Cull DL, et al. Clinical success using patient-oriented outcome measures after lower extremity bypass and endovascular intervention for ischemic tissue loss. J Vasc Surg. 2009;50(3):534-41; discussion 541. PMID: 19592193.

Tepe G, Bantleon R, Brechtel K, et al. Management of peripheral arterial interventions with mono or dual antiplatelet therapy-the MIRROR study: a randomised and double-blinded clinical trial. Eur Radiol. 2012;22(9):1998-2006. PMID: 22569995.

Timaran CH, Ohki T, Gargiulo NJ, 3rd, et al. Iliac artery stenting in patients with poor distal runoff: Influence of concomitant infrainguinal arterial reconstruction. J Vasc Surg. 2003;38(3):479-84; discussion 484-5. PMID: 12947261.

Timaran CH, Prault TL, Stevens SL, et al. Iliac artery stenting versus surgical reconstruction for TASC (TransAtlantic Inter-Society Consensus) type B and type C iliac lesions. J Vasc Surg. 2003;38(2):272-8. PMID: 12891108.

Treat-Jacobson D, Bronas UG, Leon AS. Efficacy of arm-ergometry versus treadmill exercise training to improve walking distance in patients with claudication. Vasc Med. 2009;14(3):203-13. PMID: 19651669.

Tsai JC, Chan P, Wang CH, et al. The effects of exercise training on walking function and perception of health status in elderly patients with peripheral arterial occlusive disease. J Intern Med. 2002;252(5):448-55. PMID: 12528763.

Varela C, Acin F, De Haro J, et al. Influence of surgical or endovascular distal revascularization of the lower limbs on ischemic ulcer healing. J Cardiovasc Surg (Torino). 2011;52(3):381-9. PMID: 21577193.

Varty K, Nydahl S, Butterworth P, et al. Changes in the management of critical limb ischaemia. Br J Surg. 1996;83(7):953-6. PMID: 8813785.

Varty K, Nydahl S, Nasim A, et al. Results of surgery and angioplasty for the treatment of chronic severe lower limb ischaemia. Eur J Vasc Endovasc Surg. 1998;16(2):159-63. PMID: 9728437.

Venermo M, Biancari F, Arvela E, et al. The role of chronic kidney disease as a predictor of outcome after revascularisation of the ulcerated diabetic foot. Diabetologia. 2011;54(12):2971-7. PMID: 21845468.

Whatling PJ, Gibson M, Torrie EP, et al. Iliac occlusions: stenting or crossover grafting? An examination of patency and cost. Eur J Vasc Endovasc Surg. 2000;20(1):36-40. PMID: 10906295.

Whyman MR, Fowkes FG, Kerracher EM, et al. Is intermittent claudication improved by percutaneous transluminal angioplasty? A randomized controlled trial. J Vasc Surg. 1997;26(4):551-7. PMID: 9357454.

Whyman MR, Fowkes FG, Kerracher EM, et al. Randomised controlled trial of percutaneous transluminal angioplasty for intermittent claudication. Eur J Vasc Endovasc Surg. 1996;12(2):167-72. PMID: 8760978.

Wolfle KD, Bruijnen H, Reeps C, et al. Tibioperoneal arterial lesions and critical foot ischaemia: successful management by the use of short vein grafts and percutaneous transluminal angioplasty. Vasa. 2000;29(3):207-14. PMID: 11037720.

Zdanowski Z, Troeng T, Norgren L. Outcome and influence of age after infrainguinal revascularisation in critical limb ischaemia. The Swedish Vascular Registry. Eur J Vasc Endovasc Surg. 1998;16(2):137-41. PMID: 9728433.

Study Groupings

Table D-1 presents a key to the primary and companion articles included in this report, organized alphabetically by study designation (if applicable). A full reference list follows the table.

Table D-1. Primary articles and companion articles

Study Designation	Primary Abstracted Article	Companion Articles
BASIL	Adam, 2005[1]	Bradbury, 2010[2] Bradbury, 2010[3] Bradbury, 2010[4] Bradbury, 2010[5] Bradbury, 2010[6] Forbes, 2010[7]
CAPRIE	Anonymous, 1996[8]	None
CASPAR	Belch, 2010[9]	None
CASTLE	Hiatt, 2008[10]	Stone, 2008[11]
CHARISMA	Cacoub, 2009[12]	Bhatt, 2007[13] Bhatt, 2006[14] Berger, 2010[15]
CLEVER	Murphy, 2012[16]	None
CLIPS	Catalano, 2007[17]	None
EXACT	Hobbs, 2006[18]	None
INEXACT	Hobbs, 2007[19]	None
MIMIC	Greenhalgh, 2008[20]	None
OBACT	Nylaende, 2007[21]	Nylaende, 2007[22]
POPADAD	Belch, 2008[23]	None
None	Ah Chong, 2009[24]	None
None	Beebe, 1999[25]	None
None	Belcaro, 2002[26]	None
None	Cassar, 2005[27]	None
None	Crowther, 2008[28]	None
None	Dawson, 1998[29]	None
None	Dawson, 2000[30]	None
None	De Sanctis, 2002[31]	De Sanctis, 2002[32] Cesarone, 2002[33]
None	Dorigo, 2009[34]	None
None	Dosluoglu, 2010[35]	None
None	Dosluoglu, 2012[36]	None

Study Designation	Primary Abstracted Article	Companion Articles
None	Drozdz, 2001[37]	None
None	Faglia, 2012[38]	None
None	Feinglass, 2000[39]	None
None	Fowkes, 2010[40]	None
None	Gardner, 2002[41]	None
None	Gardner, 2011[42]	None
None	Gelin, 2001[43]	Taft, 2001[44]
None	Gibellini, 2000[45]	None
None	Guigliano, 2012[46]	None
None	Horrocks, 1997[47]	None
None	Hoshino, 2010[48]	None
None	Hynes, 2004[49]	None
None	Janne d'Othee, 2008[50]	None
None	Jerabek, 2003[51]	None
None	Johnson, 1997[52]	None
None	Kamiya, 2008[53]	None
None	Kashyap, 2008[54]	None
None	Khan, 2009[55]	None
None	Koivunen, 2008[56]	None
None	Korhonen, 2011[57]	None
None	Kruidenier, 2011[58]	None
None	Kudo, 2006[59]	None
None	Laurila, 2000[60]	None
None	Lawall, 2009[61]	None
None	Lee, 2007[62]	None
None	Lepantalo, 2009[63]	None
None	Loor, 2009[64]	None
None	Mahmood, 2003[65]	None
None	Mazari, 2012[66]	Mazari, 2010[67]
None	McQuade, 2009[68]	Kedora, 2007[69] McQuade, 2010[70]
None	Minar, 1995[71]	None
None	Money, 1998[72]	None
None	Mori, 2002[73]	None
None	Nordanstig, 2011[74]	None
None	Pell, 1997[75]	None
None	Perkins, 1996[76]	None
None	Rossi, 1998[77]	None
None	Sachs, 2011[78]	None
None	Soderstrom, 2010[79]	None
None	Soga, 2009[80]	None
None	Spronk, 2009[81]	Spronk, 2008[82]
None	Stoner, 2008[83]	None
None	Strandness, 2002[84]	None
None	Sugimoto, 2010[85]	None
None	Sultan, 2009[86]	Sultan, 2011[87]
None	Taylor, 2005[88]	None

Study Designation	Primary Abstracted Article	Companion Articles
None	Taylor, 2006[89]	None
None	Taylor, 2009[90]	None
None	Tepe, 2012[91]	None
None	Timaran, 2003[92]	None
None	Timaran, 2003[93]	None
None	Treat-Jacobson, 2009[94]	Bronas, 2011[95]
None	Tsai, 2002[96]	None
None	Varela, 2011[97]	None
None	Varty, 1996[98]	Varty, 1998[99]
None	Venermo, 2011[100]	None
None	Whatling, 2000[101]	None
None	Whyman, 1997[102]	Whyman, 1996[103]
None	Wolfle, 2000[104]	None
None	Zdanowski, 1998[105]	None

References Cited in Table D-1

1. Adam DJ, Beard JD, Cleveland T, et al. Bypass versus angioplasty in severe ischaemia of the leg (BASIL): multicentre, randomised controlled trial. Lancet. 2005;366(9501):1925-34. PMID: 16325694.

2. Bradbury AW, Adam DJ, Bell J, et al. Bypass versus Angioplasty in Severe Ischaemia of the Leg (BASIL) trial: A survival prediction model to facilitate clinical decision making. J Vasc Surg. 2010;51(5 Suppl):52S-68S. PMID: 20435262.

3. Bradbury AW, Adam DJ, Bell J, et al. Bypass versus Angioplasty in Severe Ischaemia of the Leg (BASIL) trial: A description of the severity and extent of disease using the Bollinger angiogram scoring method and the TransAtlantic Inter-Society Consensus II classification. J Vasc Surg. 2010;51(5 Suppl):32S-42S. PMID: 20435260.

4. Bradbury AW, Adam DJ, Bell J, et al. Bypass versus Angioplasty in Severe Ischaemia of the Leg (BASIL) trial: Analysis of amputation free and overall survival by treatment received. J Vasc Surg. 2010;51(5 Suppl):18S-31S. PMID: 20435259.

5. Bradbury AW, Adam DJ, Bell J, et al. Bypass versus Angioplasty in Severe Ischaemia of the Leg (BASIL) trial: An intention-to-treat analysis of amputation-free and overall survival in patients randomized to a bypass surgery-first or a balloon angioplasty-first revascularization strategy. J Vasc Surg. 2010;51(5 Suppl):5S-17S. PMID: 20435258.

6. Bradbury AW, Adam DJ, Bell J, et al. Multicentre randomised controlled trial of the clinical and cost-effectiveness of a bypass-surgery-first versus a balloon-angioplasty-first revascularisation strategy for severe limb ischaemia due to infrainguinal disease. The Bypass versus Angioplasty in Severe Ischaemia of the Leg (BASIL) trial. Health Technol Assess. 2010;14(14):1-210, iii-iv. PMID: 20307380.

7. Forbes JF, Adam DJ, Bell J, et al. Bypass versus Angioplasty in Severe Ischaemia of the Leg (BASIL) trial: Health-related quality of life outcomes, resource utilization, and cost-effectiveness analysis. J Vasc Surg. 2010;51(5 Suppl):43S-51S. PMID: 20435261.

8. Anonymous. A randomised, blinded, trial of clopidogrel versus aspirin in patients at risk of ischaemic events (CAPRIE). Lancet. 1996;348(9038):1329-39. PMID: 8918275.

9. Belch JJ, Dormandy J, Biasi GM, et al. Results of the randomized, placebo-controlled clopidogrel and acetylsalicylic acid in bypass surgery for peripheral arterial disease (CASPAR) trial. J Vasc Surg. 2010;52(4):825-33, 833 e1-2. PMID: 20678878.

10. Hiatt WR, Money SR, Brass EP. Long-term safety of cilostazol in patients with peripheral artery disease: the CASTLE study (Cilostazol: A Study in Long-term Effects). J Vasc Surg. 2008;47(2):330-336. PMID: 18155871.

11. Stone WM, Demaerschalk BM, Fowl RJ, et al. Type 3 phosphodiesterase inhibitors may be protective against cerebrovascular events in patients with claudication. J Stroke Cerebrovasc Dis. 2008;17(3):129-33. PMID: 18436153.

12. Cacoub PP, Bhatt DL, Steg PG, et al. Patients with peripheral arterial disease in the CHARISMA trial. Eur Heart J. 2009;30(2):192-201. PMID: 19136484.

13. Bhatt DL, Flather MD, Hacke W, et al. Patients with prior myocardial infarction, stroke, or symptomatic peripheral arterial disease in the CHARISMA trial. J Am Coll Cardiol. 2007;49(19):1982-8. PMID: 17498584.

14. Bhatt DL, Fox KA, Hacke W, et al. Clopidogrel and aspirin versus aspirin alone for the prevention of atherothrombotic events. N Engl J Med. 2006;354(16):1706-17. PMID: 16531616.

15. Berger PB, Bhatt DL, Fuster V, et al. Bleeding complications with dual antiplatelet therapy among patients with stable vascular disease or risk factors for vascular disease: results from the Clopidogrel for High Atherothrombotic Risk and Ischemic Stabilization, Management, and Avoidance (CHARISMA) trial. Circulation. 2010;121(23):2575-83. PMID: 20516378.

16. Murphy TP, Cutlip DE, Regensteiner JG, et al. Supervised exercise versus primary stenting for claudication resulting from aortoiliac peripheral artery disease: six-month outcomes from the claudication: exercise versus endoluminal revascularization (CLEVER) study. Circulation. 2012;125(1):130-9. PMID: 22090168.

17. Catalano M, Born G, Peto R. Prevention of serious vascular events by aspirin amongst patients with peripheral arterial disease: randomized, double-blind trial. J Intern Med. 2007;261(3):276-84. PMID: 17305650.

18. Hobbs SD, Marshall T, Fegan C, et al. The constitutive procoagulant and hypofibrinolytic state in patients with intermittent claudication due to infrainguinal disease significantly improves with percutaneous transluminal balloon angioplasty. J Vasc Surg. 2006;43(1):40-6. PMID: 16414385.

19. Hobbs SD, Marshall T, Fegan C, et al. The effect of supervised exercise and cilostazol on coagulation and fibrinolysis in intermittent claudication: a randomized controlled trial. J Vasc Surg. 2007;45(1):65-70; discussion 70. PMID: 17210383.

20. Greenhalgh RM, Belch JJ, Brown LC, et al. The adjuvant benefit of angioplasty in patients with mild to moderate intermittent claudication (MIMIC) managed by supervised exercise, smoking cessation advice and best medical therapy: results from two randomised trials for stenotic femoropopliteal and aortoiliac arterial disease. Eur J Vasc Endovasc Surg. 2008;36(6):680-8. PMID: 19022184.

21. Nylaende M, Abdelnoor M, Stranden E, et al. The Oslo balloon angioplasty versus conservative treatment study (OBACT)—The 2-years results of a single centre, prospective, randomised study in patients with intermittent claudication. Eur J Vasc Endovasc Surg. 2007;33(1):3-12. PMID: 17055756.

22. Nylaende M, Kroese AJ, Morken B, et al. Beneficial effects of 1-year optimal medical treatment with and without additional PTA on inflammatory markers of atherosclerosis in patients with PAD. Results from the Oslo Balloon Angioplasty versus Conservative Treatment (OBACT) study. Vasc Med. 2007;12(4):275-83. PMID: 18048463.

23. Belch J, MacCuish A, Campbell I, et al. The prevention of progression of arterial disease and diabetes (POPADAD) trial: factorial randomised placebo controlled trial of aspirin and antioxidants in patients with diabetes and asymptomatic peripheral arterial disease. BMJ. 2008;337:a1840. PMID: 18927173.

24. Ah Chong AK, Tan CB, Wong MW, et al. Bypass surgery or percutaneous transluminal angioplasty to treat critical lower limb ischaemia due to infrainguinal arterial occlusive disease? Hong Kong Med J. 2009;15(4):249-54. PMID: 19652230.

25. Beebe HG, Dawson DL, Cutler BS, et al. A new pharmacological treatment for intermittent claudication: results of a randomized, multicenter trial. Arch Intern Med. 1999;159(17):2041-50. PMID: 10510990.

26. Belcaro G, Nicolaides AN, Griffin M, et al. Intermittent claudication in diabetics: treatment with exercise and pentoxifylline--a 6-month, controlled, randomized trial. Angiology. 2002;53 Suppl 1:S39-43. PMID: 11865835.

27. Cassar K, Ford I, Greaves M, et al. Randomized clinical trial of the antiplatelet effects of aspirin-clopidogrel combination versus aspirin alone after lower limb angioplasty. Br J Surg. 2005;92(2):159-65. PMID: 15609386.

28. Crowther RG, Spinks WL, Leicht AS, et al. Effects of a long-term exercise program on lower limb mobility, physiological responses, walking performance, and physical activity levels in patients with peripheral arterial disease. J Vasc Surg. 2008;47(2):303-9. PMID: 18241753.

29. Dawson DL, Cutler BS, Meissner MH, et al. Cilostazol has beneficial effects in treatment of intermittent claudication: results from a multicenter, randomized, prospective, double-blind trial. Circulation. 1998;98(7):678-86. PMID: 9715861.

30. Dawson DL, Cutler BS, Hiatt WR, et al. A comparison of cilostazol and pentoxifylline for treating intermittent claudication. Am J Med. 2000;109(7):523-30. PMID: 11063952.

31. De Sanctis MT, Cesarone MR, Belcaro G, et al. Treatment of intermittent claudication with pentoxifylline: a 12-month, randomized trial--walking distance and microcirculation. Angiology. 2002;53 Suppl 1:S7-12. PMID: 11865838.

32. De Sanctis MT, Cesarone MR, Belcaro G, et al. Treatment of long-distance intermittent claudication with pentoxifylline: a 12-month, randomized trial. Angiology. 2002;53 Suppl 1:S13-7. PMID: 11865829.

33. Cesarone MR, Belcaro G, Nicolaides AN, et al. Treatment of severe intermittent claudication with pentoxifylline: a 40-week, controlled, randomized trial. Angiology. 2002;53 Suppl 1:S1-5. PMID: 11865828.

34. Dorigo W, Pulli R, Marek J, et al. A comparison between open and endovascular repair in the treatment of critical limb ischemia. Ital J Vasc Endovasc Surg. 2009;16(1):17-22. PMID:

35. Dosluoglu HH, Lall P, Cherr GS, et al. Role of simple and complex hybrid revascularization procedures for symptomatic lower extremity occlusive disease. J Vasc Surg. 2010;51(6):1425-1435 e1. PMID: 20488323.

36. Dosluoglu HH, Lall P, Harris LM, et al. Long-term limb salvage and survival after endovascular and open revascularization for critical limb ischemia after adoption of endovascular-first approach by vascular surgeons. Journal of Vascular Surgery. 2012. PMID:

37. Drozdz W, Panek J, Lejman W. Red cell deformability in patients with chronic atheromatous ischemia of the legs. Med Sci Monit. 2001;7(5):933-9. PMID: 11535938.

38. Faglia E, Clerici G, Losa S, et al. Limb revascularization feasibility in diabetic patients with critical limb ischemia: results from a cohort of 344 consecutive unselected diabetic patients evaluated in 2009. Diabetes Res Clin Pract. 2012;95(3):364-71. PMID: 22104261.

39. Feinglass J, McCarthy WJ, Slavensky R, et al. Functional status and walking ability after lower extremity bypass grafting or angioplasty for intermittent claudication: results from a prospective outcomes study. J Vasc Surg. 2000;31(1 Pt 1):93-103. PMID: 10642712.

40. Fowkes FG, Price JF, Stewart MC, et al. Aspirin for prevention of cardiovascular events in a general population screened for a low ankle brachial index: a randomized controlled trial. JAMA. 2010;303(9):841-8. PMID: 20197530.

41. Gardner AW, Katzel LI, Sorkin JD, et al. Effects of long-term exercise rehabilitation on claudication distances in patients with peripheral arterial disease: a randomized controlled trial. J Cardiopulm Rehabil. 2002;22(3):192-8. PMID: 12042688.

42. Gardner AW, Parker DE, Montgomery PS, et al. Efficacy of quantified home-based exercise and supervised exercise in patients with intermittent claudication: a randomized controlled trial. Circulation. 2011;123(5):491-8. PMID: 21262997.

43. Gelin J, Jivegard L, Taft C, et al. Treatment efficacy of intermittent claudication by surgical intervention, supervised physical exercise training compared to no treatment in unselected randomised patients I: one year results of functional and physiological improvements. Eur J Vasc Endovasc Surg. 2001;22(2):107-13. PMID: 11472042.

44. Taft C, Karlsson J, Gelin J, et al. Treatment efficacy of intermittent claudication by invasive therapy, supervised physical exercise training compared to no treatment in unselected randomised patients II: one-year results of health-related quality of life. Eur J Vasc Endovasc Surg. 2001;22(2):114-23. PMID: 11472043.

45. Gibellini R, Fanello M, Bardile AF, et al. Exercise training in intermittent claudication. Int Angiol. 2000;19(1):8-13. PMID: 10853679.

46. Giugliano G, Di Serafino L, Perrino C, et al. Effects of successful percutaneous lower extremity revascularization on cardiovascular outcome in patients with peripheral arterial disease. International Journal of Cardiology. 2012. PMID:

47. Horrocks M, Horrocks EH, Murphy P, et al. The effects of platelet inhibitors on platelet uptake and restenosis after femoral angioplasty. Int Angiol. 1997(2):101-6. PMID:

48. Hoshino J, Fujimoto Y, Naruse Y, et al. Characteristics of revascularization treatment for arteriosclerosis obliterans in patients with and without hemodialysis. Circ J. 2010;74(11):2426-33. PMID: 20938099.

49. Hynes N, Akhtar Y, Manning B, et al. Subintimal angioplasty as a primary modality in the management of critical limb ischemia: comparison to bypass grafting for aortoiliac and femoropopliteal occlusive disease. J Endovasc Ther. 2004;11(4):460-71. PMID: 15298498.

50. Janne d'Othee B, Morris MF, Powell RJ, et al. Cost determinants of percutaneous and surgical interventions for treatment of intermittent claudication from the perspective of the hospital. Cardiovasc Intervent Radiol. 2008;31(1):56-65. PMID: 17973158.

51. Jerabek J, Dvorak M, Vojtisek B. Results of therapy of lower extremity ischemic disease by angiosurgery and radiointervention (PTA) methods. Bratisl Lek Listy. 2003;104(10):314-6. PMID: 15055731.

52. Johnson BF, Singh S, Evans L, et al. A prospective study of the effect of limb-threatening ischaemia and its surgical treatment on the quality of life. Eur J Vasc Endovasc Surg. 1997;13(3):306-14. PMID: 9129605.

53. Kamiya C, Sakamoto S, Tamori Y, et al. Long-term outcome after percutaneous peripheral intervention vs medical treatment for patients with superficial femoral artery occlusive disease. Circ J. 2008;72(5):734-9. PMID: 18441452.

54. Kashyap VS, Pavkov ML, Bena JF, et al. The management of severe aortoiliac occlusive disease: endovascular therapy rivals open reconstruction. J Vasc Surg. 2008;48(6):1451-7, 1457 e1-3. PMID: 18804943.

55. Khan MU, Lall P, Harris LM, et al. Predictors of limb loss despite a patent endovascular-treated arterial segment. J Vasc Surg. 2009;49(6):1440-5; discussion 1445-6. PMID: 19497503.

56. Koivunen K, Lukkarinen H. One-year prospective health-related quality-of-life outcomes in patients treated with conservative method, endovascular treatment or open surgery for symptomatic lower limb atherosclerotic disease. Eur J Cardiovasc Nurs. 2008;7(3):247-56. PMID: 18221916.

57. Korhonen M, Biancari F, Soderstrom M, et al. Femoropopliteal balloon angioplasty vs. bypass surgery for CLI: a propensity score analysis. Eur J Vasc Endovasc Surg. 2011;41(3):378-84. PMID: 21195637.

58. Kruidenier LM, Nicolai SP, Rouwet EV, et al. Additional supervised exercise therapy after a percutaneous vascular intervention for peripheral arterial disease: a randomized clinical trial. J Vasc Interv Radiol. 2011;22(7):961-8. PMID: 21571547.

59. Kudo T, Chandra FA, Kwun WH, et al. Changing pattern of surgical revascularization for critical limb ischemia over 12 years: endovascular vs. open bypass surgery. J Vasc Surg. 2006;44(2):304-13. PMID: 16890859.

60. Laurila J, Brommels M, Standertskjold-Nordenstam CG, et al. Cost-effectiveness of Percutaneous Transluminal Angioplasty (PTA) Versus Vascular Surgery in Limb-threatening Ischaemia. Int J Angiol. 2000;9(4):214-219. PMID: 11062310.

61. Lawall H, Gorriahn H, Amendt K, et al. Long-term outcomes after medical and interventional therapy of critical limb ischemia. Eur J Intern Med. 2009;20(6):616-21. PMID: 19782924.

62. Lee HL, Mehta T, Ray B, et al. A non-randomised controlled trial of the clinical and cost effectiveness of a Supervised Exercise Programme for claudication. Eur J Vasc Endovasc Surg. 2007;33(2):202-7. PMID: 17142065.

63. Lepantalo M, Laurila K, Roth WD, et al. PTFE bypass or thrupass for superficial femoral artery occlusion? A randomised controlled trial. Eur J Vasc Endovasc Surg. 2009;37(5):578-84. PMID: 19231250.

64. Loor G, Skelly CL, Wahlgren CM, et al. Is atherectomy the best first-line therapy for limb salvage in patients with critical limb ischemia? Vasc Endovascular Surg. 2009;43(6):542-50. PMID: 19640919.

65. Mahmood A, Sintler M, Edwards AT, et al. The efficacy of aspirin in patients undergoing infra-inguinal bypass and identification of high risk patients. Int Angiol. 2003;22(3):302-7. PMID: 14612858.

66. Mazari FA, Khan JA, Carradice D, et al. Randomized clinical trial of percutaneous transluminal angioplasty, supervised exercise and combined treatment for intermittent claudication due to femoropopliteal arterial disease. Br J Surg. 2012;99(1):39-48. PMID: 22021102.

67. Mazari FA, Gulati S, Rahman MN, et al. Early outcomes from a randomized, controlled trial of supervised exercise, angioplasty, and combined therapy in intermittent claudication. Ann Vasc Surg. 2010;24(1):69-79. PMID: 19762206.

68. McQuade K, Gable D, Hohman S, et al. Randomized comparison of ePTFE/nitinol self-expanding stent graft vs prosthetic femoral-popliteal bypass in the treatment of superficial femoral artery occlusive disease. J Vasc Surg. 2009;49(1):109-15, 116 e1-9; discussion 116. PMID: 19028055.

69. Kedora J, Hohmann S, Garrett W, et al. Randomized comparison of percutaneous Viabahn stent grafts vs prosthetic femoral-popliteal bypass in the treatment of superficial femoral arterial occlusive disease. J Vasc Surg. 2007;45(1):10-6; discussion 16. PMID: 17126520.

70. McQuade K, Gable D, Pearl G, et al. Four-year randomized prospective comparison of percutaneous ePTFE/nitinol self-expanding stent graft versus prosthetic femoral-popliteal bypass in the treatment of superficial femoral artery occlusive disease. J Vasc Surg. 2010;52(3):584-90; discussion 590-1, 591 e1-591 e7. PMID: 20598480.

71. Minar E, Ahmadi A, Koppensteiner R, et al. Comparison of effects of high-dose and low-dose aspirin on restenosis after femoropopliteal percutaneous transluminal angioplasty. Circulation. 1995;91(8):2167-73. PMID: 7697845.

72. Money SR, Herd JA, Isaacsohn JL, et al. Effect of cilostazol on walking distances in patients with intermittent claudication caused by peripheral vascular disease. J Vasc Surg. 1998;27(2):267-74; discussion 274-5. PMID: 9510281.

73. Mori E, Komori K, Kume M, et al. Comparison of the long-term results between surgical and conservative treatment in patients with intermittent claudication. Surgery. 2002;131(1 Suppl):S269-74. PMID: 11821823.

74. Nordanstig J, Gelin J, Hensater M, et al. Walking performance and health-related quality of life after surgical or endovascular invasive versus non-invasive treatment for intermittent claudication--a prospective randomised trial. Eur J Vasc Endovasc Surg. 2011;42(2):220-7. PMID: 21397530.

75. Pell JP, Lee AJ. Impact of angioplasty and arterial reconstructive surgery on the quality of life of claudicants. The Scottish Vascular Audit Group. Scott Med J. 1997;42(2):47-8. PMID: 9507581.

76. Perkins JM, Collin J, Creasy TS, et al. Exercise training versus angioplasty for stable claudication. Long and medium term results of a prospective, randomised trial. Eur J Vasc Endovasc Surg. 1996;11(4):409-13. PMID: 8846172.

77. Rossi E, Citterio F, Castagneto M, et al. Safety of endovascular treatment in high-cardiac-risk patients with limb-threatening ischemia. Angiology. 1998;49(6):435-40. PMID: 9631888.

78. Sachs T, Pomposelli F, Hamdan A, et al. Trends in the national outcomes and costs for claudication and limb threatening ischemia: Angioplasty vs bypass graft. J Vasc Surg. 2011;54(4):1021-1031 e1. PMID: 21880457.

79. Soderstrom MI, Arvela EM, Korhonen M, et al. Infrapopliteal percutaneous transluminal angioplasty versus bypass surgery as first-line strategies in critical leg ischemia: a propensity score analysis. Ann Surg. 2010;252(5):765-73. PMID: 21037432.

80. Soga Y, Yokoi H, Kawasaki T, et al. Efficacy of cilostazol after endovascular therapy for femoropopliteal artery disease in patients with intermittent claudication. J Am Coll Cardiol. 2009;53(1):48-53. PMID: 19118724.

81. Spronk S, Bosch JL, den Hoed PT, et al. Intermittent claudication: clinical effectiveness of endovascular revascularization versus supervised hospital-based exercise training--randomized controlled trial. Radiology. 2009;250(2):586-95. PMID: 19188327.

82. Spronk S, Bosch JL, den Hoed PT, et al. Cost-effectiveness of endovascular revascularization compared to supervised hospital-based exercise training in patients with intermittent claudication: a randomized controlled trial. J Vasc Surg. 2008;48(6):1472-80. PMID: 18771879.

83. Stoner MC, Defreitas DJ, Manwaring MM, et al. Cost per day of patency: understanding the impact of patency and reintervention in a sustainable model of healthcare. J Vasc Surg. 2008;48(6):1489-96. PMID: 18829227.

84. Strandness DE, Jr., Dalman RL, Panian S, et al. Effect of cilostazol in patients with intermittent claudication: a randomized, double-blind, placebo-controlled study. Vasc Endovascular Surg. 2002;36(2):83-91. PMID: 11951094.

85. Sugimoto I, Ohta T, Ishibashi H, et al. Conservative treatment for patients with intermittent claudication. Int Angiol. 2010;29(2 Suppl):55-60. PMID: 20357750.

86. Sultan S, Hynes N. Five-year Irish trial of CLI patients with TASC II type C/D lesions undergoing subintimal angioplasty or bypass surgery based on plaque echolucency. J Endovasc Ther. 2009;16(3):270-83. PMID: 19642779.

87. Sultan S, Hynes N. Mid-term results of subintimal angioplasty for critical limb ischemia 5-year outcomes. Vasc Dis Manage. 2011;8(9):E155-E163. PMID:

88. Taylor SM, Kalbaugh CA, Blackhurst DW, et al. Postoperative outcomes according to preoperative medical and functional status after infrainguinal revascularization for critical limb ischemia in patients 80 years and older. Am Surg. 2005;71(8):640-5; discussion 645-6. PMID: 16217945.

89. Taylor SM, Kalbaugh CA, Blackhurst DW, et al. Determinants of functional outcome after revascularization for critical limb ischemia: an analysis of 1000 consecutive vascular interventions. J Vasc Surg. 2006;44(4):747-55; discussion 755-6. PMID: 16926083.

90. Taylor SM, York JW, Cull DL, et al. Clinical success using patient-oriented outcome measures after lower extremity bypass and endovascular intervention for ischemic tissue loss. J Vasc Surg. 2009;50(3):534-41; discussion 541. PMID: 19592193.

91. Tepe G, Bantleon R, Brechtel K, et al. Management of peripheral arterial interventions with mono or dual antiplatelet therapy-the MIRROR study: a randomised and double-blinded clinical trial. Eur Radiol. 2012;22(9):1998-2006. PMID: 22569995.

92. Timaran CH, Ohki T, Gargiulo NJ, 3rd, et al. Iliac artery stenting in patients with poor distal runoff: Influence of concomitant infrainguinal arterial reconstruction. J Vasc Surg. 2003;38(3):479-84; discussion 484-5. PMID: 12947261.

93. Timaran CH, Prault TL, Stevens SL, et al. Iliac artery stenting versus surgical reconstruction for TASC (TransAtlantic Inter-Society Consensus) type B and type C iliac lesions. J Vasc Surg. 2003;38(2):272-8. PMID: 12891108.

94. Treat-Jacobson D, Bronas UG, Leon AS. Efficacy of arm-ergometry versus treadmill exercise training to improve walking distance in patients with claudication. Vasc Med. 2009;14(3):203-13. PMID: 19651669.

95. Bronas UG, Treat-Jacobson D, Leon AS. Comparison of the effect of upper body-ergometry aerobic training vs treadmill training on central cardiorespiratory improvement and walking distance in patients with claudication. J Vasc Surg. 2011;53(6):1557-64. PMID: 21515017.

96. Tsai JC, Chan P, Wang CH, et al. The effects of exercise training on walking function and perception of health status in elderly patients with peripheral arterial occlusive disease. J Intern Med. 2002;252(5):448-55. PMID: 12528763.

97. Varela C, Acin F, De Haro J, et al. Influence of surgical or endovascular distal revascularization of the lower limbs on ischemic ulcer healing. J Cardiovasc Surg (Torino). 2011;52(3):381-9. PMID: 21577193.

98. Varty K, Nydahl S, Butterworth P, et al. Changes in the management of critical limb ischaemia. Br J Surg. 1996;83(7):953-6. PMID: 8813785.

99. Varty K, Nydahl S, Nasim A, et al. Results of surgery and angioplasty for the treatment of chronic severe lower limb ischaemia. Eur J Vasc Endovasc Surg. 1998;16(2):159-63. PMID: 9728437.

100. Venermo M, Biancari F, Arvela E, et al. The role of chronic kidney disease as a predictor of outcome after revascularisation of the ulcerated diabetic foot. Diabetologia. 2011. PMID: 21845468.

101. Whatling PJ, Gibson M, Torrie EP, et al. Iliac occlusions: stenting or crossover grafting? An examination of patency and cost. Eur J Vasc Endovasc Surg. 2000;20(1):36-40. PMID: 10906295.

102. Whyman MR, Fowkes FG, Kerracher EM, et al. Is intermittent claudication improved by percutaneous transluminal angioplasty? A randomized controlled trial. J Vasc Surg. 1997;26(4):551-7. PMID: 9357454.

103. Whyman MR, Fowkes FG, Kerracher EM, et al. Randomised controlled trial of percutaneous transluminal angioplasty for intermittent claudication. Eur J Vasc Endovasc Surg. 1996;12(2):167-72. PMID: 8760978.

104. Wolfle KD, Bruijnen H, Reeps C, et al. Tibioperoneal arterial lesions and critical foot ischaemia: successful management by the use of short vein grafts and percutaneous transluminal angioplasty. Vasa. 2000;29(3):207-14. PMID: 11037720.

105. Zdanowski Z, Troeng T, Norgren L. Outcome and influence of age after infrainguinal revascularisation in critical limb ischaemia. The Swedish Vascular Registry. Eur J Vasc Endovasc Surg. 1998;16(2):137-41. PMID: 9728433.

Appendix E. Excluded Studies

All studies listed below were reviewed in their full-text version and excluded for the reason shown in bold. Reasons for exclusion signify only the usefulness of the articles for this study and are not intended as criticisms of the articles.

Non-English language

Brosa M, Garcia-Cases C, Clerch L, et al. Cost-effectiveness analysis of cilostazol vs naftidrofuryl and pentoxifylline for the treatment of intermittent claudication in Spain. Angiologia. 2011;63(3):103-7.

Bulvas M, Chochola M, Herdova J, et al. Influence of heparan sulphate on the effect of percutaneous transluminal angioplasty in vessels supplying the lower extremities. Cas Lek Cesk. 1996;135(14):445-9.

Chikiar DS, Grandjean M, Abelleyra J. Femoropopliteal bypass grafting for arterial occlusive disease. Patency and complications. Randomized retrospective study. Prensa Med Argent. 2003;90(4):338-44.

Gloor B, Wehrli E, Rotzer A, et al. Polyurethane small artery substitutes for femoropopliteal above knee bypass. Clinical and angiomorphological follow up of 20 patients in a prospective, randomized trial. Swiss Surg. 1996;(Suppl 1):13-8.

Grenacher L, Saam T, Geier A, et al. [PTA versus Palmaz stent placement in femoropopliteal artery stenoses: results of a multicenter prospective randomized study (REFSA)]. RoFo. 2004;176(9):1302-10. PMID: 15346266.

Leo W, Westrych R, Bissinger A, et al. [Effect of the acetylosalicyd acid (ASA) and ticlopidine therapy on clinical condition and parameters of blood platelets in patients with peripheral arterial occlusive disease (PAOD)]. Pol Merkuriusz Lek. 2007;23(137):335-9. PMID: 18361314.

Marinel-Lo-Roura J, Alos-Vilacrosa J, Lopez-Palencia JA, et al. Endovascular surgery of the infrapopliteal segment. Angiologia. 2003;55(Suppl 1):S175-81.

Martin-Conejero A, Serrano-Hernando FJ, Rodriguez-Gonzalez R, et al. Treatment of occlusive pathologies of the superficial femoral artery with a Viabahn(registered trademark) device. Angiologia. 2008;60(2):117-25.

Matas-Docampo M, Royo-Serrando J, Dominguez-Gonzalez JM, et al. Endovascular surgery of the distal segment: The opposite position. Angiologia. 2003;55(Suppl 1):S182-9.

Mosimann UP, Stirnemann P. Chronic critical limb ischemia: The revascularization of the isolated popliteal segment compared to the femoro-distal bypass. Vasa. 1995;24(1):49-55. PMID: 7725779.

Nasser F, Silva SGDJ, Biagioni RB, et al. Endovascular infrainguinal revascularization: Predictive factors for patency. J Vasc Bras. 2009;8(1):48-55.

Nicolai SPA, Prins MH, Teijink JaW. Supervised exercise therapy is more effective than walking advice in patients with intermittent claudication; a randomized multicenter study. Ned Tijdschr Geneeskd. 2011;155(2):55-62.

Ortigosa Mateo AB, Gutierrez Julian JM, Rivas Dominguez M, et al. Clinical results of femoropopliteal endovascular treatment in patients with critical limb ischaemia. Angiologia. 2010;62(3):103-9.

Panella-Agusti F, Berga-Fauria C, Hernandez-Osma E, et al. Iliofemoral or femorofemoral bypass. Which is the best option? A long-term follow-up study. Angiologia. 2003;55(6):526-33.

Plaza-Martinez A, Riera-Vazquez R, Diaz-Lopez M, et al. Value of endovascular treatment in the iliac sector. Angiologia. 2002;54(4):282-90.

Ramirez Saavedra OA. Sequential distal bypass: A resolved surgery in diabetic foot with TASC D gangrene and lesions. Rev Mex Angiol. 2010;38(2):46-50.

Rognoni A, Zelaschi F, Felicetti G, et al. Rehabilitation of the peripheral arterial obstructive disease: Efficacy of aerobic training. Eur Medicophys. 1995;31(4):207-13.

Schlenger R. Cilostazol therapy improves the ability to walk in patients with peripheral occlusive artery disease. Dtsch Apoth Ztg. 2007;147(10):34-6.

Stierli P, Eugster T, Hess P, et al. Occlusion of the superficial femoral artery. Choice of material for a bypass to the above-knee popliteal artery. Gefasschirurgie. 2001;6(Suppl 1):S43-6.

Tan JY, Shi WH, He J, et al. [A clinical trial of using antiplatelet therapy to prevent restenosis following peripheral artery angioplasty and stenting]. Nat Med J China. 2008;88(12):812-5. PMID: 18756983.

Tetteroo E, Van Der Graaf Y, Van Engelen AD, et al. No difference in effect on intermittent claudication between primary stent placement and primary percutaneous transluminal angioplasty followed by selective stent placement: A prospective randomized trial. Ned Tijdschr Geneeskd. 2000;144:167-71.

Trejo JMR, Sanchez IE, Ramirez NR, et al. Surgery for the rescue of critical limb ischemia. Rev Mex Angiol. 2008;36(3):88-97.

Utrilla-Fernandez F, Acin-Garcia F, March-Garcia JR, et al. Angioplasty versus angioplasty plus stent-graft in the infrainguinal segment. Results of 100 consecutive endovascular procedures. Angiologia. 2004;56(4):367-79.

Van Der Zaag ES, Prins MH, Jacobs MJ. [Treatment of intermittent claudication; prospective randomized study in the BAESIC-Trial (bypass, angioplasty or endarterectomy patients with severe intermittent claudication)]. Ned Tijdschr Geneeskd. 1996;140(14):787-8. PMID: 8668267.

Zhu BP, Fan L, Li XY. [Long-term effect and reliability of warfarin and aspirin for primary prevention of cardio-cerebral vessels events in patients with peripheral arteriosclerotic occlusive disease: a randomized, single-blind, controlled clinical trial with two-year follow-up]. Chin J Clin Rehab. 2005;9(15):10-1.

Zimmermann A, Berger H, Eckstein HH. The ABC (angioplasty or bypass surgery in intermittent claudication) trial: Background and study design. Gefasschirurgie. 2010;15(1):5-10.

Not a full publication (abstract only), not original data, not peer-reviewed literature published 1995 to present, not a clinical study (e.g., editorial, non-systematic review, letter to the editor, case series), animal study

Ahanchi SS, Chen B, Steerman S, et al. The use of reentry devices improves the technical success, safety, and patency of recanalization of chronic total occlusions of the iliac arteries. J Vasc Surg. 2012;55(6 Suppl 1):88S-89S.

Anonymous. Meta-analysis of antiplatelet trials. Pharm J. 2002;268(7180):7.

Anonymous. Stenting for peripheral artery disease of the lower extremities: An evidence-based analysis. Ont Health Technol Assess Ser. 2010;10(18):1-88. PMID: 23074395.

Atsushi T, Soga Y, Iida O, et al. Predictors of early mortality in patients with critical limb ischemia caused by isolated below-the-knee artery disease. J Am Coll Cardiol. 2012;59(13Suppl 1):E2109.

Beebe HG, Dawson DL, Cutler BS, et al. Cilostazol, a new treatment for intermittent claudication: results of a randomized, multicenter trial. Circulation. 1997;96(8):66.

Belch J, Maccuish A, Campbell I. No benefit of daily low-dose aspirin in diabetic patients with peripheral arterial disease. J Clin Outcomes Manage. 2008;15(12):575-6.

Belkin M, Donaldson MC, Whittemore AD. Composite autogenous vein grafts. Semin Vasc Surg. 1995;8(3):202-8. PMID: 8564033.

Bell J, Papp L, Bradbury AW. Bypass or angioplasty for sever ischaemia of the leg: the BASIL trial. Vascular and endovascular opportunities. 2000;485-94.

Bosch JL, Tetteroo E, Mali WP, et al. Iliac arterial occlusive disease: cost-effectiveness analysis of stent placement versus percutaneous transluminal angioplasty. Dutch Iliac Stent Trial Study Group. Radiology. 1998;208(3):641-8. PMID: 9722840.

Bradbury AW, Adam DJ, Bell J, et al. Erratum: Bypass versus Angioplasty in Severe Ischaemia of the Leg (BASIL) Trial: a description of the severity and extent of disease using the Bollinger angiogram scoring method and the TransAtlantic Inter-Society Consensus II classification. (J Vasc Surg. 2010;51(Suppl.5):32S-42S). J Vasc Surg. 2010;(6):1751.

Bradbury AW, Adam DJ, Bell J, et al. Erratum: Bypass versus Angioplasty in Severe Ischaemia of the Leg (BASIL) Trial: a survival prediction model to facilitate clinical decision making. (J Vasc Surg. 2010;51(Suppl.5):52S-68S). J Vasc Surg. 2010;(6):1751.

Bradbury AW, Adam DJ, Bell J, et al. Erratum: Bypass versus Angioplasty in Severe Ischaemia of the Leg (BASIL) Trial: an intention-to-treat analysis of amputation-free and overall survival in patients randomized to a bypass surgery-first or a balloon angioplasty-first revascularization strategy. (J Vasc Surg. 2010;51(Suppl.5):5S-17S). J Vasc Surg. 2010;(6):1751.

Bradbury AW, Adam DJ, Bell J, et al. Erratum: Bypass versus Angioplasty in Severe Ischaemia of the Leg (BASIL) Trial: analysis of amputation free and overall survival by treatment received. (J Vasc Surg. 2010;51(Suppl.5):18S-31S). J Vasc Surg. 2010;(6):1751.

Breek JC, De Vries J, Hamming JF. The Oslo Balloon Angioplasty versus Conservative Treatment Study (OBACT) - The 2-years results of a single centre, prospective, randomised study in patients with intermittent claudication. Eur J Vasc Endovasc Surg. 2007;34(3):378. PMID: 17582794.

Caro JJ, Migliaccio-Walle K. Generalizing the results of clinical trials to actual practice: the example of clopidogrel therapy for the prevention of vascular events. CAPRA (CAPRIE Actual Practice Rates Analysis) Study Group. Clopidogrel versus Aspirin in Patients at Risk of Ischaemic Events. Am J Med. 1999;107(6):568-72. PMID: 10625025.

Cassar K, Bachoo P, Ford I, et al. Variability in responsiveness to clopidogrel in patients with intermittent claudication. The Vascular Society of Great Britain & Ireland Yearbook 2005. 2005;Abstract no: 66.

Cassar K, Ford I, Greaves M, et al. The CAVA study: a double-blind randomized controlled trial of clopidogrel and aspirin vs. aspirin alone in patients with intermittent claudication undergoing peripheral percutaneous transluminal angioplasty. J Thromb Haemost. 2003;(Suppl 1):Abstract no: P2009.

Cejna M, Durakovic N, Mathies R, et al. Long-term follow-up and total cost analysis of in-hospital invasive interdisciplinary treatment of critical limb ischemia: Comparison of surgical and endovascular therapy. CardioVascular and Interventional Radiology. 2011;34(Suppl 3):528.

Clement Darling R, Mehta M, Roddy SP, et al. Distal bypass in the endovascular-first era: Is there still a need for open surgery? J Vasc Surg. 2011;54(3):922-3.

Cull DL, Langan EM, Gray BH, et al. Open versus endovascular intervention for critical limb ischemia: a population-based study. J Am Coll Surg. 2010;210(5):555-61, 561-3. PMID: 20421003.

Dardik H. Regarding "a comparative evaluation of polytetrafluoroethylene, umbilical vein, and saphenous vein bypass grafts for femoral-popliteal above-knee revascularization: a prospective randomized Department of Veterans Affairs cooperative study". J Vasc Surg. 2001;33(3):658-9. PMID: 11241144.

Dawson DL, Beebe HG, Herd JA, et al. Cilostazol or pentoxifylline for claudication. Circulation. 1998;(Suppl 1):12.

Drozdz W, Lejman W. Response to exercise training in patients with intermittent claudication. Pol Prz Chir. 2006;78(1):85-105.

Farkouh ME. 2008 -- aspirin and/or antioxidants did not prevent CV events in diabetes and peripheral arterial disease. ACP Journal Club. 2009;150:JC1-8.

Flis V, Pavlovic M, Miksic K. The value of adjunctive vein patches to improve the outcome of femorodistal polytetrafluoroethylene bypass grafts. Wien Klin Wochenschr. 2001;113(Suppl.3):5-10. PMID: 15503612.

Friedberg MW. Supervised exercise is equivalent to endovascular revascularization for the treatment of intermittent claudication. J Clin Outcomes Manage. 2009;16(8):349-50.

Gaines P. Results of bypass vs. interventional radiology for occlusive disease. Cardiovasc Intervent Radiol. 2011;34(Suppl.3):336-8.

Gardner AW, Montgomery PS, Parker DE. Optimal exercise program length for patients with claudication: A randomized controlled trial. J Cardiopulm Rehabil Prev. 2011;31(4):E4-5.

Gardner AW. Supervised exercise therapy provided by local physiotherapists improves walking distance in patients with claudication. Evid-Based Med. 2011;16(2):43-4. PMID: 21427053.

Greenhalgh J, Bagust A, Boland A, et al. Clopidogrel and modified-release dipyridamole for the prevention of occlusive vascular events (review of Technology Appraisal No. 90): a systematic review and economic analysis. Health Technol Assess. 2011;15(31):1-178. PMID: 21888837.

Grenon SM, Conte MS. Aspirin prophylaxis (100 mg daily) does not improve cardiovascular outcomes compared to placebo in asymptomatic individuals with incidental low-ankle brachial index. Evid-Based Med. 2010;15(4):106-8. PMID: 20530607.

Guest JF, Davie AM, Clegg JP. Cost effectiveness of cilostazol compared with naftidrofuryl and pentoxifylline in the treatment of intermittent claudication in the UK. Curr Med Res Opin. 2005;21(6):817-26. PMID: 15969881.

Hamburg NM, Balady GJ. Exercise rehabilitation in peripheral artery disease: functional impact and mechanisms of benefits. Circulation. 2011;123(1):87-97. PMID: 21200015.

Harker LA, Boissel JP, Pilgrim AJ, et al. Comparative safety and tolerability of clopidogrel and aspirin: results from CAPRIE. CAPRIE Steering Committee and Investigators. Clopidogrel versus aspirin in patients at risk of ischaemic events. Drug Saf. 1999;21(4):325-35. PMID: 10514023.

Hepp W, Von Bary S, Corovic D, et al. Intravenous prostaglandin E1 versus pentoxifylline: a randomized controlled study in patients with intermittent claudication. Int Angiol. 1995;(Suppl 1):280.

Hiatt WR, Cooper LT, Morgan RE, et al. Clinical effects of the phosphodiesterase inhibitor K-134 in peripheral artery disease and claudication. Circulation. 2011;124(21):A9800.

Hong JB, Jeon YS, Cho SG, et al. Endovascular treatment as a reasonable option for extensive total occlusion of iliac artery. Am J Cardiol. 2012;109(7):138S-139S.

Huber TS. Commentary. Anand, Yusuf, Xie, et al. The Warfarin Antiplatelet Vascular Evaluation Trial Investigators. Oral anticoagulation and antiplatelet therapy and peripheral arterial disease. N Engl J Med. 2007;357:217-227. Perspect Vasc Surg Endovasc Ther. 2008;20(4):383-4. PMID: 19095638.

Hunink MG, Wong JB, Donaldson MC, et al. Revascularization for femoropopliteal disease. A decision and cost-effectiveness analysis. JAMA. 1995;274(2):165-71. PMID: 7596006.

Jacomella V, Shenoy A, Mosimann K, et al. Impact of lower limb revascularization on aortic augmentation index and subendocardial viability ratio in patients with peripheral arterial disease. Atheroscler Suppl. 2011;12(1):70.

Kalani M, Apelqvist J, Blomback M, et al. Dalteparin improved chronic foot ulcers and reduced the number of amputations in diabetic peripheral arterial occlusive disease. Evid-Based Med. 2004;9(3):73.

Karnon J, Brennan A, Pandor A, et al. Modelling the long term cost effectiveness of clopidogrel for the secondary prevention of occlusive vascular events in the UK. Curr Med Res Opin. 2005;21(1):101-12. PMID: 15881481.

Killewich LA. Improving functional status and quality of life in elderly patients with peripheral arterial disease. J Am Coll Surg. 2006;202(2):345-55. PMID: 16427563.

Kruidenier LM, Nicola SP. Additional supervised exercise therapy after a percutaneous vascular intervention for peripheral arterial disease: A randomized clinical trial. J Vasc Surg. 2011;54(6):1846.

Lee HL, Mehta T, Ray B, et al. A trial of the clinical and cost-effectiveness of a supervised exercise programme for claudication. Br J Surg. 2005;92(Suppl 1):11.

Masser PA, Taylor LM, Jr., Moneta GL, et al. Technique of reversed vein bypass for lower extremity ischemia. Ann Vasc Surg. 1996;10(2):190-200. PMID: 8733873.

Mazari F, Khan J, Abdul Rahman MNA, et al. Cost utility analysis of a randomised control trial of percutaneous transluminal angioplasty (PTA), supervised exercise programme (SEP) and combined treatment (PTA+SEP) for patients with intermittent claudication (IC) due to femoropopliteal disease. The Vascular Society of Great Britain & Ireland Yearbook 2009. 2009;44.

Mehta M, Ramay F, Roddy SP, et al. Cost per day of patency: Long-term implications of patency and reinterventions after endovascular vs surgical lower extremity revascularizations. J Vasc Surg. 2011;54(4):1227-8.

Melton C. Supervised exercise program helps patients with peripheral artery disease walk longer. Clin Geriatr. 2011;19(12):17.

Mewissen MW. IX.4 direct stenting in long femoropopliteal lesions. Vascular. 2005;13(Suppl 1):S47-9.

Mohler ER, 3rd, Beebe HG, Salles-Cuhna S, et al. Effects of cilostazol on resting ankle pressures and exercise-induced ischemia in patients with intermittent claudication. Vasc Med. 2001;6(3):151-6. PMID: 11789969.

Murphy TP. Supervised exercise vs. primary stenting for claudication due to aorto-iliac peripheral artery disease: 6-month outcomes from the CLEVER Study. Eur Heart J. 2012;33(1):144-5.

Nair V, Chaisson G, Abben R. Strategies in infrapopliteal intervention: improving outcomes in challenging patients. J Interv Cardiol. 2009;22(1):27-36. PMID: 19281520.

Nordanstig J, Gelin J, Hensater M, et al. Walking performance and health-related quality of life after surgical or endovascular invasive versus non-invasive treatment for intermittent claudication - A prospective randomised trial. J Vasc Surg. 2011;54(2):584.

Pande RL, Hiatt WR, Zhang P, et al. A pooled analysis of the durability and predictors of treatment response of cilostazol in patients with intermittent claudication. Vasc Med. 2010;15(3):181-8. PMID: 20385711

Patel MR, Becker RC, Wojdyla DM, et al. Cardiovascular events in acute coronary syndrome patients with peripheral arterial disease treated with ticagrelor compared to clopidogrel: Data from the PLATO trial. Circulation. 2011;124(24):A14299.

Price JF, Leng GC, Fowkes FG. Should claudicants receive angioplasty or exercise training? Cardiovasc Surg. 1997;5(5):463-70. PMID: 9464601.

Renwick P, Johnson B, Wilkinson A, et al. Vascular surgical society of great britain and ireland: limb outcome following failed femoropopliteal polytetrafluoroethylene bypass for intermittent claudication. Br J Surg. 1999;86(5):693. PMID: 10361318.

Roitman JL. Treadmill exercise and resistance training in patients with peripheral arterial disease with and without in intermittent claudication: A randomized controlled trial. J Cardiopulm Rehabil Prev. 2010;30(1):62.

Shindelman LE. Experience with the LuMend Frontrunner CTO Catheter System for the Treatment of TASC D SFA Lesions. J Invasive Cadiol. 2004;16(Suppl B):13.

Shiraki T, Iida O, Fujita M, et al. Predictors of mortality within 2-year after endovascular therapy for patients with critical limb ischemia. J Am Coll Cardiol. 2012;59(13Suppl 1):E2103.

Singer E, Imfeld S, Hoffmann U, et al. Aspirin in peripheral arterial disease: breakthrough or pitfall? Vasa. 2006;35(3):174-7. PMID: 16941406.

Soejima H, Morimoto T, Saito Y, et al. Aspirin for the primary prevention of cardiovascular events in patients with peripheral artery disease or diabetes mellitus. Analyses from the JPAD, POPADAD and AAA trials. Thromb Haemost. 2010;104(6):1085-8. PMID: 20941462.

Sood J. Is the antiplatelet effect of aspirin sufficient in atherosclerosis? Pharm Pract. 2008;18(4):133-5.

Strandness DE, Dalman R, Panian S, et al. Two doses of Cilostazol versus placebo in the treatment of claudication: results of a randomized, multicenter trial. Circulation. 1998;17(Suppl 1):12.

Strobl F, Bantleon R, Schmehl J, et al. Management of peripheral arterial interventions with mono or dual antiplatelet therapy. MIRROR study. Eur Heart J. 2011;32(Suppl 1):1053.

Sultan S, Tawfick W. Technical superiority and clinical excellence of duplex ultrsound arterial maping (DUAM) versus magnetic resonance angiogram (MRA) as the sole imaging modality in bypass surgery (BS) and endovascular revascularization (EVR) for critical lower ischemia (CLI) patients: A six-year comparative study in a tertiary referral vascular centre. J Vasc Surg. 2012. 55(6 Suppl 1):71S.

Thomason AR, Skipwith DF. Lower extremity peripheral arterial disease. U.S. Pharm. 2007;32(2).

Thomson IA, Van Rij AM, Morrison ND, et al. A ten year randomised controlled trial of percutaneous femoropopliteal angioplasty for claudication. ANZ J Surg. 1999;69(Suppl):98.

Tovar-Pardo AE, Bernhard VM. Where the profunda femoris artery fits in the spectrum of lower limb revascularization. Semin Vasc Surg. 1995;8(3):225-35. PMID: 8564036

Tran H. Vascular viewpoint. Vasc Med. 2004;9(1):90.

Walsh SR, Tang TY, Cooper DG, et al. Remote ischemic preconditioning will reduce graft-related events after surgical infrainguinal revascularization: evidence-based surgery hypothesis. Surgery. 2010;148(5):1020-1. PMID: 20472262.

Weismantel D. Is cilostazol more effective than pentoxifylline in the treatment of symptoms of intermittent claudication? J Fam Pract. 2001;50(2):181. PMID: 11219570.

Whyman MR, Fowkes FGR, Kerracher EMG, et al. Intermittent claudication is not improved by percutaneous transluminal angioplasty - A randomised controlled trial. BJS. 1996;35

Does not include a study population of interest

Bhatt DL, Hirsch AT, Ringleb PA, et al. Reduction in the need for hospitalization for recurrent ischemic events and bleeding with clopidogrel instead of aspirin. CAPRIE investigators. Am Heart J. 2000;140(1):67-73. PMID: 10874265.

Butterfield JS, Fitzgerald JB, Razzaq R, et al. Early mobilization following angioplasty. Clin Radiol. 2000;55(11):874-7. PMID: 11069744.

Campeau L, Lesperance J, Bilodeau L, et al. Effect of cholesterol lowering and cardiovascular risk factors on the progression of aortoiliac arteriosclerosis: a quantitative cineangiography study. Angiology. 2005;56(2):191-9. PMID: 15793608.

Carroccio A, Faries PL, Morrissey NJ, et al. Predicting iliac limb occlusions after bifurcated aortic stent grafting: anatomic and device-related causes. J Vasc Surg. 2002;36(4):679-84. PMID: 12368725.

Drozdz W, Wilczek M, Gajdzinska K, et al. Mechanisms of symptomatic relief observed after conservative treatment or revascularization in patients with chronic lower limb ischemia. Pol Prz Chir. 2004;76(4):359-72.

Eikelboom JW, Hankey GJ, Thom J, et al. Incomplete inhibition of thromboxane biosynthesis by acetylsalicylic acid: determinants and effect on cardiovascular risk. Circulation. 2008;118(17):1705-12. PMID: 18838564.

Gschwandtner ME, Minar E, Ahmadi A, et al. Impact of different therapeutic alternatives in treatment of severe limb ischemia: experiences on 190 consecutive patients at a department of medical angiology. Vasa. 1999;28(4):271-8. PMID: 10611845.

Harker LA, Boissel JP, Pilgrim AJ, et al. Comparative safety and tolerability of clopidogrel and aspirin: results from CAPRIE. CAPRIE Steering Committee and Investigators. Clopidogrel versus aspirin in patients at risk of ischaemic events. Drug Saf. 1999;21(4):325-35. PMID: 10514023

Julliard W, Katzen J, Nabozny M, et al. Long-term results of endoscopic versus open saphenous vein harvest for lower extremity bypass. Ann Vasc Surg. 2011;25(1):101-7. PMID: 21172585.

Kreienberg PB, Darling RC, 3rd, Chang BB, et al. Adjunctive techniques to improve patency of distal prosthetic bypass grafts: polytetrafluoroethylene with remote arteriovenous fistulae versus vein cuffs. J Vasc Surg. 2000;31(4):696-701. PMID: 10753277.

Lee ES, Steenson CC, Trimble KE, et al. Comparing patency rates between external iliac and common iliac artery stents. J Vasc Surg. 2000;31(5):889-94. PMID: 10805878.

Leizorovicz A, Becker F. Oral buflomedil in the prevention of cardiovascular events in patients with peripheral arterial obstructive disease: a randomized, placebo-controlled, 4-year study. Circulation. 2008;117(6):816-22. PMID: 18212283.

Lepantalo M, Salenius JP, Alback A, et al. Frequency of repeated vascular surgery. A survey of 7616 surgical and endovascular Finnvasc procedures. Finnvasc Study Group. Eur J Surg. 1996;162(4):279-85. PMID: 8739414.

Lombardini R, Marchesi S, Collebrusco L, et al. The use of osteopathic manipulative treatment as adjuvant therapy in patients with peripheral arterial disease. Man Ther. 2009;14(4):439-43. PMID: 18824395.

Lopez-Galarza LA, Ray LI, Rodriguez-Lopez J, et al. Combined percutaneous transluminal angioplasty, iliac stent deployment, and femorofemoral bypass for bilateral aortoiliac occlusive disease. J Am Coll Surg. 1997;184(3):249-58. PMID: 9060920.

Louridas G, Saadia R, Spelay J, et al. The ArtAssist Device in chronic lower limb ischemia. A pilot study. Int Angiol. 2002;21(1):28-35. PMID: 11941271.

Mak KH, Bhatt DL, Shao M, et al. The influence of body mass index on mortality and bleeding among patients with or at high-risk of atherothrombotic disease. Eur Heart J. 2009;30(7):857-65. PMID: 19233855.

Milio G, Coppola G, Novo S. The effects of prostaglandin E-1 in patients with intermittent claudication. Cardiovasc Hematol Disord Drug Targets. 2006;6(2):71-6. PMID: 16787192.

Mukherjee D, Topol EJ, Moliterno DJ, et al. Extracardiac vascular disease and effectiveness of sustained clopidogrel treatment. Heart. 2006;92(1):49-51. PMID: 15845611.

Newton W. Does aspirin heal leg ulcers? J Fam Pract. 1995;40(1):93. PMID: 7807046.

Nguyen LL, Lipsitz SR, Bandyk DF, et al. Resource utilization in the treatment of critical limb ischemia: The effect of tissue loss, comorbidities, and graft-related events. J Vasc Surg. 2006;44(5):971-5; discussion 975-6. PMID: 17098527.

Oka RK, Szuba A, Giacomini JC, et al. A pilot study of L-arginine supplementation on functional capacity in peripheral arterial disease. Vasc Med. 2005;10(4):265-74. PMID: 16444855.

Pomposelli FB, Jr., Marcaccio EJ, Gibbons GW, et al. Dorsalis pedis arterial bypass: durable limb salvage for foot ischemia in patients with diabetes mellitus. J Vasc Surg. 1995;21(3):375-84. PMID: 7877219.

Presern-Strukelj M, Poredos P. The influence of electrostimulation on the circulation of the remaining leg in patients with one-sided amputation. Angiology. 2002;53(3):329-35. PMID: 12025921.

Proia RR, Walsh DB, Nelson PR, et al. Early results of infragenicular revascularization based solely on duplex arteriography. J Vasc Surg. 2001;33(6):1165-70. PMID: 11389413.

Robbs JV, Paruk N. Management of HIV vasculopathy - a South African experience. Eur J Vasc Endovasc Surg. 2010;39(Suppl 1):S25-31. PMID: 20189418.

Rodgers A, Macmahon S. Antiplatelet therapy and the prevention of thrombosis. Aust N Z J Med. 1996;26(2):210-5. PMID: 8744620.

Rustempasic N, Solakovic E, Rustempasic M, et al. Evaluation of medical and surgical management of critical extremity ischemia caused by atherothrombosis. Med Arh. 2010;64(6):328-31. PMID: 21218748.

Samson RH, Showalter DP, Yunis JP. Isolated femoropopliteal bypass graft for limb salvage after failed tibial reconstruction: a viable alternative to amputation. J Vasc Surg. 1999;29(3):409-12. PMID: 10069904.

Schleinitz MD, Weiss JP, Owens DK. Clopidogrel versus aspirin for secondary prophylaxis of vascular events: a cost-effectiveness analysis. Am J Med. 2004;116(12):797-806. PMID: 15178495.

Shukla V. Cilostazol: a replacement for pentoxifylline? Issues Emerg Health Technol. 1999;(7):1-4. PMID: 11811214.

Steinhubl SR, Bhatt DL, Brennan DM, et al. Aspirin to prevent cardiovascular disease: the association of aspirin dose and clopidogrel with thrombosis and bleeding. Ann Intern Med. 2009;150(6):379-86. PMID: 19293071.

Toursarkissian B, Shireman PK, Schoolfield J, et al. Outcomes following distal bypass graft occlusion in diabetics. Ann Vasc Surg. 2003;17(6):670-5. PMID: 14534843.

Vikram R, Ross RA, Bhat R, et al. Cutting balloon angioplasty versus standard balloon angioplasty for failing infra-inguinal vein grafts: comparative study of short- and mid-term primary patency rates. Cardiovasc Intervent Radiol. 2007;30(4):607-10. PMID: 17393055.

Visser K, De Vries SO, Kitslaar PJ, et al. Cost-effectiveness of diagnostic imaging work-up and treatment for patients with intermittent claudication in The Netherlands. Eur J Vasc Endovasc Surg. 2003;25(3):213-23. PMID: 12623332.

Yamasaki Y, Kim YS, Kawamori R. Rationale and protocol of a trial for prevention of diabetic atherosclerosis by using antiplatelet drugs: Study of Diabetic Atherosclerosis Prevention by Cilostazol (DAPC study). Cardiovasc Diabetol. 2006;5:16. PMID: 16925808.

Yeomans ND, Lanas AI, Talley NJ, et al. Prevalence and incidence of gastroduodenal ulcers during treatment with vascular protective doses of aspirin. Aliment Pharmacol Ther. 2005;22(9):795-801. PMID: 16225488.

Does not include intervention/comparators of interest

Allie DE, Hebert CJ, Lirtzman MD, et al. A safety and feasibility report of combined direct thrombin and GP IIb/IIIa inhibition with bivalirudin and tirofiban in peripheral vascular disease intervention: treating critical limb ischemia like acute coronary syndrome. J Invasive Cardiol. 2005;17(8):427-32. PMID: 16079449.

Allie DE, Hebert CJ, Lirtzman MD, et al. Combined glycoprotein IIb/IIIa and direct thrombin inhibition with eptifibatide and bivalirudin in the interventional treatment of critical limb ischemia: A safety and feasibility report. Vasc Dis Manage. 2006;3(6):368-75.

Anand S, Yusuf S, Xie C, et al. Oral anticoagulant and antiplatelet therapy and peripheral arterial disease. N Engl J Med. 2007;357(3):217-27. PMID: 17634457.

Antonicelli R, Sardina M, Scotti A, et al. Randomized trial of the effects of low-dose calcium-heparin in patients with peripheral arterial disease and claudication. Italian CAP Study Group. Am J Med. 1999;107(3):234-9. PMID: 10492316.

Aune S, Laxdal E. Above-knee prosthetic femoropopliteal bypass for intermittent claudication. Results of the initial and secondary procedures. Eur J Vasc Endovasc Surg. 2000;19(5):476-80. PMID: 10828227.

Awad S, Karkos CD, Serrachino-Inglott F, et al. The impact of diabetes on current revascularisation practice and clinical outcome in patients with critical lower limb ischaemia. Eur J Vasc Endovasc Surg. 2006;32(1):51-9. PMID: 16488631.

Badger SA, Soong CV, O'donnell ME, et al. Benefits of a supervised exercise program after lower limb bypass surgery. Vasc Endovascular Surg. 2007;41(1):27-32. PMID: 17277240.

Baldwin ZK, Pearce BJ, Curi MA, et al. Limb salvage after infrainguinal bypass graft failure. J Vasc Surg. 2004;39(5):951-7. PMID: 15111843.

Berceli SA, Hevelone ND, Lipsitz SR, et al. Surgical and endovascular revision of infrainguinal vein bypass grafts: analysis of midterm outcomes from the PREVENT III trial. J Vasc Surg. 2007;46(6):1173-9. PMID: 17950564.

Bregar U, Poredos P, Sabovic M, et al. The influence of atorvastatin on walking performance in peripheral arterial disease. Vasa. 2009;38(2):155-9. PMID: 19588303.

Cachovan M, Rogatti W, Creutzig A, et al. Treadmill testing for evaluation of claudication: comparison of constant-load and graded-exercise tests. Eur J Vasc Endovasc Surg. 1997;14(4):238-43. PMID: 9366786.

Cachovan M, Rogatti W, Woltering F, et al. Randomized reliability study evaluating constant-load and graded-exercise treadmill test for intermittent claudication. Angiology. 1999;50(3):193-200. PMID: 10088798.

Carreira JM, Reyes R, Gude F, et al. Long-term follow-up of Symphony nitinol stents in iliac arteriosclerosis obliterans. Minim Invasive Ther Allied Technol. 2008;17(1):34-42. PMID: 18270875.

Chaudhry H, Holland A, Dormandy J. Comparison of graded versus constant treadmill test protocols for quantifying intermittent claudication. Vasc Med. 1997;2(2):93-7. PMID: 9546962.

Delis KT, Nicolaides AN, Wolfe JH, et al. Improving walking ability and ankle brachial pressure indices in symptomatic peripheral vascular disease with intermittent pneumatic foot compression: a prospective controlled study with one-year follow-up. J Vasc Surg. 2000;31(4):650-61. PMID: 10753272.

Djoric P. Early individual experience with distal venous arterialization as a lower limb salvage procedure. Am Surg. 2011;77(6):726-30. PMID: 21679641.

Donas KP, Schwindt A, Pitoulias GA, et al. Endovascular treatment of internal iliac artery obstructive disease. J Vasc Surg. 2009;49(6):1447-51. PMID: 19497505.

Dosluoglu HH, Attuwaybi B, Cherr GS, et al. The management of ischemic heel ulcers and gangrene in the endovascular era. Am J Surg. 2007;194(5):600-5. PMID: 17936420.

Dosluoglu HH, Cherr GS, Lall P, et al. Peroneal artery-only runoff following endovascular revascularizations is effective for limb salvage in patients with tissue loss. J Vasc Surg. 2008;48(1):137-43. PMID: 18502081.

Duschek N, Vafaie M, Skrinjar E, et al. Comparison of enoxaparin and unfractionated heparin in endovascular interventions for the treatment of peripheral arterial occlusive disease: A randomized controlled trial. J Thromb Haemost. 2011;9(11):2159-67. PMID: 21910821.

Engelhardt M, Boos J, Bruijnen H, et al. Critical limb ischaemia: Initial treatment and predictors of amputation-free survival. Eur J Vasc Endovasc Surg. 2012;43(1):55-61. PMID: 22001150.

Esperon A, Kamaid E, Diamant M, et al. Uruguayan experience with cryopreserved arterial homografts. Transplant Proc. 2009;41(8):3500-4. PMID: 19857780.

Fernandez N, Mcenaney R, Marone LK, et al. Multilevel versus isolated endovascular tibial interventions for critical limb ischemia. J Vasc Surg. 2011;54(3):722-9. PMID: 21803523.

Fiotti N, Altamura N, Cappelli C, et al. Long term prognosis in patients with peripheral arterial disease treated with antiplatelet agents. Eur J Vasc Endovasc Surg. 2003;26(4):374-80. PMID: 14511998.

Fransson T, Thorne J. In situ saphenous vein bypass grafting - still first line treatment? A prospective study comparing surgical results between diabetic and non-diabetic populations. Vasa. 2010;39(1):59-65. PMID: 20186677.

Gardner AW, Killewich LA, Montgomery PS, et al. Response to exercise rehabilitation in smoking and nonsmoking patients with intermittent claudication. J Vasc Surg. 2004;39(3):531-8. PMID: 14981444.

Goodney PP, Schanzer A, Demartino RR, et al. Validation of the Society for Vascular Surgery's objective performance goals for critical limb ischemia in everyday vascular surgery practice. J Vasc Surg. 2011;54(1):100-8.e4. PMID: 21334173.

Gray BH, Olin JW. Limitations of percutaneous transluminal angioplasty with stenting for femoropopliteal arterial occlusive disease. Semin Vasc Surg. 1997;10(1):8-16. PMID: 9068071.

Green RM, Donarye C, Deweese JA. Autogenous venous bypass grafts and limb salvage: 5-year results in 1971 and 1991. Cardiovasc Surg. 1995;3(4):425-30. PMID: 7582999.

Gresele P, Migliacci R, Di Sante G, et al. Effect of cloricromene on intermittent claudication. A randomized, double-blind, placebo-controlled trial in patients treated with aspirin: effect on claudication distance and quality of life. CRAMPS Investigator Group. Cloricromene Randomized Arteriopathy Multicenter Prospective Study. Vasc Med. 2000;5(2):83-9. PMID: 10943584.

Gruss JD. Effects of adjuvant PGE1 therapy following profundaplasty in patients with severe limb ischaemia. Early and long-term results. Vasa. 1997;26(2):117-21. PMID: 9174388.

Heider P, Wildgruber M, Wolf O, et al. Improvement of microcirculation after percutaneous transluminal angioplasty in the lower limb with prostaglandin E1. Prostaglandins Other Lipid Mediat. 2009;88(1-2):23-30. PMID: 18832042.

Heneghan HM, Sultan S. Homocysteine, the cholesterol of the 21st century. Impact of hyperhomocysteinemia on patency and amputation-free survival after intervention for critical limb ischemia. J Endovasc Ther. 2008;15(4):399-407. PMID: 18729558.

Hiatt WR, Creager MA, Amato A, et al. Effect of propionyl-L-carnitine on a background of monitored exercise in patients with claudication secondary to peripheral artery disease. J Cardiopulm Rehabil Prev. 2011;31(2):125-32. PMID: 20861750.

Hingorani A, Ascher E, Markevich N, et al. The role of the endovascular surgeon for lower extremity ischemia. Acta Chir Belg. 2004;104(5):527-31. PMID: 15571018.

Ho GH, Moll FL, Eikelboom BC, et al. Endarterectomy of the superficial femoral artery. Semin Vasc Surg. 1995;8(3):216-24. PMID: 8564035.

Iida O, Nanto S, Uematsu M, et al. Cilostazol reduces restenosis after endovascular therapy in patients with femoropopliteal lesions. J Vasc Surg. 2008;48(1):144-9. PMID: 18482817.

Illnait J, Castano G, Alvarez E, et al. Effects of policosanol (10 mg/d) versus aspirin (100 mg/d) in patients with intermittent claudication: a 10-week, randomized, comparative study. Angiology. 2008;59(3):269-77. PMID: 18388038.

Jackson MR, Johnson WC, Williford WO, et al. The effect of anticoagulation therapy and graft selection on the ischemic consequences of femoropopliteal bypass graft occlusion: results from a multicenter randomized clinical trial. J Vasc Surg. 2002;35(2):292-8. PMID: 11854727.

Jaff MR, Dale RA, Creager MA, et al. Anti-chlamydial antibiotic therapy for symptom improvement in peripheral artery disease: prospective evaluation of rifalazil effect on vascular symptoms of intermittent claudication and other endpoints in Chlamydia pneumoniae seropositive patients (PROVIDENCE-1). Circulation. 2009;119(3):452-8. PMID: 19139383.

Jain KM, O'brien SP, Munn JS, et al. Axillobifemoral bypass: elective versus emergent operation. Ann Vasc Surg. 1998;12(3):265-9. PMID: 9588514.

Jivegard L, Drott C, Gelin J, et al. Effects of three months of low molecular weight heparin (dalteparin) treatment after bypass surgery for lower limb ischemia--a randomised placebo-controlled double blind multicentre trial. Eur J Vasc Endovasc Surg. 2005;29(2):190-8. PMID: 15649728.

Johnson WC, Williford WO. Benefits, morbidity, and mortality associated with long-term administration of oral anticoagulant therapy to patients with peripheral arterial bypass procedures: a prospective randomized study. J Vasc Surg. 2002;35(3):413-21. PMID: 11877686.

Johnson WC, Williford WO, Corson JD, et al. Hemorrhagic complications during long-term postoperative warfarin administration in patients undergoing lower extremity arterial bypass surgery. Vascular. 2004;12(6):362-8. PMID: 15895759.

Kaputin M, Ovcharenko DV, Platonov SA, et al. Comparative analysis of remote results of transluminal balloon angioplasty in treatment of lower limb critical ischaemia in groups of patients with and without diabetes mellitus. Angiol Sosud Khir. 2010;16(3):41-6. PMID: 21275231.

Kavros SJ, Delis KT, Turner NS, et al. Improving limb salvage in critical ischemia with intermittent pneumatic compression: a controlled study with 18-month follow-up. J Vasc Surg. 2008;47(3):543-9. PMID: 18295105.

Klevsgard R, Hallberg IR, Risberg B, et al. The effects of successful intervention on quality of life in patients with varying degrees of lower-limb ischaemia. Eur J Vasc Endovasc Surg. 2000;19(3):238-45. PMID: 10753686.

Klevsgard R, Risberg BO, Thomsen MB, et al. A 1-year follow-up quality of life study after hemodynamically successful or unsuccessful surgical revascularization of lower limb ischemia. J Vasc Surg. 2001;33(1):114-22. PMID: 11137931.

Ko YG, Shin S, Kim KJ, et al. Efficacy of stent-supported subintimal angioplasty in the treatment of long iliac artery occlusions. J Vasc Surg. 2011;54(1):116-22. PMID: 21334171.

Koch M, Trapp R, Hepp W. Impact of femoropopliteal bypass surgery on the survival and amputation rate of end-stage renal disease patients with critical limb ischemia. Med Klin (Munich). 2007;102(2):107-11. PMID: 17323017.

Koppensteiner R, Spring S, Amann-Vesti BR, et al. Low-molecular-weight heparin for prevention of restenosis after femoropopliteal percutaneous transluminal angioplasty: a randomized controlled trial. J Vasc Surg. 2006;44(6):1247-53. PMID: 17145426.

Kreatsoulas C, Anand SS. Disparity in outcomes of surgical revascularization for limb salvage. Race and gender are synergistic determinants of vein graft failure and limb loss. Nguyen LL, Hevelone N, Rogers SO, Bandyk DF, Clowes AW, Moneta GL, Lipsitz S, Conte MS. Circulation. 2009; 119: 123-130. Vasc Med. 2009;14(4):397-9. PMID: 19808727.

Kudo T, Chandra FA, Ahn SS. Long-term outcomes and predictors of iliac angioplasty with selective stenting. J Vasc Surg. 2005;42(3):466-75. PMID: 16171589.

Kudo T, Chandra FA, Ahn SS. The effectiveness of percutaneous transluminal angioplasty for the treatment of critical limb ischemia: a 10-year experience. J Vasc Surg. 2005;41(3):423-35; discussion 435. PMID: 15838475.

Kudo T, Rigberg DA, Reil TD, et al. The influence of the ipsilateral superficial femoral artery on iliac angioplasty. Ann Vasc Surg. 2006;20(4):502-11. PMID: 16732446.

Kumada Y, Aoyama T, Ishii H, et al. Long-term outcome of percutaneous transluminal angioplasty in chronic haemodialysis patients with peripheral arterial disease. Nephrol Dial Transplant. 2008;23(12):3996-4001. PMID: 18596131.

Kumar BN, Gambhir RP. Critical limb ischemia-need to look beyond limb salvage. Ann Vasc Surg. 2011;25(7):873-7. PMID: 21831588.

Lam RC, Shah S, Faries PL, et al. Incidence and clinical significance of distal embolization during percutaneous interventions involving the superficial femoral artery. J Vasc Surg. 2007;46(6):1155-9. PMID: 18154991.

Lantis JC, 2nd, Conte MS, Belkin M, et al. Infrainguinal bypass grafting in patients with end-stage renal disease: improving outcomes? J Vasc Surg. 2001;33(6):1171-8. PMID: 11389414.

Laxdal E, Eide GE, Wirsching J, et al. Homocysteine levels, haemostatic risk factors and patency rates after endovascular treatment of the above-knee femoro-popliteal artery. Eur J Vasc Endovasc Surg. 2004;28(4):410-7. PMID: 15350565.

Lesiak T, Mikosinski J, Piskorz L, et al. Evaluation of combined, conservative treatment impact on the clinical course, blood flow parameters and muscle perfussion in the group of patients with newly diagnosed, untreated peripheral arterial disease (PAD). Clin Exp Med Lett. 2010;51(2):123-9.

Letterstal A, Forsberg C, Olofsson P, et al. Risk attitudes to treatment among patients with severe intermittent claudication. J Vasc Surg. 2008;47(5):988-94. PMID: 18455642.

Leu AJ, Schneider E, Canova CR, et al. Long-term results after recanalisation of chronic iliac artery occlusions by combined catheter therapy without stent placement. Eur J Vasc Endovasc Surg. 1999;18(6):499-505. PMID: 10637146.

Lofberg AM, Lorelius LE, Karacagil S, et al. The use of below-knee percutaneous transluminal angioplasty in arterial occlusive disease causing chronic critical limb ischemia. Cardiovasc Intervent Radiol. 1996;19(5):317-22. PMID: 8781151.

Luther M, Lepantalo M. Arterial reconstruction to the foot arteries--a viable option? Eur J Surg. 1997;163(9):659-65. PMID: 9311472.

Luther M, Lepantalo M. Infrainguinal reconstructions: influence of surgical experience on outcome. Cardiovasc Surg. 1998;6(4):351-7. PMID: 9725513.

Luther M. Surgical treatment for chronic critical leg ischaemia: a 5 year follow-up of socioeconomic outcome. Eur J Vasc Endovasc Surg. 1997;13(5):452-9. PMID: 9166267.

Manzi M, Fusaro M, Ceccacci T, et al. Clinical results of below-the knee intervention using pedal-plantar loop technique for the revascularization of foot arteries. J Cardiovasc Surg (Torino). 2009;50(3):331-7. PMID: 19543193.

Marin ML, Veith FJ, Sanchez LA, et al. Endovascular repair of aortoiliac occlusive disease. World J Surg. 1996;20(6):679-86. PMID: 8662152.

Martens JM, Knippenberg B, Vos JA, et al. Update on PADI trial: percutaneous transluminal angioplasty and drug-eluting stents for infrapopliteal lesions in critical limb ischemia. J Vasc Surg. 2009;50(3):687-9. PMID: 19700099.

Marzelle J, Fichelle JM, Cormier F, et al. Outcome of infrainguinal endovascular revascularization procedures for limb-threatening ischemia. Ann Vasc Surg. 1995;9(Suppl):S24-31. PMID: 8688306.

Maxwell AJ, Anderson BE, Cooke JP. Nutritional therapy for peripheral arterial disease: a double-blind, placebo-controlled, randomized trial of HeartBar. Vasc Med. 2000;5(1):11-9. PMID: 10737151.

Mazari FA, Carradice D, Rahman MN, et al. An analysis of relationship between quality of life indices and clinical improvement following intervention in patients with intermittent claudication due to femoropopliteal disease. J Vasc Surg. 2010;52(1):77-84. PMID: 20471779.

Melliere D, Berrahal D, Desgranges P, et al. Influence of diabetes on revascularisation procedures of the aorta and lower limb arteries: early results. Eur J Vasc Endovasc Surg. 1999;17(5):438-41. PMID: 10329530.

Mijailovic M, Lukic S. Limb salvage procedure in occlusion of the infrapopliteal arteries. Vojnosanit Pregl. 2007;64(2):135-8. PMID: 17348466.

Mirenda F, La Spada M, Baccellieri D, et al. Iloprost infusion in diabetic patients with peripheral arterial occlusive disease and foot ulcers. Chir Ital. 2005;57(6):731-5. PMID: 16400768.

Mobin-Uddin K, Vincent GS, Evans WE. Prevention of anastomotic intimal hyperplasia in infrainguinal PTFE bypass grafts with distal arterial segment interposition. Vasc Surg. 1999;33(3):269-81.

Mohler ER, 3rd, Gainer JL, Whitten K, et al. Evaluation of trans sodium crocetinate on safety and exercise performance in patients with peripheral artery disease and intermittent claudication. Vasc Med. 2011;16(5):346-53. PMID: 22003000.

Munoz-Torrero JF, Escudero D, Suarez C, et al. Concomitant use of proton pump inhibitors and clopidogrel in patients with coronary, cerebrovascular, or peripheral artery disease in the factores de Riesgo y ENfermedad Arterial (FRENA) registry. J Cardiovasc Pharmacol. 2011;57(1):13-9. PMID: 21164357.

Nehler MR, Brass EP, Anthony R, et al. Adjunctive parenteral therapy with lipo-ecraprost, a prostaglandin E1 analog, in patients with critical limb ischemia undergoing distal revascularization does not improve 6-month outcomes. J Vasc Surg. 2007;45(5):953-60; discussion 960-1. PMID: 17350216.

Nenci GG, Gresele P, Ferrari G, et al. Treatment of intermittent claudication with mesoglycan--a placebo-controlled, double-blind study. Thromb Haemost. 2001;86(5):1181-7. PMID: 11816704.

Neri Serneri GG, Coccheri S, Marubini E, et al. Picotamide, a combined inhibitor of thromboxane A2 synthase and receptor, reduces 2-year mortality in diabetics with peripheral arterial disease: the DAVID study. Eur Heart J. 2004;25(20):1845-52. PMID: 15474700.

Neville RF, Dy B, Singh N, et al. Distal vein patch with an arteriovenous fistula: a viable option for the patient without autogenous conduit and severe distal occlusive disease. J Vasc Surg. 2009;50(1):83-8. PMID: 19563955.

Nguyen BN, Conrad MF, Guest JM, et al. Late outcomes of balloon angioplasty and angioplasty with selective stenting for superficial femoral-popliteal disease are equivalent. J Vasc Surg. 2011;54(4):1051-7 e1. PMID: 21636240

Nguyen LL, Hevelone N, Rogers SO, et al. Disparity in outcomes of surgical revascularization for limb salvage: race and gender are synergistic determinants of vein graft failure and limb loss. Circulation. 2009;119(1):123-30. PMID: 19103988.

Nguyen LL, Moneta GL, Conte MS, et al. Prospective multicenter study of quality of life before and after lower extremity vein bypass in 1404 patients with critical limb ischemia. J Vasc Surg. 2006;44(5):977-83; discussion 983-4. PMID: 17098529.

Ogawa H, Nakayama M, Morimoto T, et al. Low-dose aspirin for primary prevention of atherosclerotic events in patients with type 2 diabetes: a randomized controlled trial. JAMA. 2008;300(18):2134-41. PMID: 18997198.

Oka RK, Altman M, Giacomini JC, et al. Abnormal cardiovascular response to exercise in patients with peripheral arterial disease: Implications for management. J Vasc Nurs. 2005;23(4):130-6; quiz 137-8. PMID: 16326331.

Ortmann J, Gahl B, Diehm N, et al. Survival benefits of revascularization in patients with critical limb ischemia and renal insufficiency. J Vasc Surg. 2012;56(3):737-45.e1. PMID: 22677008.

Ortmann J, Nesch E, Cajori G, et al. Benefit of immediate revascularization in women with critical limb ischemia in an intention-to-treat analysis. J Vasc Surg. 2011;54(6):1668-78.e1. PMID: 22035761.

Oser RF, Picus D, Hicks ME, et al. Accuracy of DSA in the evaluation of patency of infrapopliteal vessels. J Vasc Interv Radiol. 1995;6(4):589-94. PMID: 7579870.

Owens CD, Ho KJ, Kim S, et al. Refinement of survival prediction in patients undergoing lower extremity bypass surgery: stratification by chronic kidney disease classification. J Vasc Surg. 2007;45(5):944-52. PMID: 17391900.

Panchenko E, Eshkeeva A, Dobrovolsky A, et al. Effects of indobufen and pentoxifylline on walking capacity and hemostasis in patients with intermittent claudication: results of six months of treatment. Angiology. 1997;48(3):247-54. PMID: 9071201.

Panneton JM, Gloviczki P, Bower TC, et al. Pedal bypass for limb salvage: impact of diabetes on long-term outcome. Ann Vasc Surg. 2000;14(6):640-7. PMID: 11128460.

Passman MA, Marston WA, Carlin RE, et al. Long-term results of infrapopliteal bypass using polytetrafluoroethylene and Taylor vein patch for critical lower extremity ischemia. Vasc Surg. 2000;34(6):569-76.

Paumier A, Abraham P, Mahe G, et al. Functional outcome of hypogastric revascularisation for prevention of buttock claudication in patients with peripheral artery occlusive disease. Eur J Vasc Endovasc Surg. 2010;39(3):323-9. PMID: 19910224.

Peeters P, Verbist J, Deloose K, et al. Results with heparin bonded polytetrafluoroethylene grafts for femorodistal bypasses. J Cardiovasc Surg (Torino). 2006;47(4):407-13. PMID: 16953160.

Peregrin JH, Smirova S, Koznar B, et al. Self-expandable stent placement in infrapopliteal arteries after unsuccessful angioplasty failure: one-year follow-up. Cardiovasc Intervent Radiol. 2008;31(5):860-4. PMID: 18236105.

Plate G, Qvarfordt P, Oredsson S, et al. Obturator bypass to the distal profunda femoris artery using a medial approach--long-term results. Eur J Vasc Endovasc Surg. 1998;16(2):164-8. PMID: 9728438.

Plecha EJ, Lee C, Hye RJ. Factors influencing the outcome of paramalleolar bypass grafts. Ann Vasc Surg. 1996;10(4):356-60. PMID: 8879390.

Pomposelli FB, Jr., Arora S, Gibbons GW, et al. Lower extremity arterial reconstruction in the very elderly: successful outcome preserves not only the limb but also residential status and ambulatory function. J Vasc Surg. 1998;28(2):215-25. PMID: 9719316.

Rabellino M, Aragon-Sanchez J, Gonzalez G, et al. Is endovascular revascularisation worthwhile in diabetic patients with critical limb ischemia who also have end-stage renal disease? Diabetes Res Clin Pract. 2010;90(3):e79-81. PMID: 21030104.

Raffetto JD, Chen MN, Lamorte WW, et al. Factors that predict site of outflow target artery anastomosis in infrainguinal revascularization. J Vasc Surg. 2002;35(6):1093-9. PMID: 12042719.

Ramaswami G, D'ayala M, Hollier LH, et al. Rapid foot and calf compression increases walking distance in patients with intermittent claudication: results of a randomized study. J Vasc Surg. 2005;41(5):794-801. PMID: 15886663.

Randon C, Jacobs B, De Ryck F, et al. Fifteen years of infrapopliteal arterial reconstructions with cryopreserved venous allografts for limb salvage. J Vasc Surg. 2010;51(4):869-77. PMID: 20347683.

Rastan A, Schwarzwalder U, Noory E, et al. Primary use of sirolimus-eluting stents in the infrapopliteal arteries. J Endovasc Ther. 2010;17(4):480-7. PMID: 20681763.

Rauwerda JA. Surgical treatment of the infected diabetic foot. Diabetes Metab Res Rev. 2004;20(Suppl 1):S41-4. PMID: 15150813.

Ray SA, Buckenham TM, Belli AM, et al. The predictive value of laser Doppler fluxmetry and transcutaneous oximetry for clinical outcome in patients undergoing revascularisation for severe leg ischaemia. Eur J Vasc Endovasc Surg. 1997;13(1):54-9. PMID: 9046915.

Ray SA, Rowley MR, Bevan DH, et al. Hypercoagulable abnormalities and postoperative failure of arterial reconstruction. Eur J Vasc Endovasc Surg. 1997;13(4):363-70. PMID: 9133987.

Rhee SY, Kim YS, Chon S, et al. Long-term effects of cilostazol on the prevention of macrovascular disease in patients with type 2 diabetes mellitus. Diabetes Res Clin Pract. 2011;91(1):e11-4. PMID: 20934769.

Rossi PJ, Skelly CL, Meyerson SL, et al. Redo infrainguinal bypass: factors predicting patency and limb salvage. Ann Vasc Surg. 2003;17(5):492-502. PMID: 12958672.

Rzucidlo EM, Powell RJ, Zwolak RM, et al. Early results of stent-grafting to treat diffuse aortoiliac occlusive disease. J Vasc Surg. 2003;37(6):1175-80. PMID: 12764261.

Sarkar R, Ro KM, Obrand DI, et al. Lower extremity vascular reconstruction and endovascular surgery without preoperative angiography. Am J Surg. 1998;176(2):203-7. PMID: 9737633.

Scatena A, Petruzzi P, Ferrari M, et al. Outcomes of three years of teamwork on critical limb ischemia in patients with diabetes and foot lesions. Int J Low Extrem Wounds. 2012;11(2):113-9. PMID: 22665920.

Schmidt A, Piorkowski M, Werner M, et al. First experience with drug-eluting balloons in infrapopliteal arteries: restenosis rate and clinical outcome. J Am Coll Cardiol. 2011;58(11):1105-9. PMID: 21884945.

Schneider PA, Abcarian PW, Ogawa DY, et al. Should balloon angioplasty and stents have any role in operative intervention for lower extremity ischemia? Ann Vasc Surg. 1997;11(6):574-80. PMID: 9363302.

Schneider PA, Caps MT, Nelken N. Infrainguinal vein graft stenosis: cutting balloon angioplasty as the first-line treatment of choice. J Vasc Surg. 2008;47(5):960-6; discussion 966. PMID: 18372146.

Schneider PA, Caps MT, Ogawa DY, et al. Intraoperative superficial femoral artery balloon angioplasty and popliteal to distal bypass graft: an option for combined open and endovascular treatment of diabetic gangrene. J Vasc Surg. 2001;33(5):955-62. PMID: 11331834.

Schneider PA, Ogawa DY, Rush MP. Lower extremity revascularization without contrast arteriography: a prospective study of operation based upon duplex mapping. Cardiovasc Surg. 1999;7(7):699-703. PMID: 10639043.

Scott EC, Biuckians A, Light RE, et al. Subintimal angioplasty for the treatment of claudication and critical limb ischemia: 3-year results. J Vasc Surg. 2007;46(5):959-64. PMID: 17905560.

Scott EC, Biuckians A, Light RE, et al. Subintimal angioplasty: Our experience in the treatment of 506 infrainguinal arterial occlusions. J Vasc Surg. 2008;48(4):878-84. PMID: 18586445.

Seabrook GR, Cambria RA, Freischlag JA, et al. Health-related quality of life and functional outcome following arterial reconstruction for limb salvage. Cardiovasc Surg. 1999;7(3):279-86. PMID: 10386743.

Shah AP, Klein AJ, Sterrett A, et al. Clinical outcomes using aggressive approach to anatomic screening and endovascular revascularization in a veterans affairs population with critical limb ischemia. Catheter Cardiovasc Interv. 2009;74(1):11-9. PMID: 19360870.

Shammas NW, Dippel EJ, Amidon C, et al. In-hospital complications in treating chronic limb ischemia: The feasibility of alternative anticoagulation therapy to unfractionated heparin. Vasc Dis Manage. 2006;3(6):376-8.

Sigvant B, Henriksson M, Lundin F, et al. Asymptomatic peripheral arterial disease: is pharmacological prevention of cardiovascular risk cost-effective? Eur J Cardiovasc Prev Rehabil. 2011;18(2):254-61. PMID: 21450673.

Simo G, Banga P, Darabos G, et al. Stent-assisted Remote Iliac Artery Endarterectomy: An Alternative Approach to Treating Combined External Iliac and Common Femoral Artery Disease. Eur J Vasc Endovasc Surg. 2011;42(5):648-55. PMID: 21704539.

Simsir SA, Cabellon A, Kohlman-Trigoboff D, et al. Factors influencing limb salvage and survival after amputation and revascularization in patients with end-stage renal disease. Am J Surg. 1995;170(2):113-7. PMID: 7631913.

Smeets L, Ho GH, Hagenaars T, et al. Remote endarterectomy: first choice in surgical treatment of long segmental SFA occlusive disease? Eur J Vasc Endovasc Surg. 2003;25(6):583-9. PMID: 12787704.

Soder HK, Manninen HI, Jaakkola P, et al. Prospective trial of infrapopliteal artery balloon angioplasty for critical limb ischemia: angiographic and clinical results. J Vasc Interv Radiol. 2000;11(8):1021-31. PMID: 10997465.

Soder HK, Manninen HI, Rasanen HT, et al. Failure of prolonged dilation to improve long-term patency of femoropopliteal artery angioplasty: results of a prospective trial. J Vasc Interv Radiol. 2002;13(4):361-9. PMID: 11932366.

Soga Y, Iida O, Hirano K, et al. Impact of cilostazol after endovascular treatment for infrainguinal disease in patients with critical limb ischemia. J Vasc Surg. 2011;54(6):1659-67. PMID: 21872419.

Soga Y, Iida O, Hirano K, et al. Restenosis after stent implantation for superficial femoral artery disease in patients treated with cilostazol. Catheter Cardiovasc Interv. 2011;79(4):541-8. PMID: 21805619.

Spinosa DJ, Harthun NL, Bissonette EA, et al. Subintimal arterial flossing with antegrade-retrograde intervention (SAFARI) for subintimal recanalization to treat chronic critical limb ischemia. J Vasc Interv Radiol. 2005;16(1):37-44. PMID: 15640408.

Stanisic M, Winckiewicz M and Majewska N. Evaluation of the criteria influencing certification regarding the ability to work on patients after open or endovascular operations on the arterial system of lower limbs. Acta Angiolog. 2008;14(1):9-17.

Stone PA, Armstrong PA, Bandyk DF, et al. Duplex ultrasound criteria for femorofemoral bypass revision. J Vasc Surg. 2006;44(3):496-502. PMID: 16950423.

Strano A. Propionyl-L-carnitine versus pentoxifylline: Improvement in walking capacity in patients with intermittent claudication. Clin Drug Invest. 2002;22(Suppl 1):1-6.

Suding PN, Mcmaster W, Hansen E, et al. Increased endovascular interventions decrease the rate of lower limb artery bypass operations without an increase in major amputation rate. Ann Vasc Surg. 2008;22(2):195-9. PMID: 18346571.

Szyma, ska J, Nowotny J, et al. The effect of high tone power therapy on gait range in patients with chronic lower limb ischaemia. Ortop Traumatol Rehabil. 2011;13(3):279-92. PMID: 21750358.

Taylor MD, Napolitano LM. Methicillin-resistant Staphylococcus aureus infections in vascular surgery: increasing prevalence. Surg Infect (Larchmt). 2004;5(2):180-7. PMID: 15353115.

Taylor SM, Kalbaugh CA, Blackhurst DW, et al. A comparison of percutaneous transluminal angioplasty versus amputation for critical limb ischemia in patients unsuitable for open surgery. J Vasc Surg. 2007;45(2):304-10; discussion 310-1. PMID: 17264008.

Taylor SM, Kalbaugh CA, Healy MG, et al. Do current outcomes justify more liberal use of revascularization for vasculogenic claudication? A single center experience of 1,000 consecutively treated limbs. J Am Coll Surg. 2008;206(5):1053-62; discussion 1062-4. PMID: 18471755.

Taylor SM, Langan EM, 3rd, Snyder BA, et al. Superficial femoral artery eversion endarterectomy: a useful adjunct for infrainguinal bypass in the presence of limited autogenous vein. J Vasc Surg. 1997;26(3):439-45; discussion 445-6. PMID: 9308589.

Tebbutt N, Robinson L, Todhunter J, et al. A plantar flexion device exercise programme for patients with peripheral arterial disease: a randomised prospective feasibility study. Physiotherapy. 2011;97(3):244-9. PMID: 21820543.

Thorne J, Danielsson G, Danielsson P, et al. Intraoperative angioscopy may improve the outcome of in situ saphenous vein bypass grafting: a prospective study. J Vasc Surg. 2002;35(4):759-65. PMID: 11932676.

Tielbeek AV, Vroegindeweij D, Buth J, et al. Comparison of intravascular ultrasonography and intraarterial digital subtraction angiography after directional atherectomy of short lesions in femoropopliteal arteries. J Vasc Surg. 1996;23(3):436-45. PMID: 8601885.

Tisi PV, Mirnezami A, Baker S, et al. Role of subintimal angioplasty in the treatment of chronic lower limb ischaemia. Eur J Vasc Endovasc Surg. 2002;24(5):417-22. PMID: 12435341.

Tonnesen KH, Holstein P, Rordam L, et al. Early results of percutaneous transluminal angioplasty (PTA) of failing below-knee bypass grafts. Eur J Vasc Endovasc Surg. 1998;15(1):51-6. PMID: 9519000.

Treiman GS, Schneider PA, Lawrence PF, et al. Does stent placement improve the results of ineffective or complicated iliac artery angioplasty? J Vasc Surg. 1998;28(1):104-12; discussion 113-4. PMID: 9685136.

Treiman GS, Treiman R, Whiting J. Results of percutaneous subintimal angioplasty using routine stenting. J Vasc Surg. 2006;43(3):513-9. PMID: 16520165.

Ubbink DT, Tulevski, Ii, Legemate DA, et al. Diabetes mellitus is not a contra-indication for peripheral vascular intervention in patients with leg ischemia. Vasa. 1997;26(1):39-42. PMID: 9163236.

Uccioli L, Gandini R, Giurato L, et al. Long-term outcomes of diabetic patients with critical limb ischemia followed in a tertiary referral diabetic foot clinic. Diabetes Care. 2010;33(5):977-82. PMID: 20200304.

Van Dijk LC, Van Urk H, Du Bois NA, et al. A new "closed" in situ vein bypass technique results in a reduced wound complication rate. Eur J Vasc Endovasc Surg. 1995;10(2):162-7. PMID: 7655967.

Virkkunen J, Heikkinen M, Lepantalo M, et al. Diabetes as an independent risk factor for early postoperative complications in critical limb ischemia. J Vasc Surg. 2004;40(4):761-7. PMID: 15472606.

Voellinger DG, Jordan Jr WD. Video-assisted vein harvest: A single institution's experience of 103 peripheral bypass cases. Vasc Surg. 1998;32(6):545-57.

Vouyouka AG, Egorova NN, Salloum A, et al. Lessons learned from the analysis of gender effect on risk factors and procedural outcomes of lower extremity arterial disease. J Vasc Surg. 2010;52(5):1196-202. PMID: 20674247.

Wann-Hansson C, Hallberg IR, Risberg B, et al. A comparison of the Nottingham Health Profile and Short Form 36 Health Survey in patients with chronic lower limb ischaemia in a longitudinal perspective. Health Qual Life Outcomes. 2004;2:9. PMID: 14969590.

Weaver FA, Comerota AJ, Youngblood M, et al. Surgical revascularization versus thrombolysis for nonembolic lower extremity native artery occlusions: results of a prospective randomized trial. The STILE Investigators. Surgery versus Thrombolysis for Ischemia of the Lower Extremity. J Vasc Surg. 1996;24(4):513-21; discussion 521-3. PMID: 8911400.

Welten GM, Schouten O, Hoeks SE, et al. Long-term prognosis of patients with peripheral arterial disease: a comparison in patients with coronary artery disease. J Am Coll Cardiol. 2008;51(16):1588-96. PMID: 18420103.

Werneck CC, Lindsay TF. Tibial angioplasty for limb salvage in high-risk patients and cost analysis. Ann Vasc Surg. 2009;23(5):554-9. PMID: 19632085.

Wilson YG, Davies AH, Currie IC, et al. Vein graft stenosis: incidence and intervention. Eur J Vasc Endovasc Surg. 1996;11(2):164-9. PMID: 8616647.

Wixon CL, Mills JL, Westerband A, et al. An economic appraisal of lower extremity bypass graft maintenance. J Vasc Surg. 2000;32(1):1-12. PMID: 10876201.

Yoshida RDA, Matida CK, Sobreira ML, et al. Comparative study of evolution and survival of patients with intermittent claudication, with or without limitation for exercises, followed in a specific outpatient setting. J Vasc Bras. 2008;7(2):112-22.

Zachry WM, Wilson JP, Lawson KA, et al. Procedure costs and outcomes associated with pharmacologic management of peripheral arterial disease in the Department of Defense. Clin Ther. 1999;21(8):1358-69. PMID: 10485507.

Zukauskas G, Ulevicius H. Simultaneous versus two-stage multisegmental reconstruction for critical lower limb ischemia. Ann Saudi Med. 1995;15(4):333-8. PMID: 17590601.

Zukauskas G, Ulevicius H, Janusauskas E. Re-do operations after failed multisegmental reconstructive arterial surgery for critical limb ischaemia. Cardiovasc Surg. 1997;5(4):419-23. PMID: 9350799.

Does not include primary or secondary outcomes of interest

Berger K, Hessel F, Kreuzer J, et al. Clopidogrel versus aspirin in patients with atherothrombosis: CAPRIE-based calculation of cost-effectiveness for Germany. Curr Med Res Opin. 2008;24(1):267-74. PMID: 18053318.

Bradbury A, Wilmink T, Lee AJ, et al. Bypass versus angioplasty to treat severe limb ischemia: factors that affect treatment preferences of UK surgeons and interventional radiologists. J Vasc Surg. 2004;39(5):1026-32. PMID: 15111856.

Bramer SL, Forbes WP, Mallikaarjun S. Cilostazol pharmacokinetics after single and multiple oral doses in healthy males and patients with intermittent claudication resulting from peripheral arterial disease. Clin Pharmacokinet. 1999;37(Suppl 2):1-11. PMID: 10702882.

Cleanthis M, Bhattacharya V, Smout J, et al. Combined aspirin and cilostazol treatment is associated with reduced platelet aggregation and prevention of exercise-induced platelet activation. Eur J Vasc Endovasc Surg. 2009;37(5):604-10. PMID: 19297212.

Cleanthis M, Smout J, Bhattacharya V, et al. Treadmill exercise in claudicants on aspirin results in improved antioxidant status but only minimal platelet activation. Platelets. 2005;16(8):446-52. PMID: 16287611.

Cox MH, Robison JG, Brothers TE, et al. Contemporary analysis of outcomes following lower extremity bypass in patients with end-stage renal disease. Ann Vasc Surg. 2001;15(3):374-82. PMID: 11414090.

Crowther RG, Spinks WL, Leicht AS, et al. The influence of a long term exercise program on lower limb movement variability and walking performance in patients with peripheral arterial disease. Hum Mov Sci. 2009;28(4):494-503. PMID: 19435644.

Duscha BD, Robbins JL, Jones WS, et al. Angiogenesis in Skeletal Muscle Precede Improvements in Peak Oxygen Uptake in Peripheral Artery Disease Patients. Arterioscler Thromb Vasc Biol. 2011;31(11):2742-8. PMID: 21868709.

Heredero AF, Acin F, March JR, et al. Impact of endovascular surgery on management of critical lower-limb ischemia in a vascular surgery department. Vasc Endovascular Surg. 2005;39(5):429-35. PMID: 16193216.

Hiatt WR, Regensteiner JG, Wolfel EE, et al. Effect of exercise training on skeletal muscle histology and metabolism in peripheral arterial disease. J Appl Physiol. 1996;81(2):780-8. PMID: 8872646.

Huisinga JM, Pipinos, Ii, Johanning JM, et al. The effect of pharmacological treatment on gait biomechanics in peripheral arterial disease patients. J Neuroeng Rehabil. 2010;7:25. PMID: 20529284.

Incandela L, De Sanctis MT, Cesarone MR, et al. Short-range intermittent claudication and rest pain: microcirculatory effects of pentoxifylline in a randomized, controlled trial. Angiology. 2002;53(Suppl 1)S27-30. PMID: 11865832.

Singh S, Evans L, Datta D, et al. The costs of managing lower limb-threatening ischaemia. Eur J Vasc Endovasc Surg. 1996;12(3):359-62. PMID: 8896481.

Smout JD, Mikhailidis DP, Shenton BK, et al. Combination antiplatelet therapy in patients with peripheral vascular bypass grafts. Clin Appl Thromb Hemost. 2004;10(1):9-18. PMID: 14979400.

Sung RS, Althoen M, Howell TA, et al. Peripheral vascular occlusive disease in renal transplant recipients: risk factors and impact on kidney allograft survival. Transplantation. 2000;70(7):1049-54. PMID: 11045641.

Taft C, Sullivan M, Lundholm K, et al. Predictors of treatment outcome in intermittent claudication. Eur J Vasc Endovasc Surg. 2004;27(1):24-32. PMID: 14652833.

Van Asselt AD, Nicolai SP, Joore MA, et al. Cost-effectiveness of exercise therapy in patients with intermittent claudication: supervised exercise therapy versus a 'go home and walk' advice. Eur J Vasc Endovasc Surg. 2011;41(1):97-103. PMID: 21159527.

Van Dijk LC, Seerden R, Van Urk H, et al. Comparison of cost affecting parameters and costs of the "closed" and "open" in situ bypass technique. Eur J Vasc Endovasc Surg. 1997;13(5):460-3. PMID: 9166268.

Varela C, Acin F, De Haro J, et al. The role of foot collateral vessels on ulcer healing and limb salvage after successful endovascular and surgical distal procedures according to an angiosome model. Vasc Endovascular Surg. 2010;44(8):654-60. PMID: 20675308.

Wilhite DB, Comerota AJ, Schmieder FA, et al. Managing PAD with multiple platelet inhibitors: the effect of combination therapy on bleeding time. J Vasc Surg. 2003;38(4):710-3. PMID: 14560218.

Wyttenbach R, Gallino A, Alerci M, et al. Effects of percutaneous transluminal angioplasty and endovascular brachytherapy on vascular remodeling of human femoropopliteal artery by noninvasive magnetic resonance imaging. Circulation. 2004;110(9):1156-61. PMID: 15326071.

Zeltsman D, Kerstein MD. Sociology of care in patients with severe peripheral vascular disease. Am Surg. 1998;64(2):175-7. PMID: 9486893.

Ziegler S, Maca T, Alt E, et al. Monitoring of antiplatelet therapy with the PFA-100 in peripheral angioplasty patients. Platelets. 2002;13(8):493-7. PMID: 12487783.

Single treatment strategy comparison

Abou-Zamzam AM, Jr., Moneta GL, Lee RW, et al. Peroneal bypass is equivalent to inframalleolar bypass for ischemic pedal gangrene. Arch Surg. 1996;131(8):894-8; discussion 988-9. PMID: 8712916.

Aburahma AF, Hayes JD, Flaherty SK, et al. Primary iliac stenting versus transluminal angioplasty with selective stenting. J Vasc Surg. 2007;46(5):965-70. PMID: 17905559.

Albers M, Fratezi AC, De Luccia N. Walking ability and quality of life as outcome measures in a comparison of arterial reconstruction and leg amputation for the treatment of vascular disease. Eur J Vasc Endovasc Surg. 1996;11(3):308-14. PMID: 8601241.

Alexandrescu V, Vincent G, Azdad K, et al. A reliable approach to diabetic neuroischemic foot wounds: below-the-knee angiosome-oriented angioplasty. J Endovasc Ther. 2011;18(3):376-87. PMID: 21679080.

Alimi Y, Di Mauro P, Barthelemy P, et al. Iliac transluminal angioplasty and distal surgical revascularisation can be performed in a one-step technique. Int Angiol. 1997;16(2):83-7. PMID: 9257667.

Allen BT, Reilly JM, Rubin BG, et al. Femoropopliteal bypass for claudication: vein vs. PTFE. Ann Vasc Surg. 1996;10(2):178-85. PMID: 8733871.

Allen JD, Stabler T, Kenjale A, et al. Plasma nitrite flux predicts exercise performance in peripheral arterial disease after 3months of exercise training. Free Radic Biol Med. 2010;49(6):1138-44. PMID: 20620208.

Amighi J, Schillinger M, Dick P, et al. De novo superficial femoropopliteal artery lesions: peripheral cutting balloon angioplasty and restenosis rates--randomized controlled trial. Radiology. 2008;247(1):267-72. PMID: 18270378.

Anonymous. PTFE bypass to below-knee arteries: distal vein collar or not? A prospective randomised multicentre study. Eur J Vasc Endovasc Surg. 2010;39(6):747-54. PMID: 20236841.

Arnold TE, Kerstein MD. Secondary distal extension of infrainguinal bypass: long-term limb and patient survival. Ann Vasc Surg. 2000;14(5):450-6. PMID: 10990553.

Bacourt F. Prospective randomized study of carbon-impregnated polytetrafluoroethylene grafts for below-knee popliteal and distal bypass: results at 2 years. The Association Universitaire de Recherche en Chirurgie. Ann Vasc Surg. 1997;11(6):596-603. PMID: 9363305.

Bakken AM, Saad WE, Davies MG. Cryoballoon angioplasty broadens the role of primary angioplasty and reduces adjuvant stenting in complex superficial femoral artery lesions. J Am Coll Surg. 2008;206(3):524-32. PMID: 18308225.

Ballotta E, Renon L, De Rossi A, et al. Prospective randomized study on reversed saphenous vein infrapopliteal bypass to treat limb-threatening ischemia: common femoral artery versus superficial femoral or popliteal and tibial arteries as inflow. J Vasc Surg. 2004;40(4):732-40. PMID: 15472602.

Ballotta E, Renon L, Toffano M, et al. Prospective randomized study on bilateral above-knee femoropopliteal revascularization: Polytetrafluoroethylene graft versus reversed saphenous vein. J Vasc Surg. 2003;38(5):1051-5. PMID: 14603216.

Bastounis E, Georgopoulos S, Maltezos C, et al. PTFE-vein composite grafts for critical limb ischaemia: a valuable alternative to all-autogenous infrageniculate reconstructions. Eur J Vasc Endovasc Surg. 1999;18(2):127-32. PMID: 10426969.

Battaglia G, Tringale R, Monaca V. Retrospective comparison of a heparin bonded ePTFE graft and saphenous vein for infragenicular bypass: implications for standard treatment protocol. J Cardiovasc Surg (Torino). 2006;47(1):41-7. PMID: 16434944.

Becquemin JP, Favre JP, Marzelle J, et al. Systematic versus selective stent placement after superficial femoral artery balloon angioplasty: a multicenter prospective randomized study. J Vasc Surg. 2003;37(3):487-94. PMID: 12618680.

Bonvini R, Baumgartner I, Do DD, et al. Late acute thrombotic occlusion after endovascular brachytherapy and stenting of femoropopliteal arteries. J Am Coll Cardiol. 2003;41(3):409-12. PMID: 12575967.

Bosch JL, Van Der Graaf Y, Hunink MG. Health-related quality of life after angioplasty and stent placement in patients with iliac artery occlusive disease: results of a randomized controlled clinical trial. The Dutch Iliac Stent Trial Study Group. Circulation. 1999;99(24):3155-60. PMID: 10377079.

Bosiers M, Hart JP, Deloose K, et al. Endovascular therapy as the primary approach for limb salvage in patients with critical limb ischemia: experience with 443 infrapopliteal procedures. Vascular. 2006;14(2):63-9. PMID: 16956473.

Bosiers M, Peeters P, D'archambeau O, et al. AMS INSIGHT--absorbable metal stent implantation for treatment of below-the-knee critical limb ischemia: 6-month analysis. Cardiovasc Intervent Radiol. 2009;32(3):424-35. PMID: 19093148.

Bosiers M, Scheinert D, Peeters P, et al. Randomized comparison of everolimus-eluting versus bare-metal stents in patients with critical limb ischemia and infrapopliteal arterial occlusive disease. J Vasc Surg. 2012;55(2):390-8. PMID: 22169682.

Boufi M, Dona B, Orsini B, et al. A comparison of the standard bolia technique versus subintimal recanalization plus Viabahn stent graft in the management of femoro-popliteal occlusions. J Vasc Surg. 2010;52(5):1211-7. PMID: 20692789.

Brass EP, Cooper LT, Morgan RE, et al. A phase II dose-ranging study of the phosphodiesterase inhibitor K-134 in patients with peripheral artery disease and claudication. J Vasc Surg. 2012;55(2):381-9.e1. PMID: 22119244.

Brothers TE, Robison JG, Elliott BM. Diabetes mellitus is the major risk factor for African Americans who undergo peripheral bypass graft operation. J Vasc Surg. 1999;29(2):352-9. PMID: 9950993.

Burger DH, Kappetein AP, Van Bockel JH, et al. A prospective randomized trial comparing vein with polytetrafluoroethylene in above-knee femoropopliteal bypass grafting. J Vasc Surg. 2000;32(2):278-83. PMID: 10917987.

Carmeli E, Barchad S, Masharawi Y, et al. Impact of a walking program in people with down syndrome. J Strength Cond Res. 2004;18(1):180-4. PMID: 14971963.

Cejna M, Thurnher S, Illiasch H, et al. PTA versus Palmaz stent placement in femoropopliteal artery obstructions: a multicenter prospective randomized study. J Vasc Interv Radiol. 2001;12(1):23-31. PMID: 11200349.

Cheetham DR, Burgess L, Ellis M, et al. Does supervised exercise offer adjuvant benefit over exercise advice alone for the treatment of intermittent claudication? A randomised trial. Eur J Vasc Endovasc Surg. 2004;27(1):17-23. PMID: 14652832.

Chew DK, Nguyen LL, Owens CD, et al. Comparative analysis of autogenous infrainguinal bypass grafts in African Americans and Caucasians: the association of race with graft function and limb salvage. J Vasc Surg. 2005;42(4):695-701. PMID: 16242557.

Ciocon JO, Galindo-Ciocon D, Galindo DJ. A comparison between aspirin and pentoxifylline in relieving claudication due to peripheral vascular disease in the elderly. Angiology. 1997;48(3):237-40. PMID: 9071199.

Collins EG, Edwin Langbein W, Orebaugh C, et al. PoleStriding exercise and vitamin E for management of peripheral vascular disease. Med Sci Sports Exerc. 2003;35(3):384-93. PMID: 12618567.

Collins EG, Langbein WE, Orebaugh C, et al. Cardiovascular training effect associated with polestriding exercise in patients with peripheral arterial disease. J Cardiovasc Nurs. 2005;20(3):177-85. PMID: 15870588.

Creager MA, Pande RL, Hiatt WR. A randomized trial of iloprost in patients with intermittent claudication. Vasc Med. 2008;13(1):5-13. PMID: 18372433.

Davidovic L, Jakovljevic N, Radak D, et al. Dacron or ePTFE graft for above-knee femoropopliteal bypass reconstruction. A bi-centre randomised study. Vasa. 2010;39(1):77-84. PMID: 20186679.

Degischer S, Labs KH, Hochstrasser J, et al. Physical training for intermittent claudication: a comparison of structured rehabilitation versus home-based training. Vasc Med. 2002;7(2):109-15. PMID: 12402991.

Derubertis BG, Vouyouka A, Rhee SJ, et al. Percutaneous intervention for infrainguinal occlusive disease in women: equivalent outcomes despite increased severity of disease compared with men. J Vasc Surg. 2008;48(1):150-7; discussion 157-8. PMID: 18589232.

Devine C, Mccollum C. Heparin-bonded Dacron or polytetrafluorethylene for femoropopliteal bypass: five-year results of a prospective randomized multicenter clinical trial. J Vasc Surg. 2004;40(5):924-31. PMID: 15557906.

Devine C, Hons B, Mccollum C. Heparin-bonded Dacron or polytetrafluoroethylene for femoropopliteal bypass grafting: a multicenter trial. J Vasc Surg. 2001;33(3):533-9. PMID: 11241124

Di Salvo MM, Ardita G, Giani L, et al. Comparison between intravenous iloprost and vasoactive drugs in limb ischemia IIB severe. A retrospective analysis. Minerva Cardioangiol. 2006;54(3):377-81. PMID: 16733512.

Dick P, Wallner H, Sabeti S, et al. Balloon angioplasty versus stenting with nitinol stents in intermediate length superficial femoral artery lesions. Catheter Cardiovasc Interv. 2009;74(7):1090-5. PMID: 19859954.

Dorigo W, Pulli R, Castelli P, et al. A multicentric comparison between autologous saphenous vein and heparin-bonded expanded polytetrafluoroethylene (ePTFE) graft in the treatment of critical limb ischemia in diabetics. J Vasc Surg. 2011;54(5):1332-8. PMID: 21840151.

Duda SH, Bosiers M, Lammer J, et al. Drug-eluting and bare nitinol stents for the treatment of atherosclerotic lesions in the superficial femoral artery: long-term results from the SIROCCO trial. J Endovasc Ther. 2006;13(6):701-10. PMID: 17154704.

Duda SH, Bosiers M, Lammer J, et al. Sirolimus-eluting versus bare nitinol stent for obstructive superficial femoral artery disease: the SIROCCO II trial. J Vasc Interv Radiol. 2005;16(3):331-8. PMID: 15758128.

Duda SH, Pusich B, Richter G, et al. Sirolimus-eluting stents for the treatment of obstructive superficial femoral artery disease: six-month results. Circulation. 2002;106(12):1505-9. PMID: 12234956.

Eiberg JP, Roder O, Stahl-Madsen M, et al. Fluoropolymer-coated dacron versus PTFE grafts for femorofemoral crossover bypass: randomised trial. Eur J Vasc Endovasc Surg. 2006;32(4):431-8. PMID: 16807001.

Fakhry F, Spronk S, De Ridder M, et al. Long-term effects of structured home-based exercise program on functional capacity and quality of life in patients with intermittent claudication. Arch Phys Med Rehabil. 2011;92(7):1066-73. PMID: 21704786.

Fisher CM, Fletcher JP, May J, et al. No additional benefit from laser in balloon angioplasty of the superficial femoral artery. Eur J Vasc Endovasc Surg. 1996;11(3):349-52. PMID: 8601248.

Fowler B, Jamrozik K, Norman P, et al. Improving maximum walking distance in early peripheral arterial disease: randomised controlled trial. Aust J Physiother. 2002;48(4):269-75. PMID: 12443521.

Gardner AW, Montgomery PS. The Baltimore activity scale for intermittent claudication: a validation study. Vasc Endovascular Surg. 2006;40(5):383-91. PMID: 17038572.

Gardner AW, Katzel LI, Sorkin JD, et al. Exercise rehabilitation improves functional outcomes and peripheral circulation in patients with intermittent claudication: a randomized controlled trial. J Am Geriatr Soc. 2001;49(6):755-62. PMID: 11454114.

Gardner AW, Montgomery PS, Flinn WR, et al. The effect of exercise intensity on the response to exercise rehabilitation in patients with intermittent claudication. J Vasc Surg. 2005;42(4):702-9. PMID: 16242558.

Gisbertz SS, Ramzan M, Tutein Nolthenius RP, et al. Short-term results of a randomized trial comparing remote endarterectomy and supragenicular bypass surgery for long occlusions of the superficial femoral artery [the REVAS trial]. Eur J Vasc Endovasc Surg. 2009;37(1):68-76. PMID: 18990592.

Gisbertz SS, Tutein Nolthenius RP, De Borst GJ, et al. Remote endarterectomy versus supragenicular bypass surgery for long occlusions of the superficial femoral artery: medium-term results of a randomized controlled trial (the REVAS trial). Ann Vasc Surg. 2010;24(8):1015-23. PMID: 21035693.

Green RM, Abbott WM, Matsumoto T, et al. Prosthetic above-knee femoropopliteal bypass grafting: five-year results of a randomized trial. J Vasc Surg. 2000;31(3):417-25. PMID: 10709052.

Grimm J, Muller-Hulsbeck S, Jahnke T, et al. Randomized study to compare PTA alone versus PTA with Palmaz stent placement for femoropopliteal lesions. J Vasc Interv Radiol. 2001;12(8):935-42. PMID: 11487673.

Grizzo Cucato G, De Moraes Forjaz CL, Kanegusuku H, et al. Effects of walking and strength training on resting and exercise cardiovascular responses in patients with intermittent claudication. Vasa. 2011;40(5):390-7. PMID: 21948782.

Gupta AK, Bandyk DF, Cheanvechai D, et al. Natural history of infrainguinal vein graft stenosis relative to bypass grafting technique. J Vasc Surg. 1997;25(2):211-20; discussion 220-5. PMID: 9052556.

Hamsho A, Nott D, Harris PL. Prospective randomised trial of distal arteriovenous fistula as an adjunct to femoro-infrapopliteal PTFE bypass. Eur J Vasc Endovasc Surg. 1999;17(3):197-201. PMID: 10092890.

Hepp W, Von BaE, Corovic I, et al. Clinical efficacy of IV prostaglandin E1 and IV pentoxifylline in patients with arterial occlusive disease of Fontaine stage IIb: A multicenter, randomized comparative study. Int J Angiol. 1996;5(1):32-7.

Hertzer NR, Bena JF, Karafa MT. A personal experience with direct reconstruction and extra-anatomic bypass for aortoiliofemoral occlusive disease. J Vasc Surg. 2007;45(3):527-35; discussion 535. PMID: 17321340.

Hertzer NR, Bena JF, Karafa MT. A personal experience with the influence of diabetes and other factors on the outcome of infrainguinal bypass grafts for occlusive disease. J Vasc Surg. 2007;46(2):271-9. PMID: 17600656.

Hodges LD, Sandercock GR, Das SK, et al. Randomized controlled trial of supervised exercise to evaluate changes in cardiac function in patients with peripheral atherosclerotic disease. Clin Physiol Funct Imaging. 2008;28(1):32-7. PMID: 18005078.

Hoedt MT, Van Urk H, Hop WC, et al. A comparison of distal end-to-side and end-to-end anastomoses in femoropopliteal bypasses. Eur J Vasc Endovasc Surg. 2001;21(3):266-70. PMID: 11352686.

Huisinga JM, Pipinos, Ii, Stergiou N, et al. Treatment with pharmacological agents in peripheral arterial disease patients does not result in biomechanical gait changes. J Appl Biomech. 2010;26(3):341-8. PMID: 20841626.

Hultgren R, Olofsson P, Wahlberg E. Gender differences in patients treated for critical limb ischemia. Eur J Vasc Endovasc Surg. 2005;29(3):295-300. PMID: 15694804.

Imfeld S, Singer L, Degischer S, et al. Quality of life improvement after hospital-based rehabilitation or home-based physical training in intermittent claudication. Vasa. 2006;35(3):178-84. PMID: 16941407.

Ishii H, Kumada Y, Toriyama T, et al. Effects of oral cilostazol 100 mg BID on long-term patency after percutaneous transluminal angioplasty in patients with femoropopliteal disease undergoing hemodialysis: a retrospective chart review in Japanese patients. Clin Ther. 2010;32(1):24-33. PMID: 20171408.

Izquierdo-Porrera AM, Gardner AW, Powell CC, et al. Effects of exercise rehabilitation on cardiovascular risk factors in older patients with peripheral arterial occlusive disease. J Vasc Surg. 2000;31(4):670-7. PMID: 10753274.

Jackson MR, Ali AT, Bell C, et al. Aortofemoral bypass in young patients with premature atherosclerosis: is superficial femoral vein superior to Dacron? J Vasc Surg. 2004;40(1):17-23. PMID: 15218456.

Jackson MR, Belott TP, Dickason T, et al. The consequences of a failed femoropopliteal bypass grafting: comparison of saphenous vein and PTFE grafts. J Vasc Surg. 2000;32(3):498-504; 504-5. PMID: 10957656.

Jensen LP, Lepantalo M, Fossdal JE, et al. Dacron or PTFE for above-knee femoropopliteal bypass. a multicenter randomised study. Eur J Vasc Endovasc Surg. 2007;34(1):44-9. PMID: 17400486.

Johnson WC, Lee KK. Comparative evaluation of externally supported Dacron and polytetrafluoroethylene prosthetic bypasses for femorofemoral and axillofemoral arterial reconstructions. Veterans Affairs Cooperative Study #141. J Vasc Surg. 1999;30(6):1077-83. PMID: 10587392.

Jones PP, Skinner JS, Smith LK, et al. Functional improvements following StairMaster vs. treadmill exercise training for patients with intermittent claudication. J Cardiopulm Rehabil. 1996;16(1):47-55. PMID: 8907442.

Kakkos SK, Geroulakos G, Nicolaides AN. Improvement of the walking ability in intermittent claudication due to superficial femoral artery occlusion with supervised exercise and pneumatic foot and calf compression: a randomised controlled trial. Eur J Vasc Endovasc Surg. 2005;30(2):164-75. PMID: 15890545.

Kapfer X, Meichelboeck W, Groegler FM. Comparison of carbon-impregnated and standard ePTFE prostheses in extra-anatomical anterior tibial artery bypass: a prospective randomized multicenter study. Eur J Vasc Endovasc Surg. 2006;32(2):155-68. PMID: 16617028.

Karnabatidis D, Spiliopoulos S, Diamantopoulos A, et al. Primary everolimus-eluting stenting versus balloon angioplasty with bailout bare metal stenting of long infrapopliteal lesions for treatment of critical limb ischemia. J Endovasc Ther. 2011;18(1):1-12. PMID: 21314342.

Killewich LA, Macko RF, Montgomery PS, et al. Exercise training enhances endogenous fibrinolysis in peripheral arterial disease. J Vasc Surg. 2004;40(4):741-5. PMID: 15472603.

Kimura H, Miyata T, Sato O, et al. Infrainguinal arterial reconstruction for limb salvage in patients with end-stage renal disease. Eur J Vasc Endovasc Surg. 2003;25(1):29-34. PMID: 12525808.

Klein WM, Van Der Graaf Y, Seegers J, et al. Long-term cardiovascular morbidity, mortality, and reintervention after endovascular treatment in patients with iliac artery disease: The Dutch Iliac Stent Trial Study. Radiology. 2004;232(2):491-8. PMID: 15286319.

Klinkert P, Schepers A, Burger DH, et al. Vein versus polytetrafluoroethylene in above-knee femoropopliteal bypass grafting: five-year results of a randomized controlled trial. J Vasc Surg. 2003;37(1):149-55. PMID: 12514593.

Kobayashi M, Hida K, Shikata H, et al. Long term outcome of femoropopliteal bypass for claudication and critical ischemia. Asian Cardiovasc Thorac Ann. 2004;12(3):208-12. PMID: 15353457.

Koscielny A, Putz U, Willinek W, et al. Case-control comparison of profundaplasty and femoropopliteal supragenicular bypass for peripheral arterial disease. Br J Surg. 2010;97(3):344-8. PMID: 20101647.

Koskela VK, Salenius J, Suominen V. Peripheral arterial disease in octogenarians and nonagenarians: factors predicting survival. Ann Vasc Surg. 2011;25(2):169-76. PMID: 20926240.

Krajcer Z, Sioco G, Reynolds T. Comparison of Wallgraft and Wallstent for treatment of complex iliac artery stenosis and occlusion. Preliminary results of a prospective randomized study. Tex Heart Inst J. 1997;24(3):193-9. PMID: 9339507.

Krankenberg H, Schluter M, Steinkamp HJ, et al. Nitinol stent implantation versus percutaneous transluminal angioplasty in superficial femoral artery lesions up to 10 cm in length: the femoral artery stenting trial (FAST). Circulation. 2007;116(3):285-92. PMID: 17592075.

Kreienberg PB, Darling RC, 3rd, Chang BB, et al. Early results of a prospective randomized trial of spliced vein versus polytetrafluoroethylene graft with a distal vein cuff for limb-threatening ischemia. J Vasc Surg. 2002;35(2):299-306. PMID: 11854728.

Laird JR, Katzen BT, Scheinert D, et al. Nitinol stent implantation versus balloon angioplasty for lesions in the superficial femoral artery and proximal popliteal artery: twelve-month results from the RESILIENT randomized trial. Circ Cardiovasc Interv. 2010;3(3):267-76. PMID: 20484101.

Langbein WE, Collins EG, Orebaugh C, et al. Increasing exercise tolerance of persons limited by claudication pain using polestriding. J Vasc Surg. 2002;35(5):887-93. PMID: 12021703.

Larena-Avellaneda A, Russmann S, Fein M, et al. Prophylactic use of the silver-acetate-coated graft in arterial occlusive disease: a retrospective, comparative study. J Vasc Surg. 2009;50(4):790-8. PMID: 19660894.

Laurila K, Lepantalo M, Teittinen K, et al. Does an adjuvant AV-fistula improve the patency of a femorocrural PTFE bypass with distal vein cuff in critical leg ischaemia?--a prospective randomised multicentre trial. Eur J Vasc Endovasc Surg. 2004;27(2):180-5. PMID: 14718901.

Lawson JA, Tangelder MJ, Algra A, et al. The myth of the in situ graft: superiority in infrainguinal bypass surgery? Eur J Vasc Endovasc Surg. 1999;18(2):149-57. PMID: 10428752.

Lee TM, Su SF, Tsai CH, et al. Differential effects of cilostazol and pentoxifylline on vascular endothelial growth factor in patients with intermittent claudication. Clin Sci (Lond). 2001;101(3):305-11. PMID: 11524048.

Lindholt JS, Gottschalksen B, Johannesen N, et al. The Scandinavian Propaten((R)) trial - 1-year patency of PTFE vascular prostheses with heparin-bonded luminal surfaces compared to ordinary pure PTFE vascular prostheses - a randomised clinical controlled multi-centre trial. Eur J Vasc Endovasc Surg. 2011;41(5):668-73. PMID: 21376643.

Lu CH, Chang J, Lai ST, et al. Comparative evaluation of stretch and non-stretch polytetrafluorethylene (PTFE) prosthetic grafts for femoro-popliteal bypass. Zhonghua Yi Xue Za Zhi (Taipei). 2002;65(5):200-4. PMID: 12166763.

Madiba TE, Mars M, Robbs JV. Aorto-iliac occlusive disease in the different population groups--clinical pattern, risk profile and results of reconstruction. S Afr Med J. 1999;89(12):1288-92. PMID: 10678200.

Madiba TE, Mars M, Robbs JV. Choosing the proximal anastomosis in aortobifemoral bypass. Br J Surg. 1997;84(10):1416-8. PMID: 9361602.

Manfredini F, Malagoni AM, Mascoli F, et al. Training rather than walking: the test in -train out program for home-based rehabilitation in peripheral arteriopathy. Circ J. 2008;72(6):946-52. PMID: 18503221.

Martinez CA, Carmeli E, Barak S, et al. Changes in pain-free walking based on time in accommodating pain-free exercise therapy for peripheral arterial disease. J Vasc Nurs. 2009;27(1):2-7. PMID: 19217538.

Matarazzo A, Rosati Tarulli V, Florio A, et al. Chronic critical ischaemia of the lower extremities. G Ital Chir Vasc. 2000;7(4):309-15.

Matsubara J, Sakamoto S, Yamamoto K, et al. Externally Supported, Noncoated, Knitted Dacron Graft and Gelatin-Coated Knitted Dacron Graft with Rings for Peripheral Arterial Reconstruction. Int J Angiol. 2000;9(2):103-6. PMID: 10758206.

Matzke S, Pitkanen J, Lepantalo M. Does saphenous vein arterialisation prevent major amputation in critical leg ischaemia? A comparative study. J Cardiovasc Surg (Torino). 1999;40(6):845-7. PMID: 10776715.

Mcdermott MM, Ades P, Guralnik JM, et al. Treadmill exercise and resistance training in patients with peripheral arterial disease with and without intermittent claudication: a randomized controlled trial. JAMA. 2009;301(2):165-74. PMID: 19141764.

Mcdermott MM, Liu K, Ferrucci L, et al. Physical performance in peripheral arterial disease: a slower rate of decline in patients who walk more. Ann Intern Med. 2006;144(1):10-20. PMID: 16389250.

Mcdermott MM, Tiukinhoy S, Greenland P, et al. A pilot exercise intervention to improve lower extremity functioning in peripheral arterial disease unaccompanied by intermittent claudication. J Cardiopulm Rehabil. 2004;24(3):187-96. PMID: 15235301.

Meister RH, Schweiger H, Lang W. Knitted double-velour Dacron prostheses in aortobifemoral position--long-term performance of different coating materials. Vasa. 1998;27(4):236-9. PMID: 9859745

Meneses AL, De Lima GH, Forjaz CL, et al. Impact of a supervised strength training or walking training over a subsequent unsupervised therapy period on walking capacity in patients with claudication. J Vasc Nurs. 2011;29(2):81-6. PMID: 21558030.

Mika P, Spodaryk K, Cencora A, et al. Experimental model of pain-free treadmill training in patients with claudication. Am J Phys Med Rehabil. 2005;84(10):756-62. PMID: 16205431.

Mika P, Spodaryk K, Cencora A, et al. Red blood cell deformability in patients with claudication after pain-free treadmill training. Clin J Sport Med. 2006;16(4):335-40. PMID: 16858218.

Nawaz S, Walker RD, Wilkinson CH, et al. The inflammatory response to upper and lower limb exercise and the effects of exercise training in patients with claudication. J Vasc Surg. 2001;33(2):392-9. PMID: 11174795.

Nicolai SP, Hendriks EJ, Prins MH, et al. Optimizing supervised exercise therapy for patients with intermittent claudication. J Vasc Surg. 2010;52(5):1226-33. PMID: 20692797.

Nicolai SP, Teijink JA and Prins MH. Multicenter randomized clinical trial of supervised exercise therapy with or without feedback versus walking advice for intermittent claudication. J Vasc Surg. 2010;52(2):348-55. PMID: 20478681.

Oderich GS, Panneton JM, Yagubyan M, et al. Comparison of precuffed and vein-cuffed expanded polytetrafluoroethylene grafts for infragenicular arterial reconstructions: a case-matched study. Ann Vasc Surg. 2005;19(1):49-55. PMID: 15714367.

O'donnell ME, Badger SA, Sharif MA, et al. The effects of cilostazol on exercise-induced ischaemia-reperfusion injury in patients with peripheral arterial disease. Eur J Vasc Endovasc Surg. 2009;37(3):326-35. PMID: 19112032.

O'donnell ME, Badger SA, Sharif MA, et al. The vascular and biochemical effects of cilostazol in patients with peripheral arterial disease. J Vasc Surg. 2009;49(5):1226-34. PMID: 19217745.

Onohara T, Komori K, Kume M, et al. Multivariate analysis of long-term results after an axillobifemoral and aortobifemoral bypass in patients with aortoiliac occlusive disease. J Cardiovasc Surg (Torino). 2000;41(6):905-10. PMID: 11232974.

Oostenbrink JB, Tangelder MJ, Busschbach JJ, et al. Cost-effectiveness of oral anticoagulants versus aspirin in patients after infrainguinal bypass grafting surgery. J Vasc Surg. 2001;34(2):254-62. PMID: 11496277.

Palumbo N, Cevolani M, Paragona O, et al. Revascularization of the peroneal artery in chronic critical leg ischemia. G Ital Chir Vasc. 2000;7(2):105-13.

Panayiotopoulos YP, Taylor PR. A paper for debate: vein versus PTFE for critical limb ischaemia--an unfair comparison? Eur J Vasc Endovasc Surg. 1997;14(3):191-4. PMID: 9345238.

Panneton JM, Hollier LH, Hofer JM. Multicenter randomized prospective trial comparing a pre-cuffed polytetrafluoroethylene graft to a vein cuffed polytetrafluoroethylene graft for infragenicular arterial bypass. Ann Vasc Surg. 2004;18(2):199-206. PMID: 15253256.

Parr BM, Noakes TD, Derman EW. Peripheral arterial disease and intermittent claudication: efficacy of short-term upper body strength training, dynamic exercise training, and advice to exercise at home. S Afr Med J. 2009;99(11):800-4. PMID: 20218480.

Passman MA, Taylor LM, Moneta GL, et al. Comparison of axillofemoral and aortofemoral bypass for aortoiliac occlusive disease. J Vasc Surg. 1996;23(2):263-9; discussion 269-71. PMID: 8637103.

Pinto BM, Marcus BH, Patterson RB, et al. On-site versus home exercise programs: psychological benefits for individuals with arterial claudication. J Aging Phys Act. 1997;5(4):311-28.

Plecha EJ, Freischlag JA, Seabrook GR, et al. Femoropopliteal bypass revisited: an analysis of 138 cases. Cardiovasc Surg. 1996;4(2):195-9. PMID: 8861436.

Ponec D, Jaff MR, Swischuk J, et al. The Nitinol SMART stent vs Wallstent for suboptimal iliac artery angioplasty: CRISP-US trial results. J Vasc Interv Radiol. 2004;15(9):911-8. PMID: 15361558.

Pozzi Mucelli F, Fisicaro M, Calderan L, et al. Percutaneous revascularization of femoropopliteal artery disease: PTA and PTA plus stent. Results after six years' follow-up. Radiol Med. 2003;105(4):339-49. PMID: 12835627.

Pullatt R, Brothers TE, Robison JG, et al. Compromised bypass graft outcomes after minimal-incision vein harvest. J Vasc Surg. 2006;44(2):289-94; discussion 294-5. PMID: 16890856.

Rabellino M, Zander T, Baldi S, et al. Clinical follow-up in endovascular treatment for TASC C-D lesions in femoro-popliteal segment. Catheter Cardiovasc Interv. 2009;73(5):701-5. PMID: 19309709.

Rand T, Basile A, Cejna M, et al. PTA versus carbofilm-coated stents in infrapopliteal arteries: pilot study. Cardiovasc Intervent Radiol. 2006;29(1):29-38. PMID: 16252079.

Rand T, Lammer J, Rabbia C, et al. Percutaneous transluminal angioplasty versus turbostatic carbon-coated stents in infrapopliteal arteries: InPeria II trial. Radiology. 2011;261(2):634-42. PMID: 22012905.

Randon C, Jacobs B, De Ryck F, et al. Angioplasty or primary stenting for infrapopliteal lesions: results of a prospective randomized trial. Cardiovasc Intervent Radiol. 2010;33(2):260-9. PMID: 19957178.

Raouf AA, Rouleau Y, Clement A, et al. Stentgraft and concomitant infrainguinal revascularization in complex iliac occlusive disease: A retrospective study and follow-up in 22 cases. Chirurgia. 2008;21(2):57-61.

Raptis S, Miller JH. Influence of a vein cuff on polytetrafluoroethylene grafts for primary femoropopliteal bypass. Br J Surg. 1995;82(4):487-91. PMID: 7613892.

Rastan A, Tepe G, Krankenberg H, et al. Sirolimus-eluting stents vs. bare-metal stents for treatment of focal lesions in infrapopliteal arteries: a double-blind, multi-centre, randomized clinical trial. Eur Heart J. 2011;32(18):2274-81. PMID: 21622669.

Regensteiner JG, Meyer TJ, Krupski WC, et al. Hospital vs home-based exercise rehabilitation for patients with peripheral arterial occlusive disease. Angiology. 1997;48(4):291-300. PMID: 9112877.

Regensteiner JG, Steiner JF, Hiatt WR. Exercise training improves functional status in patients with peripheral arterial disease. J Vasc Surg. 1996;23(1):104-15. PMID: 8558725.

Ricco JB, Probst H. Long-term results of a multicenter randomized study on direct versus crossover bypass for unilateral iliac artery occlusive disease. J Vasc Surg. 2008;47(1):45-53; discussion 53-4. PMID: 17997269.

Ritti-Dias RM, Wolosker N, De Moraes Forjaz CL, et al. Strength training increases walking tolerance in intermittent claudication patients: randomized trial. J Vasc Surg. 2010;51(1):89-95. PMID: 19837534.

Robinson BI, Fletcher JP. Fluoropolymer coated Dacron or polytetrafluoroethylene for femoropopliteal bypass grafting: a multicentre trial. ANZ J Surg. 2003;73(3):95-9. PMID: 12608965.

Robinson BI, Fletcher JP, Tomlinson P, et al. A prospective randomized multicentre comparison of expanded polytetrafluoroethylene and gelatin-sealed knitted Dacron grafts for femoropopliteal bypass. Cardiovasc Surg. 1999;7(2):214-8. PMID: 10353674.

Sabeti S, Czerwenka-Wenkstetten A, Dick P, et al. Quality of life after balloon angioplasty versus stent implantation in the superficial femoral artery: findings from a randomized controlled trial. J Endovasc Ther. 2007;14(4):431-7. PMID: 17696615.

Sabeti S, Schillinger M, Amighi J, et al. Primary patency of femoropopliteal arteries treated with nitinol versus stainless steel self-expanding stents: propensity score-adjusted analysis. Radiology. 2004;232(2):516-21. PMID: 15286322.

Sadek M, Ellozy SH, Turnbull IC, et al. Improved outcomes are associated with multilevel endovascular intervention involving the tibial vessels compared with isolated tibial intervention. J Vasc Surg. 2009;49(3):638-43; discussion 643-4. PMID: 19268768.

Sala F, Hassen-Khodja R, Lecis A, et al. Long-term outcome of femoral above-knee popliteal artery bypass using autologous saphenous vein versus expanded polytetrafluoroethylene grafts. Ann Vasc Surg. 2003;17(4):401-7. PMID: 14670018.

Sanderson B, Askew C, Stewart I, et al. Short-term effects of cycle and treadmill training on exercise tolerance in peripheral arterial disease. J Vasc Surg. 2006;44(1):119-27. PMID: 16828435.

Sarac TP, Huber TS, Back MR, et al. Warfarin improves the outcome of infrainguinal vein bypass grafting at high risk for failure. J Vasc Surg. 1998;28(3):446-57. PMID: 9737454.

Savage P, Ricci MA, Lynn M, et al. Effects of home versus supervised exercise for patients with intermittent claudication. J Cardiopulm Rehabil. 2001;21(3):152-7. PMID: 11409225.

Saxon RR, Coffman JM, Gooding JM, et al. Long-term results of ePTFE stent-graft versus angioplasty in the femoropopliteal artery: single center experience from a prospective, randomized trial. J Vasc Interv Radiol. 2003;14(3):303-11. PMID: 12631634.

Saxon RR, Dake MD, Volgelzang RL, et al. Randomized, multicenter study comparing expanded polytetrafluoroethylene-covered endoprosthesis placement with percutaneous transluminal angioplasty in the treatment of superficial femoral artery occlusive disease. J Vasc Interv Radiol. 2008;19(6):823-32. PMID: 18503895.

Saxton JM, Zwierska I, Blagojevic M, et al. Upper- versus lower-limb aerobic exercise training on health-related quality of life in patients with symptomatic peripheral arterial disease. J Vasc Surg. 2011;53(5):1265-73. PMID: 21215558.

Sayers RD, Raptis S, Berce M, et al. Long-term results of femorotibial bypass with vein or polytetrafluoroethylene. Br J Surg. 1998;85(7):934-8. PMID: 9692567.

Schillinger M, Sabeti S, Dick P, et al. Sustained benefit at 2 years of primary femoropopliteal stenting compared with balloon angioplasty with optional stenting. Circulation. 2007;115(21):2745-9. PMID: 17502568.

Schillinger M, Sabeti S, Loewe C, et al. Balloon angioplasty versus implantation of nitinol stents in the superficial femoral artery. N Engl J Med. 2006;354(18):1879-88. PMID: 16672699.

Schlager O, Dick P, Sabeti S, et al. Long-segment SFA stenting--the dark sides: in-stent restenosis, clinical deterioration, and stent fractures. J Endovasc Ther. 2005;12(6):676-84. PMID: 16363897.

Schmieder GC, Richardson AI, Scott EC, et al. Selective stenting in subintimal angioplasty: analysis of primary stent outcomes. J Vasc Surg. 2008;48(5):1175-80; discussion 1180-1. PMID: 18778911.

Semaan E, Hamburg N, Nasr W, et al. Endovascular management of the popliteal artery: comparison of atherectomy and angioplasty. Vasc Endovascular Surg. 2010;44(1):25-31. PMID: 19942598.

Setacci F, Sirignano P, Raucci A, et al. Below the knee endovascular revascularization strategy for limb salvage in diabetic patients. Ital J Vasc Endovasc Surg. 2010;17(3):189-94.

Siablis D, Karnabatidis D, Katsanos K, et al. Infrapopliteal application of sirolimus-eluting versus bare metal stents for critical limb ischemia: analysis of long-term angiographic and clinical outcome. J Vasc Interv Radiol. 2009;20(9):1141-50. PMID: 19620014.

Siablis D, Karnabatidis D, Katsanos K, et al. Sirolimus-eluting versus bare stents after suboptimal infrapopliteal angioplasty for critical limb ischemia: enduring 1-year angiographic and clinical benefit. J Endovasc Ther. 2007;14(2):241-50. PMID: 17484536.

Siablis D, Kraniotis P, Karnabatidis D, et al. Sirolimus-eluting versus bare stents for bailout after suboptimal infrapopliteal angioplasty for critical limb ischemia: 6-month angiographic results from a nonrandomized prospective single-center study. J Endovasc Ther. 2005;12(6):685-95. PMID: 16363898.

Singer E, Imfeld S, Staub D, et al. Effect of aspirin versus clopidogrel on walking exercise performance in intermittent claudication-a double-blind randomized multicenter trial. J Am Heart Assoc. 2012;1(1):51-6. PMID: 23130118.

Singh S, Singh H, Kohli A, et al. Effects of cilostazole and pentoxifylline on claudication distance and lipid profile in patients with occlusive peripheral arterial disease: A comparative trial. Indian J Thorac Cardiovasc Surg. 2009;25(2):45-8.

Slim H, Tiwari A, Ahmed A, et al. Distal versus ultradistal bypass grafts: amputation-free survival and patency rates in patients with critical leg ischaemia. Eur J Vasc Endovasc Surg. 2011;42(1):83-8. PMID: 21514854.

Slordahl SA, Wang E, Hoff J, et al. Effective training for patients with intermittent claudication. Scand Cardiovasc J. 2005;39(4):244-9. PMID: 16118073.

Smeets L, Ho GH, Tangelder MJ, et al. Outcome after occlusion of infrainguinal bypasses in the Dutch BOA Study: comparison of amputation rate in venous and prosthetic grafts. Eur J Vasc Endovasc Surg. 2005;30(6):604-9. PMID: 16098774.

Smeets L, Van Der Horn G, Gisbertz SS, et al. Does conversion of intended remote iliac artery endarterectomy alter the early and long-term outcome? Vascular. 2005;13(6):336-42. PMID: 16390651.

Solakovic E, Totic D, Solakovic S. Femoro-popliteal bypass above knee with saphenous vein vs synthetic graft. Bosn J Basic Med Sci. 2008;8(4):367-72. PMID: 19125710.

Spiliopoulos S, Katsanos K, Karnabatidis D, et al. Cryoplasty versus conventional balloon angioplasty of the femoropopliteal artery in diabetic patients: long-term results from a prospective randomized single-center controlled trial. Cardiovasc Intervent Radiol. 2010;33(5):929-38. PMID: 20574796.

Sultan S, Tawfick W, Hynes N. Cool excimer laser-assisted angioplasty vs tibial balloon angioplasty in management of infragenicular tibial arterial occlusion in critical lower limb ischemia TASC D. Vasc Dis Manage. 2011;8(11):E187-97.

Tetteroo E, Van Der Graaf Y, Bosch JL, et al. Randomised comparison of primary stent placement versus primary angioplasty followed by selective stent placement in patients with iliac-artery occlusive disease. Dutch Iliac Stent Trial Study Group. Lancet. 1998;351(9110):1153-9. PMID: 9643685.

Tew G, Nawaz S, Zwierska I, et al. Limb-specific and cross-transfer effects of arm-crank exercise training in patients with symptomatic peripheral arterial disease. Clin Sci (Lond). 2009;117(12):405-13. PMID: 19388883.

Thompson MM, Sayers RD, Reid A, et al. Quality of life following infragenicular bypass and lower limb amputation. Eur J Vasc Endovasc Surg. 1995;9(3):310-3. PMID: 7620957.

Tielbeek AV, Vroegindeweij D, Buth J, et al. Comparison of balloon angioplasty and Simpson atherectomy for lesions in the femoropopliteal artery: angiographic and clinical results of a prospective randomized trial. J Vasc Interv Radiol. 1996;7(6):837-44. PMID: 8951750.

Timaran CH, Stevens SL, Freeman MB, et al. External iliac and common iliac artery angioplasty and stenting in men and women. J Vasc Surg. 2001;34(3):440-6. PMID: 11533595.

Tofigh AM, Warnier De Wailly G, Rhissassi B. Comparing vein with collagen impregnated woven polyester prosthesis in above-knee femoropopliteal bypass grafting. Int J Surg. 2007;5(2):109-13. PMID: 17448975.

Townley WA, Carrell TW, Jenkins MP, et al. Critical limb ischemia in the dialysis-dependent patient: infrainguinal vein bypass is justified. Vasc Endovascular Surg. 2006;40(5):362-6. PMID: 17038569.

Treat-Jacobson D, Henly SJ, Bronas UG, et al. The pain trajectory during treadmill testing in peripheral artery disease. Nurs Res. 2011;60(3 Suppl):S38-49. PMID: 21543960.

Troisi N, Dorigo W, Pratesi G, et al. Below-knee revascularization in patients with critical limb ischemia: long-term comparison of redo vs primary interventions. J Cardiovasc Surg (Torino). 2008;49(4):489-95. PMID: 18665112.

Unni NM, Mandalam KR, Rao VR, et al. Balloon angioplasty of the femoro-popliteal segment: follow up results from southern India. Natl Med J India. 1995;8(3):105-13. PMID: 7780349.

Urayama H, Ohtake H, Yokoi K, et al. Long-term results of endarterectomy, anatomic bypass and extraanatomic bypass for aortoiliac occlusive disease. Surg Today. 1998;28(2):151-5. PMID: 9525003.

Van Det RJ, Vriens BH, Van Der Palen J, et al. Dacron or ePTFE for femoro-popliteal above-knee bypass grafting: short- and long-term results of a multicentre randomised trial. Eur J Vasc Endovasc Surg. 2009;37(4):457-63. PMID: 19231253.

Volpe P, Conti B, Palazzo V, et al. Suprageniculate standard femoropopliteal bypass and popliteotibial angioplasty: An option for simultaneous combined open and endovascular treatment in limb salvage. Ital J Vasc Endovasc Surg. 2009;16(1):23-9.

Vroegindeweij D, Tielbeek AV, Buth J, et al. Directional atherectomy versus balloon angioplasty in segmental femoropopliteal artery disease: two-year follow-up with color-flow duplex scanning. J Vasc Surg. 1995;21(2):255-68; discussion 268-9. PMID: 7853599.

Vroegindeweij D, Vos LD, Tielbeek AV, et al. Balloon angioplasty combined with primary stenting versus balloon angioplasty alone in femoropopliteal obstructions: A comparative randomized study. Cardiovasc Intervent Radiol. 1997;20(6):420-5. PMID: 9354709.

Walker RD, Nawaz S, Wilkinson CH, et al. Influence of upper- and lower-limb exercise training on cardiovascular function and walking distances in patients with intermittent claudication. J Vasc Surg. 2000;31(4):662-9. PMID: 10753273.

Walluscheck KP, Bierkandt S, Brandt M, et al. Infrainguinal ePTFE vascular graft with bioactive surface heparin bonding. First clinical results. J Cardiovasc Surg (Torino). 2005;46(4):425-30. PMID: 16160689.

Wang E, Hoff J, Loe H, et al. Plantar flexion: an effective training for peripheral arterial disease. Eur J Appl Physiol. 2008;104(4):749-56. PMID: 18726111.

Watelet J, Soury P, Menard JF, et al. Femoropopliteal bypass: in situ or reversed vein grafts? Ten-year results of a randomized prospective study. Ann Vasc Surg. 1997;11(5):510-9. PMID: 9302064.

Wijesinghe LD, Beardsmore DM, Scott DJ. Polytetrafluoroethylene (PTFE) femorodistal grafts with a distal vein cuff for critical ischaemia. Eur J Vasc Endovasc Surg. 1998;15(5):449-53. PMID: 9633503.

Wilson YG, Davies AH, Currie IC, et al. Angioscopically-assisted in situ saphenous vein bypass for infrainguinal revascularisation. Eur J Vasc Endovasc Surg. 1996;12(2):223-9. PMID: 8760987.

Wolosker N, Nakano L, Rosoky RA, et al. Evaluation of walking capacity over time in 500 patients with intermittent claudication who underwent clinical treatment. Arch Intern Med. 2003;163(19):2296-300. PMID: 14581248.

Yasa H, Cakir C, Tetik O, et al. Bypass grafting for infrapopliteal occlusive disease with poor distal flow on angiography. Anadolu Kardiyol Derg. 2008;8(6):444-8. PMID: 19103541.

Yilmaz S, Sindel T, Yegin A, et al. Subintimal angioplasty of long superficial femoral artery occlusions. J Vasc Interv Radiol. 2003;14(8):997-1010. PMID: 12902557.

Zdanowski Z, Albrechtsson U, Lundin A, et al. Percutaneous transluminal angioplasty with or without stenting for femoropopliteal occlusions? A randomized controlled study. Int Angiol. 1999;18(4):251-5. PMID: 10811511.

Zukauskas G, Ulevicius H, Janusauskas E. An optimal inflow procedure for multi-segmental occlusive arterial disease: ilio-femoral versus aorto-bifemoral bypass. Cardiovasc Surg. 1998;6(3):250-5. PMID: 9705096.

Zwierska I, Walker RD, Choksy SA, et al. Upper- vs lower-limb aerobic exercise rehabilitation in patients with symptomatic peripheral arterial disease: a randomized controlled trial. J Vasc Surg. 2005;42(6):1122-30. PMID: 16376202.

No outcomes of interest ≥30 days

Burdess A, Nimmo AF, Garden OJ, et al. Randomized controlled trial of dual antiplatelet therapy in patients undergoing surgery for critical limb ischemia. Ann Surg. 2010;252(1):37-42. PMID: 20562608

Printed in Great Britain
by Amazon